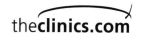

ENDOCRINOLOGY AND METABOLISM CLINICS OF NORTH AMERICA

Thyroid Tumors

GUEST EDITORS
Shereen Ezzat, MD
Sylvia L. Asa, MD, PhD

CONSULTING EDITOR
Derek LeRoith, MD, PhD

June 2008 • Volume 37 • Number 2

SAUNDERS

An Imprint of Elsevier, Inc.
PHILADELPHIA   LONDON   TORONTO   MONTREAL   SYDNEY   TOKYO

W.B. SAUNDERS COMPANY
A Division of Elsevier Inc.

1600 John F. Kennedy Boulevard • Suite 1800 • Philadelphia, Pennsylvania 19103-2899

http://www.theclinics.com

ENDOCRINOLOGY AND METABOLISM	Volume 37, Number 2
CLINICS OF NORTH AMERICA	ISSN 0889-8529
June 2008	ISBN-13: 978-1-4160-5859-5
Editor: Rachel Glover	ISBN-10: 1-4160-5859-1

The ideas and opinions expressed in *Endocrinology and Metabolism Clinics of North America* do not necessarily reflect those of the Publisher. The Publisher does not assume any responsibility for any injury and/or damage to persons or property arising out of or related to any use of the material contained in this periodical. The reader is advised to check the appropriate medical literature and the product information currently provided by the manufacturer of each drug to be administered to verify the dosage, the method and duration of administration, or contraindications. It is the responsibility of the treating physician or other health care professional, relying on independent experience and knowledge of the patient, to determine drug dosages and the best treatment for the patient. Mention of any product in this issue should not be construed as endorsement by the contributors, editors, or the Publisher of the product or manufacturers' claims.

Endocrinology and Metabolism Clinics of North America (ISSN 0889-8529) is published quarterly by Elsevier Inc., 360 Park Avenue South, New York, NY 10010-1710. Months of publication are March, June, September, and December. Business and editorial offices: 1600 John F. Kennedy Boulevard, Suite 1800, Philadelphia, PA 19103-2899. Customer Service Office: 6277 Sea Harbor Drive, Orlando, FL 32887-4800. Periodicals postage paid at New York, NY and additional mailing offices. Subscription prices are USD 220 per year for US individuals, USD 364 per year for US institutions, USD 113 per year for US students and residents, USD 276 per year for Canadian individuals, USD 437 per year for Canadian institutions, USD 301 per year for international individuals, USD 437 per year for international institutions and USD 157 per year for Canadian and foreign students/residents. To receive student/resident rate, orders must be accompanied by name of affiliated institution, date of term, and the *signature* of program/residency coordinator on institution letterhead. Orders will be billed at individual rate until proof of status is received. Foreign air speed delivery is included in all *Clinics* subscription prices. All prices are subject to change without notice. POSTMASTER: Send address changes to *Endocrinology and Metabolism Clinics of North America*, Elsevier Periodicals Customer Service, 6277 Sea Harbor Drive, Orlando, FL 32887-4800. **Customer Service: 1-800-654-2452 (US). From outside of the US: 1-407-563-6020. Fax: 1-407-363-9661. E-mail: JournalsCustomer Service-usa@elsevier.com.**

Reprints. For copies of 100 or more, of articles in this publication, please contact the Commercial Rights Department, Elsevier Inc., 360 Park Avenue South, New York, NY 10010-1710; phone: (+1) 212-633-3813; fax: (+1) 212-462-1935; e-mail: reprints@elsevier.com.

Endocrinology and Metabolism Clinics of North America is covered in *Index Medicus, EMBASE/Excerpta Medica, Current Contents/Clinical Medicine, Current Contents/Life Sciences, Science Citation Index, ISI/BIOMED, BIOSIS, and Chemical Abstracts.*

Printed in the United States of America.

CONSULTING EDITOR

DEREK LEROITH, MD, PhD, Chief, Division of Endocrinology, Metabolism, and Bone Diseases, Mount Sinai School of Medicine, New York, New York

GUEST EDITORS

SHEREEN EZZAT, MD, Professor of Medicine and Oncology, Department of Medicine, University of Toronto; and Head, Endocrine Oncology Site Group, Princess Margaret Hospital, Toronto, Ontario, Canada

SYLVIA L. ASA, MD, PhD, Professor, Department of Laboratory Medicine and Pathobiology, University of Toronto; Pathologist-in-Chief, University Health Network and Toronto Medical Laboratories; and Senior Scientist, Ontario Cancer Institute, Toronto, Ontario, Canada

CONTRIBUTORS

SYLVIA L. ASA, MD, PhD, Professor, Department of Laboratory Medicine and Pathobiology, University of Toronto; Pathologist-in-Chief, University Health Network and Toronto Medical Laboratories; and Senior Scientist, Ontario Cancer Institute, Toronto, Ontario, Canada

ZUBAIR W. BALOCH, MD, PhD, Professor of Pathology and Laboratory Medicine, Department of Pathology and Laboratory Medicine, University of Pennsylvania Medical Center, Philadelphia, Pennsylvania

JAMES D. BRIERLEY, MBBS, FRCP, FRCR, FRCP(C), Associate Professor, Department of Radiation Oncology, University of Toronto, Princess Margaret Hospital, Toronto, Ontario, Canada

KENNETH D. BURMAN, MD, Director, Endocrine Section, Washington Hospital Center, Washington, DC

MARIA DOMENICA CASTELLONE, MD, PhD, Instituto di Endocrinologia e Oncologia Sperimentale del CNR "G. Salvatore," Dipartmento di Biologia e Patologia Cellulare e Molecolare, Universita di Napoli Federico II, Naples, Italy

PATRICIA CASTRO, PhD, Researcher, Institute of Molecular Pathology and Immunology of the University of Porto, Porto, Portugal

ORLO H. CLARK, MD, Professor, University of California, San Francisco, Mt. Zion Medical Center, San Francisco, California

SHEREEN EZZAT, MD, Professor of Medicine and Oncology, Department of Medicine, University of Toronto; and Head, Endocrine Oncology Site Group, Princess Margaret Hospital, Toronto, Ontario, Canada

WILLIAM B. FARRAR, MD, Chief, Department of Surgery, Division of Surgical Oncology, The Ohio State University, The Arthur G. James Cancer Hospital and Richard J. Solove Research Institute, Columbus, Ohio

STEPHANIE A. FISH, MD, Assistant Professor of Medicine, Department of Medicine, University of Pennsylvania School of Medicine, Philadelphia, Pennsylvania

AMIRAM GAFNI, PhD, Department of Clinical Epidemiology and Biostatistics, McMaster University; and Centre for Health Economics and Policy Analysis, Hamilton, Ontario, Canada

ROBERT F. GAGEL, MD, Professor and Head, Division of Internal Medicine, Department of Endocrine Neoplasia and Hormonal Disorders, The University of Texas M.D. Anderson Cancer Center, Houston, Texas

THOMAS J. GIORDANO, MD, PhD, Associate Professor, Department of Pathology, University of Michigan Health System, Ann Arbor, Michigan

DAVID P. GOLDSTEIN, MD, FRCSC, Department of Otolaryngology Head and Neck Surgery, University Health Network; and University of Toronto, Toronto, Ontario, Canada

JESSICA E. GOSNELL, MD, Assistant Professor of Surgery, University of California, San Francisco, Mt. Zion Medical Center, San Francisco, California

MIMI I-NAN HU, MD, Assistant Professor, Department of Endocrine Neoplasia and Hormonal Disorders, The University of Texas M.D. Anderson Cancer Center, Houston, Texas

CAMILO JIMÉNEZ, MD, Assistant Professor, Department of Endocrine Neoplasia and Hormonal Disorders, The University of Texas M.D. Anderson Cancer Center, Houston, Texas

RICHARD T. KLOOS, MD, Professor, Departments of Internal Medicine and Radiology, Divisions of Endocrinology, Diabetes, and Metabolism, and Nuclear Medicine, The Ohio State University, The Arthur G. James Cancer Hospital and Richard J. Solove Research Institute; and The Ohio State University Comprehensive Cancer Center, Columbus, Ohio

TETSUO KONDO, MD, PhD, Assistant Professor, Department of Pathology, University of Yamanashi, Japan

JILL E. LANGER, MD, Associate Professor of Radiology, Department of Radiology, University of Pennsylvania School of Medicine, Philadelphia, Pennsylvania

REBECCA LEBOEUF, MD, Assistant Professor of Medicine, Joan and Sanford I. Weill Medical College of Cornel University; and Assistant Attending, Memorial Sloan-Kettering Cancer Center, New York, New York

JORGE LIMA, PhD, Researcher, Institute of Molecular Pathology and Immunology of the University of Porto, Porto, Portugal

VIRGINIA A. LIVOLSI, MD, Professor of Pathology and Laboratory Medicine, Department of Pathology and Laboratory Medicine, University of Pennsylvania Medical Center, Philadelphia, Pennsylvania

SUSAN J. MANDEL, MD, MPH, Associate Professor of Medicine, Department of Medicine, University of Pennsylvania School of Medicine; and Director of Clinical Endocrinology, Diabetes, and Metabolism, University of Pennsylvania Health System, Philadelphia, Pennsylvania

VALDEMAR MÁXIMO, PhD, Researcher, Institute of Molecular Pathology and Immunology of the University of Porto; and Associate Professor, Department of Pathology, University of Porto, Porto, Portugal

RYAN L. NEFF, MD, Fellow, Department of Surgery, Division of Surgical Oncology, The Ohio State University, Arthur G. James Cancer Hospital and Richard J. Solove Research Institute, Columbus, Ohio

JOHN E. PAES, DO, Clinical Fellow, Division of Endocrinology, Diabetes, and Metabolism, The Ohio State University Medical Center, The Ohio State University, Columbus, Ohio

ANA PRETO, PhD, Researcher, Institute of Molecular Pathology and Immunology of the University of Porto, Porto; and Assistant Professor, Department of Biology, University of Minho, Braga, Portugal

MATTHEW D. RINGEL, MD, Professor of Medicine, Division of Endocrinology, Diabetes, and Metabolism, The Ohio State University Medical Center; and Arthur G. James Comprehensive Cancer Center, The Ohio State University, Columbus, Ohio

ANA SOFIA ROCHA, PhD, Researcher, Institute of Molecular Pathology and Immunology of the University of Porto, Porto, Portugal

LORNE ROTSTEIN, MD, FRCSC, Department of Surgery, University Health Network; and Department of Surgery, University of Toronto, Toronto, Ontario, Canada

MASSIMO SANTORO, MD, PhD, Dipartmento di Biologia e Patologia Cellulare e Molecolare, Universita di Napoli Federico II, Naples, Italy

ANNA M. SAWKA, MD, PhD, FRCPC, Division of Endocrinology, Department of Medicine, University Health Network; and Division of Endocrinology, Department of Medicine, University of Toronto, Toronto, Ontario, Canada

STEVEN I. SHERMAN, MD, Professor and Chair, Department of Endocrine Neoplasia and Hormonal Disorders, Division of Internal Medicine, The University of Texas M.D. Anderson Cancer Center, Houston, Texas

PAULA SOARES, PhD, Researcher, Institute of Molecular Pathology and Immunology of the University of Porto; and Associate Professor, Department of Pathology, University of Porto, Porto, Portugal

MANUEL SOBRINHO-SIMÕES, MD, PhD, Director, Institute of Molecular Pathology and Immunology of the University of Porto; Professor and Director, Department of Pathology, University of Porto; and Chief of Service, Department of Anatomic Pathology, Hospital S. Joao, Porto, Portugal

SHARON STRAUS, MD, MSc, FRCPC, Department of Knowledge Translation, University of Toronto, Toronto, Ontario; Division of Geriatrics, Department of Medicine, University of Calgary, Calgary, Alberta, Canada

LEHANA THABANE, PhD, Department of Clinical Epidemiology and Biostatistics, McMaster University; and Centre for Evaluation of Medicines, St. Joseph's Healthcare, Hamilton, Ontario, Canada

VITOR TROVISCO, PhD, Institute of Molecular Pathology and Immunology of the University of Porto, Porto, Portugal

RICHARD W. TSANG, MD, FRCP(C), Associate Professor, Department of Radiation Oncology, University of Toronto, Princess Margaret Hospital, Toronto, Ontario, Canada

R. MICHAEL TUTTLE, MD, Associate Professor of Medicine, Joan and Sanford I. Weill Medical College of Cornell University; and Associate Attending, Memorial Sloan-Kettering Cancer Center, New York, New York

CONTENTS

Thyroid neoplasms are classified into three major categories: epithelial, nonepithelial, and secondary. Most primary epithelial tumors of thyroid are derived from follicular cells. These include follicular adenoma and carcinoma (Hürthle and non-Hürthle), and papillary carcinoma and its variants. Other primary epithelial tumors include medullary carcinoma, mixed medullary and follicular carcinomas, insular and poorly differentiated carcinoma, anaplastic carcinoma, and the least common squamous carcinoma and related tumors. The nonepithelial tumors are rare; the most common include malignant lymphoma and tumors arising from the mesenchymal elements. The secondary tumors represent metastatic tumors to the thyroid usually originating in lung, kidney, and breast. In this article, the authors review the unusual tumors of the thyroid, their morphologic features, and clinical and prognostic implications.

There is much interest in the application of genome biology to the field of thyroid neoplasia, despite the relatively low mortality rate associated with thyroid cancer in general. The principal reason for this interest is that the field of thyroid neoplasia stands to benefit from the application of genomic information to address a variety of pathologic and clinical issues. In addition to practical patient care issues, there is an excellent opportunity of expand the basic understanding of thyroid carcinogenesis. In this article, the most relevant genomic work on thyroid tumors performed to date is reviewed along with some general comments about the potential impact of genomic biology on thyroid pathology and the management of patients with thyroid nodules and cancer.

The close genotype-phenotype relationship that characterizes thyroid oncology stimulated the authors to address this article by using a mixed, genetic and phenotypic approach. As such, this article addresses the following aspects of intragenic mutations in thyroid cancer: thyroid stimulating hormone receptor and guanine-nucleotide-binding proteins of the stimulatory family mutations in hyperfunctioning tumors; mutations in RAS and other genes and aneuploidy; PAX8-PPARγ rearrangements; BRAF mutations; mutations in oxidative phosphorylation and Krebs cycle genes in Hürthle cell tumors; mutations in succinate dehydrogenase genes in medullary carcinoma and C-cell hyperplasia; and mutations in TP53 and other genes in poorly differentiated and anaplastic carcinomas.

Numerous biologic processes and such diseases as cancer depend on activation of tyrosine kinase receptors. The RET tyrosine kinase receptor was discovered two decades ago as a transforming gene and was subsequently implicated in the formation of papillary and medullary thyroid carcinoma. This article examines the data about the mechanism of activation of downstream signal transduction pathways by RET oncoproteins. Collectively, these findings have advanced the understanding of the processes underlying thyroid carcinoma formation.

The phosphatidylinositol 3-kinase (PI3K) signaling pathway is an important regulator of many cellular events, including apoptosis, proliferation, and motility. Enhanced activation of this pathway can occur through several mechanisms, such as inactivation of its negative regulator, phosphatase and tensin homolog deleted on chromosome ten (*PTEN*), and activating mutations and gene amplification of the gene encoding the catalytic subunit of PI3K

(*PIK3CA*). These genetic abnormalities have been particularly associated with follicular thyroid neoplasia and anaplastic thyroid cancer, suggesting an important role for PI3K signaling in these disorders. In this article, the role of PI3K pathway activation in thyroid cancer is discussed, with a focus on recent advances.

Gain-of-function mutations in oncogenes have aided our understanding of the molecular mechanisms of thyroid carcinogenesis. Mutations or deletions cause inactivation of tumor suppressor genes in thyroid carcinomas. However, recent advances have disclosed the significance of epigenetic events in the development and progression of human tumorigenesis. Indeed, various tumor-suppressor genes and thyroid hormone–related genes are epigenetically silenced in thyroid tumors. This article reviews the evidence for epigenetic gene dysregulation in follicular cell–derived thyroid carcinomas including papillary thyroid carcinoma, follicular thyroid carcinoma, and undifferentiated thyroid carcinoma. The authors also discuss future applications of epigenetics as ancillary diagnostic tools and in the design of targeted therapies for thyroid cancer.

The initial application of sonography for the evaluation of the neck, more than 30 years ago, was to differentiate cystic and solid thyroid nodules. With improvements in technology, ultrasound has been applied to characterize distinct features in the appearance of thyroid nodules. More recently, its function has been expanded to assess cervical lymph nodes for metastatic thyroid cancer. This article discusses the sonographic features of thyroid nodules associated with malignancy and the role of ultrasound in the management of patients with thyroid cancer.

The primary goal in the follow up of thyroid cancer patients is to identify and treat persistent and recurrent disease at a time that minimizes morbidity and disease specific mortality. This article presents a risk-adapted follow-up paradigm to guide both intensity and methodology of follow-up testing based on initial risk stratification, ongoing risk stratification, and secondary risk stratification that incorporates each of the well-known risk factors for recurrence and death from thyroid cancer, with a response to therapy variable as well as duration of disease-free survival. With a proper understanding of the biology of the disease and with accurate assessments of response to therapy, clinicians are better able to tailor a risk-appropriate follow-up approach to individual patients, minimizing excessive testing while still providing adequate testing to detect clinically significant disease recurrence in a timely fashion.

this disease before development of metastasis. Thanks to this discovery, we can now establish the association of MTC with other tumors in the context of MEN2 syndrome; determine adequate follow-up, prognosis, and treatment for patients with hereditary disease; and use this information to develop new therapies against both sporadic and hereditary MTCs.

FORTHCOMING ISSUES

RECENT ISSUES

ENDOCRINOLOGY
AND METABOLISM
CLINICS
OF NORTH AMERICA

Endocrinol Metab Clin N Am
37 (2008) xiii–xv

Foreword

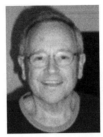

Derek LeRoith, MD, PhD
Consulting Editor

In this issue of *Endocrinology and Metabolism Clinics of North America*, Drs. Ezzat and Asa have compiled a remarkable list of authors and topics on thyroid tumors. The articles cover all of the aspects from a basic and practical point of view.

Drs. Baloch and LiVolsi describe the pathology of unusual thyroid tumors, both benign and malignant. Though papillary and follicular tumors are the most common, with medullary and anaplastic being the less common tumors, there is a large variety of very uncommon tumors, mostly nonepithelial thyroid tumors or secondary from other tissues.

As discussed by Giordano, there is a growing interest in genetic studies involving thyroid cancer. Genetic analysis allows for improving clinical diagnosis where the pathology may be confusing. Pharmacogenetics enables investigators to determine which patients will respond appropriately to certain therapies. Furthermore, genetic analysis enhances the possibility of identifying new therapeutic targets. There are examples of each of these in regard to thyroid cancer, including the over-expression of the MET oncogene in papillary tumors and the mutations of the Ret oncogene; the latter are a target for a specific tyrosine kinase inhibitor now in clinical trials. Molecular profiling should also be able to identify those well-differentiated tumors that are at high risk for recurrence and metastasis. Thus, the possibilities for the use of genetics are endless.

Extending the discussion on genetic mutations in various thyroid cancer types, Soares and coauthors present information on thyroid stimulating hormone receptor and Gs protein mutations in hyperfunctioning tumors, mutations in the *RAS* and *BRAF* genes, rearrangements of *PAX8-PPAR*γ,

doi:10.1016/j.ecl.2008.03.003
endo.theclinics.com

mutations in OXPHOS and Krebs cycle genes in Hürthle cell tumors, mutations in *SDH* genes in medullary carcinoma and C-cell hyperplasia, and mutations in *TP53* and other genes in poorly differentiated and anaplastic carcinomas. Each of these tumors demonstrates a genotype-phenotype relationship with the associated genes.

The RET tyrosine kinase is dysregulated in papillary and medullary cancers. Papillary thyroid carcinoma is associated with RET/PTC chromosomal rearrangements, whereas MTC features RET germline or somatic point mutations. Grb7/10 binding, inhibition of the tyrosine phosphatase SHP-1, and activation of phospholipase Cγ are some of the major signaling pathways in the RET oncogenic transformation of thyroid cells that result in tumor development. Castellone and Santoro, in addition to describing the above mechanisms of action, also discuss in detail other important pathways involved.

Paes and Ringel, on the other hand, describe in their article how the enhanced activation of the PI3K/Akt pathway is seen in follicular and anaplastic thyroid cancers. This may occur through several mechanisms, such as inactivation of its negative regulator, phosphatase and tensin homolog deleted on chromosome ten (*PTEN*), and activating mutations and gene amplification of the gene encoding the catalytic subunit of PI3K (*PIK3CA*).

Kondo, Asa, and Ezzat describe the epigenetic silencing of tumor-suppressor and thyroid-related genes in thyroid tumors. The effect may be seen with follicular-cell derived thyroid carcinomas, including papillary thyroid carcinoma, follicular thyroid carcinoma, and undifferentiated thyroid carcinoma. Now that DNA methylation inhibitors with histone deacetylase inhibitors have demonstrated utility in other tumors by re-expression of tumor suppressor genes, their use in certain thyroid cancers is a distinct possibility.

Tuttle and Leboeuf describe the evidence behind the rationale for the different approaches in the monitoring of patients who have differentiated thyroid cancer. They emphasize the role of thyroglobulin detection and the emerging utility of PET/CT imaging in identifying residual disease.

Thyroid sonography technology and usage has progressed enormously. As described by Fish, Langer, and Mandel, it is used today to characterize distinct features in the appearance of thyroid nodules to aid in the diagnosis, and to assess cervical lymph nodes, for metastatic thyroid cancer. In the former instance, characteristic sonographic appearance of a nodule can be helpful in determining which nodules should undergo fine needle aspiration, especially when the nodule is small or there are multiple nodules present. In the latter case, a heterogeneous appearance with calcifications or peripheral vascularity strongly suggests metastatic disease.

The use of tyrosine kinase inhibitors has proven to be partially effective in clinical trials in patients who have differentiated and medullary thyroid cancers. Most of the inhibitors affect the vascular endothelial growth factor receptor (VEGFR), and some also inhibit the RET protein. Their effectiveness suggests that the VEGFR may be more important than the RET. As Sherman points out, the partial effectiveness of the available agents, when used in combination therapy and their ineffectiveness when used alone, requires that more specific and better agents be developed.

Medullary carcinoma and its therapy are described in the article by Jiménez, Hu, and Gagel. The presence of the RET oncogene mutations in the index cases, together with the use of serum calcitonin levels, has made the diagnosis of children with the disease much easier and allows for early preemptive therapy. Surgery is still the mainstay of treatment, and cases are followed using serum calcitonin levels to identify those with metastatic disease. Recently, the tyrosine kinase inhibitors have proven useful as inhibitors of the tumors, and there is hope that newer agents will be developed.

Neff, Farrar, and Kloos discuss anaplastic carcinomas. As is well known, it is a rapidly fatal disorder, often within six months of pathologic diagnosis, with no current therapy. Fortunately, it is rare. Apparently, it may develop out of a papillary (PTC) or follicular (FTC) cancer and is therefore the cause of death in certain cases of PTC and FTC. Though surgery may be necessary to protect the airway, and radiation therapy and chemotherapy are used, no therapy is currently of any real value. The authors plead for some new clinical trials to attempt to find some therapeutic modality that can alter the prognosis.

Sawka and coauthors reexamine the value of radioactive iodine for ablation of remnant thyroid in cases of well-differentiated cancer and find that the results are inconclusive and warrant controlled trials. External beam radiotherapy may be used to treat well-differentiated thyroid cancer, medullary, and anaplastic thyroid cancer. It can be used to control residual well-differentiated cancers after surgery and radioactive iodine, or may be the only effective therapy in some cases of anaplastic thyroid cancer and may be useful in metastatic thyroid cancer. However, as pointed out by Brierley and Tsang, controlled trials to determine its effectiveness have not been carried out.

Surgery is an important component of the therapy of thyroid tumors. Many centers with experienced and skilled surgeons show an extremely low rate of recurrent nerve palsy or hypoparathyroidism. Consequently, Gosnell and Clark suggest that total thyroidectomy should be considered even in patients who have benign disease. They argue that this avoids the necessity of repeat surgery and the inherent morbidity, and the ease of using replacement thyroid medication.

As the reader can see, the issue is extremely comprehensive and will become an important landmark for a number of years, thanks to the hard work of Drs. Ezzat and Asa, and the authors of each impressive article.

Derek LeRoith, MD, PhD
Division of Endocrinology, Metabolism, and Bone Diseases
Mount Sinai School of Medicine
One Gustave L. Levy Place
Box 1055, Altran 4-36
New York, NY 10029, USA

E-mail address: derek.leroith@mssm.edu

ELSEVIER
SAUNDERS

Endocrinol Metab Clin N Am
37 (2008) xvii–xviii

ENDOCRINOLOGY
AND METABOLISM
CLINICS
OF NORTH AMERICA

Preface

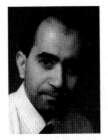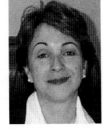

Shereen Ezzat, MD   Sylvia L. Asa, MD, PhD
Guest Editors

Thyroid cancer is the most common malignancy arising from hormone-producing glands. It is one of the few cancers that are increasing in incidence in North America, affecting mainly the young adult female population. In the United States, thyroid cancer is the sixth most common malignancy diagnosed in women aged 20 to 49 years (5.4% of incident cancers) and 58% of subjects are younger than 50 years of age (median 46 years of age) [1,2].

The vast majority of these tumors are thyroid carcinomas derived from follicular epithelial cells that represent a model of malignant transformation. They comprise a broad spectrum of neoplastic phenotypes: well-differentiated papillary thyroid carcinoma (PTC) and follicular thyroid carcinoma (FTC), representing more than 90% of thyroid malignancies; a cancer of intermediate aggression—poorly differentiated thyroid carcinoma (PDTC), representing almost 5% of thyroid cancers; and the rare but typically rapidly lethal anaplastic (or undifferentiated) thyroid carcinoma (ATC).

Several genetic molecular abnormalities have been associated with human thyroid carcinoma. Mouse models have verified that these genetic alterations are involved in malignant transformation; however, the models do not authentically recapitulate invasive and metastatic growth. Furthermore, genotypic–phenotypic correlations in human specimens of well-differentiated thyroid carcinoma do not predict invasion or metastasis. Thus, the large group of well-differentiated carcinomas in young patients that have a low risk of metastasis cannot be easily separated from the rare high-risk tumors in this population.

Given the increasing frequency with which small thyroid nodules are being detected by a variety of imaging modalities, the identification of markers of clinically-relevant disease has become more important.

The management of thyroid cancer is also controversial with several unanswered questions concerning the role and extent of surgery, and indications for adjunctive radioactive iodine treatment in low-risk well-differentiated carcinomas. Clearly the more aggressive tumors require aggressive management, but these tend to be dedifferentiated carcinomas that have lost the capacity for selective uptake of radioactive iodine, and this has led to the search for novel therapeutic agents.

In this issue of the *Endocrinology and Metabolism Clinics of North America*, we have gathered experts from around the world who share their perspectives on the latest advances in our understanding of this disease. They address controversies surrounding these topics and review the latest data in each area, in an attempt to bridge the gap between basic, translational, and clinical studies. We trust that the reader will find it useful to be updated on the most current findings, which summarize the weight of evidence and provide a clearer rationale for management options and surveillance strategies for patients with thyroid cancer.

Shereen Ezzat, MD
Princess Margaret Hospital
610 University Avenue
#8-327
Toronto, ON M5P 2S3, Canada

E-mail address: shereen.ezzat@utoronto.ca

Sylvia L. Asa, MD, PhD
University of Toronto
200 Elizabeth Street
11th Floor
Toronto, ON M5G 2C4, Canada

E-mail address: sylvia.asa@uhn.on.ca

References

[1] Hayat MJ, Howlader N, Reichman E, et al. Cancer statistics, trends, and multiple primary cancers from the Surveillance, Epidemiology, and End Results (SEER) Program. Oncologist 2007;12:20–37.
[2] Edwards BK, Howe HL, Ries LA, et al. Annual report to the nation on the status of cancer, 1973-1999, featuring implications of age and aging on U.S. cancer burden. Cancer 2002; 94(10):2766–92.

ELSEVIER
SAUNDERS

Endocrinol Metab Clin N Am
37 (2008) 297–310

ENDOCRINOLOGY
AND METABOLISM
CLINICS
OF NORTH AMERICA

Unusual Tumors of the Thyroid Gland

Zubair W. Baloch, MD, PhD, Virginia A. LiVolsi, MD*

*Department of Pathology and Laboratory Medicine, University of Pennsylvania
Medical Center, 3400 Spruce Street, 6 Founders Pavilion, Philadelphia, PA 19104, USA*

Thyroid neoplasms can be classified into three major categories: epithelial, nonepithelial, and secondary [1–3]. Most primary epithelial tumors of thyroid are derived from follicular cells. These include follicular adenoma and carcinoma (Hürthle and non-Hürthle), and papillary carcinoma and its variants. Other primary epithelial tumors include medullary carcinoma, mixed medullary and follicular carcinomas, insular and poorly differentiated carcinoma, anaplastic carcinoma, and the least common squamous carcinoma and related tumors. The nonepithelial tumors are rare; the most common in this category includes malignant lymphoma and tumors arising from the mesenchymal elements. The secondary tumors represent metastatic tumors to the thyroid usually originating in lung, kidney, and breast [3].

In this article we review the unusual tumors of the thyroid, their morphologic features, and clinical and prognostic implications.

Primary epithelial thyroid tumors, follicular derived: papillary group

Papillary Hürthle cell carcinoma with lymphocytic stroma 'Warthin-like tumor' of the thyroid

This variant of papillary cancer displays peculiar morphology that closely resembles the papillary cystadenoma lymphomatosum or "Warthin's tumor" of the salivary gland. It is usually seen in the thyroids affected by chronic lymphocytic thyroiditis. The key histologic features (Fig. 1) include oncocytic follicular epithelium arranged in papillae with nuclear features of papillary carcinoma and a brisk infiltrate of lymphocytes and plasma cells in the cores of papillary stalks [4].

The fine-needle aspiration (FNA) specimens from such tumors show oncocytic cells with nuclear features of papillary carcinoma with an admixture

---

* Corresponding author.
E-mail address: linus@mail.med.upenn.edu (V.A. LiVolsi).

0889-8529/08/$ - see front matter © 2008 Elsevier Inc. All rights reserved.
doi:10.1016/j.ecl.2007.12.001   *endo.theclinics.com*

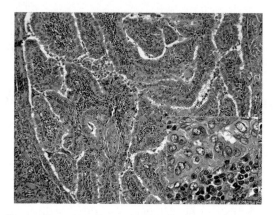

Fig. 1. Warthin-like papillary thyroid carcinoma showing oncocytic follicular epithelium arranged in papillae with nuclear features of papillary carcinoma and a brisk infiltrate of lymphocytes and plasma cells in the cores of papillary stalks (*inset*) (hematoxylin & eosin, original magnification ×40 [inset, ×100]).

of lymphocytes. The FNA specimen and the histologic sections from Warthin-like papillary carcinoma can pose difficulties in distinguishing these lesions from florid chronic thyroiditis itself, Hürthle cell nodules in chronic lymphocytic thyroiditis, Hürthle cell tumors, tall cell variant of papillary carcinoma (PTC), and oncocytic variant of medullary carcinoma [5].

The biologic behavior of these Warthin-like tumors is similar to usual papillary carcinoma when compared for tumor size and stage [4].

Macrofollicular variant of papillary carcinoma

Follicular variant represents the most common subtype of papillary carcinoma. It is a follicular patterned tumor that may grow in an infiltrative manner or be encapsulated or partially encapsulated; it shows nuclear features of papillary carcinoma [6].

Albores-Saavedra and colleagues [6] described 17 cases of follicular variant that is entirely composed of large colloid filled follicles, ie, macrofollicles growth pattern. Characteristically this particular variant lacks diffuse distribution of features of papillary carcinoma; because of this it can be mistaken for a macrofollicular adenoma and hyperplastic/adenomatous goiter. This tumor shows follicles with random distribution of cells with and without nuclear features of papillary carcinoma. Therefore a careful histologic examination is necessary to diagnose this variant of papillary carcinoma.

Similarly, the cytologic samples from the macrofollicular variant of papillary carcinoma can be diagnostically challenging [7,8].

Most of these tumors are large in size; however, despite their size, lymph node metastases or extrathyroidal extension are rare. Interestingly, the nodal metastases also show a macrofollicular growth pattern. Thus, at this time with a limited number of cases reported it is postulated that when compared with conventional papillary carcinoma and follicular variant of papillary carcinoma these tumors behave in a less aggressive fashion [6].

In a separate publication, Albores-Saavedra and colleagues [9] described five cases of macrofollicular variant of papillary carcinoma, which showed a minor (less than 5%) component of insular growth pattern. Two cases from this series showed nodal and distant (lungs and bone) metastasis, and interestingly only the macrofollicular component was present in the metastatic deposits. All patients were alive at follow-up (6 months to 5 years). Thus, the authors felt that the insular component did not worsen the prognosis in this series. However, a 40% incidence of distant metastasis would be highly unusual in classic papillary cancer.

Papillary carcinoma with spindle cell metaplasia

Spindle cell proliferations can occur in association with papillary carcinoma. These occur as either diffuse or nodular involvement of the tumor, may show rare mitoses without any evidence of necrosis, and express cytokeratin and thyroglobulin. In rare cases the spindle cells may show loss of keratin immunoreactivity with acquired immunoreactivity against smooth muscle actin, suggesting a metaplastic transformation of thyroid follicular epithelium [10].

Appropriate identification of metaplastic spindle cell proliferations of the thyroid arising within papillary carcinomas can avoid confusion with more aggressive spindle cell processes such as anaplastic carcinoma.

Papillary carcinoma with nodular fasciitis-like stroma

Chan and colleagues [11] described an unusual morphologic variant of papillary carcinoma. The stromal component in this tumor is similar to that seen in cases of nodular fasciitis and is composed of spindle cells arranged in irregular fascicles in a background of vascularized fibromyxoid stroma. The tumor cells are usually arranged in anastomosing cords, tubules, and papillae with nuclear features of papillary carcinoma and may exhibit squamous metaplasia.

Clinically, these tumors behave similarly to classic papillary carcinoma; interestingly the lymph node metastases from this tumor only show the carcinomatous element without the stromal component. Thus, this reactive fibroblastic response is only limited to the thyroid, which raises the possibility of this being a peculiar host response to tumor [11].

This variant of papillary carcinoma should be distinguished from benign fibroproliferative lesions of the thyroid such as fibrosing Hashimoto's thyroiditis and Reidel's disease, as well as anaplastic carcinoma.

Cribriform-morular variant of papillary carcinoma

This unusual variant of papillary carcinoma has been described in patients with familial adenomatous polyposis (FAP). Almost all tumors occur in females and are characterized by "multifocality" and a cribriform solid and/or spindle cell growth pattern (Fig. 2). However, the tumors are grouped as papillary cancer based on appropriate nuclear features and immunoreactivity for thyroglobulin, although this is focal [12]. About 10% of reported cases have shown metastases outside the neck. The molecular genetic relationships between these tumors and the known genetic mutations in FAP remain to be elucidated. It is also unclear if tumors with this unusual morphology may occur sporadically unassociated with colonic polyposis [13,14]. It has been shown that these tumors exhibit mutations in the beta catenin gene. Various amino acid substitutions have been described. The pathologic corollary of these changes is the finding of strong nuclear immunoreactivity for beta catenin in these tumors [14].

Encapsulated columnar-cell carcinoma

Evans [15] first described two cases of this clinically aggressive thyroid tumor with unique histologic features of papillary formation and nuclear stratification. These tumors commonly occur in men, show extrathyroidal extension, and both regional and distant metastasis, which may lead to fatal outcome.

Evans [16] also described four cases of encapsulated variant of columnar cell neoplasm, three of which occurred in women. These tumors were thickly encapsulated and showed capsular invasion only (Fig. 3). Follow-up on all these patients for up to 112 months failed to reveal any evidence of recurrence or metastasis. Similar observations were reported by Wenig and colleagues [17].

Therefore, the spectrum of this rare variant has been broadened; when one includes tumors that are predominantly encapsulated and are confined within the thyroid, the adverse prognosis originally reported does not appear to be present.

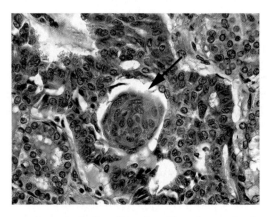

Fig. 2. Cribriform-morular variant of papillary thyroid carcinoma showing focal spindle cell nests (morules [*arrow*]) formation in papillary carcinoma (hematoxylin & eosin, original magnification ×100).

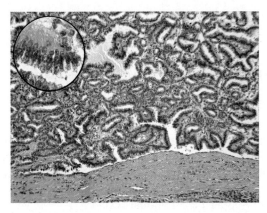

Fig. 3. Encapsulated columnar cell carcinoma showing papillae lined by tumor cells with pseu-dostratification (*inset*) (hematoxylin & eosin, original magnification ×40 [inset, ×100]).

Solid variant of papillary carcinoma and radiation-induced pediatric thyroid cancer

The association between thyroid cancer and radiation is well established. Duffy and Fitzgerald first documented an account of this occurrence in 1950; later numerous reports followed, confirming radiation as being one inducer of thyroid cancer [18].

We are including this category in our review because recent literature contains several references to radiation-induced thyroid cancer seen in children after the "Chernobyl Disaster." Nikiforov and Gnepp [19] published a detailed clinicopathologic account of various forms of pediatric thyroid cancer seen in this population. Their study included 84 cases; papillary carcinoma was found in 83 patients and medullary carcinoma in one. Solid variant of papillary carcinoma was the most common, followed by follicu-lar, classic, mixed, and diffuse sclerosing variants.

In a retrospective analysis of pediatric thyroid cancer in the United King-dom, which covered a 30-year period, the Cambridge group noted a pattern they termed as solid-follicular variant. This pattern was seen in very young children; this subtype has also been described from the affected patients in the post-Chernobyl epidemic. It is been referred to as solid if most of the tumor showed that morphology [20].

Studies from the Chernobyl pathology panel have shown an association of the morphology with iodine deficiency since it is rare (unknown?) in pediatric papillary cancers occurring in Japan (which has a high-iodine diet) [19]. In addition, the solid variant may occur in adults wherein it often arises in thyroid gland with chronic lymphocytic thyroiditis. In our experi-ence, it frequently occurs in patients with systemic autoimmune disease (rheumatoid arthritis, lupus erythematosus). A study from the Mayo Clinic [21] and a recent report from Italy [22] indicate the solid variant behaves clinically in a similar fashion to classical papillary carcinoma. This tumor should not be considered as a poorly differentiated thyroid carcinoma.

Primary epithelial tumors: follicular-derived nonpapillary

Poorly differentiated thyroid carcinoma

According to the World Health Organization, poorly differentiated thyroid carcinoma (PDTC) is defined as "a tumor of follicular cell origin with morphologic and biological attributes intermediate between differentiated and anaplastic carcinoma of the thyroid"[23]. It clinically behaves more aggressively than well-differentiated carcinoma; however, it does not follow a fatal course of anaplastic carcinoma [22].

By light microscopy, these tumors display a solid, insular, and trabecular growth pattern associated with convoluted nuclei, mitotic figures ($\geq 3 \times 10$ high power field [HPF]), abnormal mitoses, and/or areas of tumor necrosis (not in areas of FNA tracks). These less differentiated areas can be intermixed with otherwise recognizable papillary or follicular cancers indicating transformation of well-differentiated tumor to an aggressive phenotype [22,24].

Recently, an unusual aggressive variant of PDTC "the rhabdoid phenotype" has been described. These tumors show characteristic eccentric eosinophilic cytoplasmic deposits/inclusions that are thyroglobulin and cytokeratin negative and are positive for vimentin, indicating the presence of intermediate filaments [25,26].

Spindle cell squamous carcinoma of thyroid

Many thyroid neoplasms can exhibit focal or extensive squamous differentiation. Bronner and LiVolsi [27] reported five cases of a tall cell variant of papillary carcinoma that were associated with a spindle cell squamous anaplastic carcinoma. This latter component was analogous to that seen in sarcomatoid squamous cell carcinomas of breast and oropharynx. Four cases in this series had angioinvasion and all showed extrathyroidal invasion. Lymph node metastases were present in two cases and consisted of only the papillary component. By immunostaining, the squamous and the spindle cell component are negative for thyroglobulin and positive for high-molecular-weight cytokeratins [27].

Paucicellular variant of anaplastic carcinoma

Anaplastic carcinoma of the thyroid is a highly malignant tumor. Usually the pathologic diagnosis of anaplastic carcinoma of thyroid is not a problem because of its clinical presentation, microscopic picture, and immunohistochemical profile [28].

LiVolsi and colleagues [29], and later Wan and colleagues [30], described a variant of anaplastic carcinoma, which, by light microscopy, the tumors was paucicellular and showed large areas of sclerotic and infarcted tissue and spindle cells arranged in fascicular or storiform patterns (Fig. 4). The tumor cells stain positive for epithelial membrane antigen and muscle-specific actin in both cases and one case was positive for keratin.

The histologic picture in this variant of anaplastic carcinoma may mimic Riedel's thyroiditis clinically and morphologically: presentation of a neck mass with compressive symptoms, sclerosis, spindle cell proliferation, and lack of obvious anaplasia [30].

Hyalinizing trabecular neoplasm

Carney and colleagues [31] first described hyalinizing trabecular neoplasm (HTN) in thyroid as a benign encapsulated follicular neoplasm composed of elongated cells arranged around capillaries in a background of hyaline and occasionally in a calcified extracellular matrix. The individual tumor cells show nuclear features of papillary thyroid carcinoma (Fig. 5) [31]. Some authors believe that HTN is benign, since most of these cases show an encapsulated neoplasm with lack of capsular and/or vascular invasion or distant metastasis. Others believe that HTN is a type of papillary carcinoma; this assumption is based on the similar cytologic characteristics, frequent coexistence, and similar immunohistochemical and molecular profile; however, to date no cases of HTN are found to harbor BRAF oncogene mutations [32–34].

Primary "epithelial" tumors: nonfollicular derivation

Thyroid paraganglioma

Thyroid paragangliomas are rare. In the reported cases, the tumors ranged in size from 1.5 to 10 cm, presented as solitary masses, and all

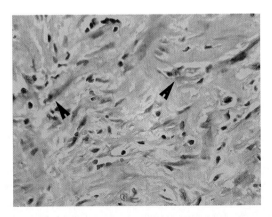

Fig. 4. Paucicellular variant of anaplastic carcinoma showing rare pleomorphic tumor cells (*arrowheads*) embedded within densely sclerotic tissue (hematoxylin & eosin, original magnification ×100).

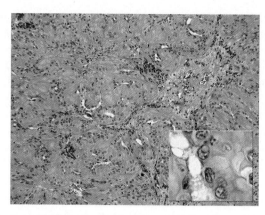

Fig. 5. Hyalinizing trabecular neoplasm containing elongated tumor cells arranged around capillaries in a background of hyaline matrix. The tumor cells show features of papillary carcinoma (*inset*) (hematoxylin & eosin, original magnification ×20 [inset, ×100]).

occurred in women. These tumors can present as circumscribed masses limited to the thyroid or can show extrathyroidal extension into the neighboring structures. By light microscopy they display the typical nesting (Zellballen) pattern seen in sites other than the thyroid. They stain positive for neuron specific-enolase (NSE), chromogranin and synaptophysin, and S-100 positive sustentacular cells and are negative for thyroglobulin, calcitonin, and carcinoembryonic antigen [35,36].

Tumors with thymic or related branchial pouch differentiation

This peculiar group of thyroid tumors shows histologic, immunohistochemical, and ultrastructural features that are consistent with thymic or related branchial pouch differentiation.

Spindle epithelial tumor with thymus-like differentiation

SETTLE (spindle epithelial tumor with thymus-like differentiation) tumors mainly occur in children and young adults and present as solitary circumscribed thyroid masses. According to the reported cases, these tumors do not behave as aggressive tumors and are characterized by slow growth and late local recurrences and distant metastasis (lung and kidney) [37].

The tumors consist of both spindle cells and epithelioid cells; however, the spindle cells usually predominate. The spindle elements are often arranged in a storiform configuration and show bland nuclear cytology. The epithelial cells show papillary, trabecular, or sheet arrangement; occasionally squamous differentiation reminiscent of Hassall's corpuscles can be seen. Angiolymphatic invasion or invasion into the surrounding parenchyma can be seen in some cases [37,38]. Immunohistochemically, the spindle cells stain positive with cytokeratins, smooth muscle actin, muscle-specific actin, and MIC-2, and stain negative with thyroglobulin and calcitonin [38,39].

Carcinoma showing thymus-like differentiation

The other terms used for CASTLE (carcinoma showing thymus-like differentiation) tumors include lymphoepithelioma-like carcinoma of the thyroid and intrathyroidal epithelial thymoma. CASTLE usually arises in the middle to lower third of the thyroid in adults between 40 and 50 years of age and often shows extrathyroidal extensions. By light microscopy and immunohistochemically these tumors closely resemble thymic carcinoma. In contrast to lymphoepithelioma-like carcinomas occurring in other sites such as nasopharynx, CASTLEs are negative for Epstein-Barr Virus (EBV) by in situ hybridization techniques [40–42].

Mucoepidermoid carcinoma of thyroid gland

Two distinct entities have been described under the umbrella of this term: mucoepidermoid carcinoma (MEC) and sclerosing mucoepidermoid carcinoma with eosinophilia (SMECE) [43].

Mucoepidermoid carcinoma

MEC tumors are common in women and present as painless solitary nodules. Microscopically, the tumors are circumscribed and unencapsulated with focal areas of infiltration into the surrounding thyroid parenchyma, and show both squamous features and mucin production. The background stroma is usually fibrotic and can exhibit foci of psammomatous calcification. These tumors are positive for thyroglobulin, thyroid transcription factor (TTF)-1, and cytokeratin and negative for calcitonin [43–45].

Sclerosing mucoepidermoid carcinoma with eosinophilia

SMECE tumors are very similar in their clinical presentation and biologic behavior to MEC of thyroid. However, there are distinct morphologic and immunohistochemical differences between these two entities that make this tumor distinct [43].

These tumors occur almost exclusively in women, and present as a painless solitary thyroid mass. The tumor cells show both squamous and glandular differentiation; occasionally there is prominent mucin production and mucous cyst formation. The background of this tumor is unique and demonstrates prominent hyaline stroma and a mixed inflammatory infiltrate with prominent eosinophilia (Fig. 6). The normal thyroid parenchyma surrounding the tumor displays chronic lymphocytic thyroiditis. Immunohistochemically the tumor cells are usually negative for thyroglobulin and calcitonin and positive for cytokeratins, TTF-1, and p63 [43, 46–48].

Almost all of MEC and SMECE cases reported in the literature have followed an indolent clinical course. There is propensity toward lymph node metastasis and some cases can show extrathyroidal extension and rarely distant metastases [43].

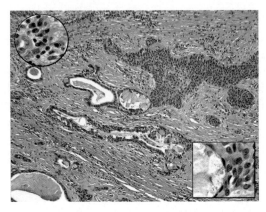

Fig. 6. Sclerosing mucoepidermoid carcinoma with eosinophilia showing squamous and glandular differentiation (*square inset*) in a background of densely sclerotic matrix and inflammatory infiltrate with prominent eosinophilia (*round inset*) (hematoxylin & eosin, original magnification ×40 [insets, ×100]).

Primary nonepithelial tumors

Mesenchymal tumors of the thyroid gland

Primary mesenchymal tumors of the thyroid are rare. The diagnosis of a primary mesenchymal tumor in thyroid should only be made after excluding metastases from another primary source, since those are more common then a primary thyroid origin.

Smooth muscle tumors of thyroid

After excluding metastatic tumors, to date fewer than 20 cases of benign and malignant primary smooth muscle tumors of the thyroid have been reported in the literature.

Leiomyomas occur exclusively in women and present as an isolated encapsulated mass confined to the thyroid and is treated by lobectomy or partial thyroidectomy. The histologic, immunohistochemical, and ultrastructural features are consistent with smooth muscle origin [49,50].

Leiomyosarcomas are more commonly seen in older patients and do not show any specific gender predilection. Their presentation is usually that of a large mass showing features of malignancy [49–51].

Tulbah and colleagues [52] reported a case of leiomyosarcoma of thyroid in a child with congenital immunodeficiency disease. This tumor was found to express large amounts of EBV messenger RNA similar to seen in pediatric smooth muscle tumors associated with AIDS and after organ transplantation.

Solitary fibrous tumor

Solitary fibrous tumor is a mesenchymal tumor that predominantly shows fibroblastic differentiation; in addition, some cases may reveal a focal or predominant myofibroblastic component. Universally this tumor stains positive with CD34.

Fewer than 10 cases of solitary fibrous tumors of the thyroid have been reported in the literature. All these reported cases have behaved in a benign fashion with no local recurrences or distant metastasis, even if the tumors extend extrathyroidally at initial surgery [50,53].

Vascular tumors

The vascular tumors of the thyroid as other mesenchymal tumors are rare. The list of reported vascular tumor in thyroid includes hemangioma, epithelioid hemangioendothelioma, and angiosarcoma [54,55]. From this list, angiosarcoma is the most notable one. Most cases have been reported from European Alpine regions, where it makes up approximately 4% of all thyroid malignancies. In these cases it is usually seen in a gland affected by nodular goiter [56].

Granular cell tumor

Granular cell tumor is a rare tumor of usually Schwann cell origin. Approximately 50% of the cases have been reported in the head and neck region. They can occur in other organs, including respiratory tract, gastrointestinal tract, genitourinary tract, vulva, and breast. Rarely these tumors can occur in thyroid or adjacent to the thyroid and clinically present as thyroid masses. Most reported tumors in the thyroid occurred in women, behaved in a benign fashion, and can be treated with lobectomy [57,58].

MALTomas of the thyroid

Most primary thyroid lymphomas are of B-cell phenotype and can represent small- or large-cell tumors [59,60]. Most primary lymphomas of the thyroid are variants of MALT (mucosa-associated lymphoid tissue) lymphomas.

Recognition of MALT lymphomas by immunophenotyping, or molecular or cytogenetic analyses is important since other B-cell lymphomas in the thyroid most likely represent secondary neoplasms and have a different clinical behavior. Primary thyroid lymphomas have a very good 5-year survival (70% to 100%) with small-cell lymphomas, especially those showing plasmacytic differentiation (common in MALTomas) having an excellent prognosis [60–62].

References

[1] Murray D. The thyroid gland. In: Kovacs K, Asa SA, editors. Functional endocrinology. Malden (MA): Blackwell Science; 1998. p. 295–380.
[2] LiVolsi VA. Surgical pathology of the thyroid. Philadelphia: WB. Saunders; 1990.
[3] Rosai J, Carcangui ML, DeLellis RA. Tumors of the thyroid gland. In: Rosai J, Sobin LE, editors. Washington, DC: Armed Forces Institute of Pathology; 1992.

[4] Apel RL, Asa SL, LiVolsi VA. Papillary Hurthle cell carcinoma with lymphocytic stroma. "Warthin-like tumor" of the thyroid. Am J Surg Pathol 1995;19(7):810–4.

[5] Baloch ZW, LiVolsi VA. Warthin-like papillary carcinoma of the thyroid. Arch Pathol Lab Med 2000;124(8):1192–5.

[6] Albores-Saavedra J GE, Vardaman C, Vuitch F. The macrofollicular variant of papillary thyroid carcinoma: a study of 17 cases. Hum Pathol 1991;22:1195–205.

[7] Woyke S, al-Jassar AK, al-Jazzaf H. Macrofollicular variant of papillary thyroid carcinoma diagnosed by fine needle aspiration biopsy: a case report. Acta Cytol 1998; 42(5):1184–8.

[8] Chan JK, Tsang WY. Endocrine malignancies that may mimic benign lesions. Semin Diagn Pathol 1995;12(1):45–63.

[9] Albores-Saavedra J, Housini I, Vuitch F, et al. Macrofollicular variant of papillary thyroid carcinoma with minor insular component. Cancer 1997;80(6):1110–6.

[10] Vergilio J, Baloch ZW, LiVolsi VA. Spindle cell metaplasia of the thyroid arising in association with papillary carcinoma and follicular adenoma. Am J Clin Pathol 2002; 117(2):199–204.

[11] Chan JK, Carcangiu ML, Rosai J. Papillary carcinoma of thyroid with exuberant nodular fasciitis-like stroma. Report of three cases. Am J Clin Pathol 1991;95(3):309–14.

[12] Cetta F, Toti P, Petracci M, et al. Thyroid carcinoma associated with familial adenomatous polyposis. Histopathology 1997;31(3):231–6.

[13] Cetta F, Olschwang S, Petracci M, et al. Genetic alterations in thyroid carcinoma associated with familial adenomatous polyposis: clinical implications and suggestions for early detection. World J Surg 1998;22(12):1231–6.

[14] Xu B, Yoshimoto K, Miyauchi A, et al. Cribriform-morular variant of papillary thyroid carcinoma: a pathological and molecular genetic study with evidence of frequent somatic mutations in exon 3 of the beta-catenin gene. J Pathol 2003;199(1):58–67.

[15] Evans HL. Columnar-cell carcinoma of the thyroid. A report of two cases of an aggressive variant of thyroid carcinoma. Am J Clin Pathol 1986;85:77–80.

[16] Evans HL. Encapsulated columnar-cell carcinoma of the thyroid. A report of four cases suggesting a favorable outcome. Am J Surg Pathol 1996;20:1205–11.

[17] Wenig BM, Thompson LDR, Adair CF, et al. Thyroid papillary carcinoma of columnar cell type. A clinicopathologic study of 16 cases. Cancer 1998;82:740–53.

[18] Duffy BJ, Fitzgerald PJ. Cancer of the thyroid in children: a report of 28 cases. J Clin Endocrinol Metab 1950;10:1296–308.

[19] Nikiforov YE, Gnepp DR. Pathomorphology of thyroid gland lesions associated with radiation exposure: the Chernobyl experience and review of the literature. Adv Anat Pathol 1999;6(2):78–91.

[20] Harach HR, Williams ED. Childhood thyroid cancer in England and Wales. Br J Cancer 1995;72(3):777–83.

[21] Nikiforov YE, Erickson LA, Nikiforova MN, et al. Solid variant of papillary thyroid carcinoma: incidence, clinical- pathologic characteristics, molecular analysis, and biologic behavior. Am J Surg Pathol 2001;25(12):1478–84.

[22] Volante M, Collini P, Nikiforov YE, et al. Poorly differentiated thyroid carcinoma: the Turin proposal for the use of uniform diagnostic criteria and an algorithmic diagnostic approach. Am J Surg Pathol 2007;31(8):1256–64.

[23] DeLellis RA, Lloyd RD, Heitz PU, et al, editors. WHO: pathology and genetics. tumours of endocrine organs. Lyon (France): IARC Press; 2004.

[24] Hiltzik D, Carlson DL, Tuttle RM, et al. Poorly differentiated thyroid carcinomas defined on the basis of mitosis and necrosis: a clinicopathologic study of 58 patients. Cancer 2006; 106(6):1286–95.

[25] Agarwal S, Sharma MC, Aron M, et al. Poorly differentiated thyroid carcinoma with rhabdoid phenotype: a diagnostic dilemma–report of a rare case. Endocr Pathol 2006; 17(4):399–405.

[26] Albores-Saavedra J, Sharma S. Poorly differentiated follicular thyroid carcinoma with rhabdoid phenotype: a clinicopathologic, immunohistochemical and electron microscopic study of two cases. Mod Pathol 2001;14(2):98–104.

[27] Bronner MP, LiVolsi VA. Spindle cell squamous carcinoma of the thyroid: an unusual anaplastic tumor associated with tall cell papillary cancer. Mod Pathol 1991;4(5):637–43.

[28] Carcangiu ML, Steeper T, Zampi G, et al. Anaplastic thyroid carcinoma. A study of 70 cases. Am J Clin Pathol 1985;83(2):135–58.

[29] LiVolsi VA, Brooks JJ, Arendash-Durand B. Anaplastic thyroid tumors. Immunohistology. Am J Clin Pathol 1987;87(4):434–42.

[30] Wan SK, Chan JK, Tang SK. Paucicellular variant of anaplastic thyroid carcinoma. A mimic of Reidel's thyroiditis. Am J Clin Pathol 1996;105(4):388–93.

[31] Carney JA, Ryan J, Goellner JR. Hyalinizing trabecular adenoma of the thyroid gland. Am J Surg Pathol 1987;11(8):583–91.

[32] Papotti M, Riella P, Montemurro F, et al. Immunophenotypic heterogeneity of hyalinizing trabecular tumours of the thyroid. Histopathology 1997;31(6):525–33.

[33] Cheung CC, Boerner SL, MacMillan CM, et al. Hyalinizing trabecular tumor of the thyroid: a variant of papillary carcinoma proved by molecular genetics. Am J Surg Pathol 2000; 24(12):1622–6.

[34] Salvatore G, Chiappetta G, Nikiforov YE, et al. Molecular profile of hyalinizing trabecular tumours of the thyroid: high prevalence of RET/PTC rearrangements and absence of B-raf and N-ras point mutations. Eur J Cancer 2005;41(5):816–21.

[35] LaGuette J, Matias-Guiu X, Rosai J. Thyroid paraganglioma: a clinicopathologic and immunohistochemical study of three cases. Am J Surg Pathol 1997;21(7):748–53.

[36] Yano Y, Nagahama M, Sugino K, et al. Paraganglioma of the thyroid: report of a male case with ultrasonographic imagings, cytologic, histologic, and immunohistochemical features. Thyroid 2007;17(6):575–8.

[37] Cheuk W, Jacobson AA, Chan JK. Spindle epithelial tumor with thymus-like differentiation (SETTLE): a distinctive malignant thyroid neoplasm with significant metastatic potential. Mod Pathol 2000;13(10):1150–5.

[38] Kirby PA, Ellison WA, Thomas PA. Spindle epithelial tumor with thymus-like differentiation (SETTLE) of the thyroid with prominent mitotic activity and focal necrosis. Am J Surg Pathol 1999;23(6):712–6.

[39] Abrosimov AY, LiVolsi VA. Spindle epithelial tumor with thymus-like differentiation (SETTLE) of the thyroid with neck lymph node metastasis: a case report. Endocr Pathol 2005;16(2):139–43.

[40] Chow SM, Chan JK, Tse LL, et al. Carcinoma showing thymus-like element (CASTLE) of thyroid: combined modality treatment in 3 patients with locally advanced disease. Eur J Surg Oncol 2007;33(1):83–5.

[41] Reimann JD, Dorfman DM, Nose V. Carcinoma showing thymus-like differentiation of the thyroid (CASTLE): a comparative study: evidence of thymic differentiation and solid cell nest origin. Am J Surg Pathol 2006;30(8):994–1001.

[42] Chan JK, Rosai J. Tumors of the neck showing thymic or related branchial pouch differentiation: a unifying concept. Hum Pathol 1991;22(4):349–67.

[43] Baloch ZW, Solomon AC, LiVolsi VA. Primary mucoepidermoid carcinoma and sclerosing mucoepidermoid carcinoma with eosinophilia of the thyroid gland: a report of nine cases. Mod Pathol 2000;13(7):802–7.

[44] Katoh R, Sugai T, Ono S, et al. Mucoepidermoid carcinoma of the thyroid gland. Cancer 1990;65(9):2020–7.

[45] Cameselle-Teijeiro J. Mucoepidermoid carcinoma and solid cell nests of the thyroid. Hum Pathol 1996;27(8):861–3.

[46] Solomon AC, Baloch ZW, Salhany KE, et al. Thyroid sclerosing mucoepidermoid carcinoma with eosinophilia: mimic of Hodgkin disease in nodal metastases. Arch Pathol Lab Med 2000;124(3):446–9.

[47] Hunt JL, LiVolsi VA, Barnes EL. p63 expression in sclerosing mucoepidermoid carcinomas with eosinophilia arising in the thyroid. Mod Pathol 2004;17(5):526–9.

[48] Albores-Saavedra J, Gu X, Luna MA. Clear cells and thyroid transcription factor I reactivity in sclerosing mucoepidermoid carcinoma of the thyroid gland. Ann Diagn Pathol 2003;7(6): 348–53.

[49] Thompson LD, Wenig BM, Adair CF, et al. Primary smooth muscle tumors of the thyroid gland. Cancer 1997;79(3):579–87.

[50] Papi G, Corrado S, LiVolsi VA. Primary spindle cell lesions of the thyroid gland: an overview. Am J Clin Pathol 2006;125(Suppl):S95–123.

[51] Chetty R, Clark SP, Dowling JP. Leiomyosarcoma of the thyroid: immunohistochemical and ultrastructural study. Pathology 1993;25(2):203–5.

[52] Tulbah A, Al-Dayel F, Fawaz I, et al. Epstein-Barr virus-associated leiomyosarcoma of the thyroid in a child with congenital immunodeficiency: a case report. Am J Surg Pathol 1999; 23(4):473–6.

[53] Rodriguez I, Ayala E, Caballero C, et al. Solitary fibrous tumor of the thyroid gland: report of seven cases. Am J Surg Pathol 2001;25(11):1424–8.

[54] Shamim M. Haemangioma of thyroid with calcification. J R Coll Surg Edinb 1978;23(4): 226–9.

[55] Kumar R, Gupta R, Khullar S, et al. Thyroid hemangioma: a case report with a review of the literature. Clin Nucl Med 2000;25(10):769–71.

[56] Maiorana A, Collina G, Cesinaro AM, et al. Epithelioid angiosarcoma of the thyroid. Clinicopathological analysis of seven cases from non-Alpine areas. Virchows Arch 1996; 429(2–3):131–7.

[57] Milias S, Hytiroglou P, Kourtis D, et al. Granular cell tumour of the thyroid gland. Histopathology 2004;44(2):190–1.

[58] Baloch ZW, Martin S, Livolsi VA. Granular cell tumor of the thyroid: a case report. Int J Surg Pathol 2005;13(3):291–4.

[59] Wirtzfeld DA, Winston JS, Hicks WL Jr, et al. Clinical presentation and treatment of non-Hodgkin's lymphoma of the thyroid gland. Ann Surg Oncol 2001;8(4):338–41.

[60] Thieblemont C, Mayer A, Dumontet C, et al. Primary thyroid lymphoma is a heterogeneous disease. J Clin Endocrinol Metab 2002;87(1):105–11.

[61] Mack LA, Pasieka JL. An evidence-based approach to the treatment of thyroid lymphoma. World J Surg 2007;31(5):978–86.

[62] Niitsu N, Okamoto M, Nakamura N, et al. Clinicopathologic correlations of stage IE/IIE primary thyroid diffuse large B-cell lymphoma. Ann Oncol 2007;18(7):1203–8.

ELSEVIER
SAUNDERS

Endocrinol Metab Clin N Am
37 (2008) 311–331

ENDOCRINOLOGY
AND METABOLISM
CLINICS
OF NORTH AMERICA

Genome-Wide Studies in Thyroid Neoplasia

Thomas J. Giordano, MD, PhD

*Department of Pathology, 1150 West Medical Center Drive, MSRB-2, C570D,
University of Michigan Health System, Ann Arbor, MI 48109, USA*

There is much interest in the application of genome biology to the field of thyroid neoplasia, despite the relatively low mortality rate associated with thyroid cancer in general. The principal reason for this interest is that one can persuasively argue the field of thyroid neoplasia stands to benefit greatly from the intelligent application of genomic information to address a variety of pathologic and clinical issues. These include (1) improved pathologic evaluation through more informative and accurate diagnoses (ie, improved tumor classification), (2) improved identification of aggressive forms of differentiated thyroid cancer, (3) prediction of response to therapy such as radioactive iodine (RAI), and (4) identification of novel therapeutic targets. In addition to these practical patient care issues, there is an excellent opportunity of expand our basic understanding of thyroid carcinogenesis.

The pathologic evaluation of thyroid nodules can be difficult and subjective. This is observed at both the cytologic and histologic levels and has been documented in several multiobserver studies [1–3]. Specifically, the evaluation of pure follicular-patterned nodules presents a differential diagnosis of follicular adenoma (FA), adenomatoid nodule of multinodular goiter, follicular carcinoma (FC), and the follicular variant of papillary carcinoma (FVPC). Thus, there is ample room for disagreement among pathologists on challenging cases. While genotyping for the common mutations present in thyroid tumors (eg, *BRAF* V600E point mutations in PC [4–12]) can assist in diagnosis, successful application of a genomic approach to the diagnostic arena of follicular-patterned nodules would represent a significant clinical advance.

E-mail address: Giordano@umich.edu

Most differentiated thyroid cancers are successfully managed with surgery and RAI [13,14]. Yet, a small subset of cancers will recur and metastasize [15,16], potentially leading to significant morbidity [17–19]. Our current ability to identify these cases is limited [20] and could be effectively supplemented with genomic information.

Assessment of response to RAI is sometimes problematic and there is some disagreement among clinicians about its effectiveness in some situations [21]. The ability to select those patients who will receive the most benefit from RAI therapy based on some intrinsic molecular parameter of a tumor would represent a true clinical advance and embodies the promise of personalized genomic medicine for patients with thyroid cancer [22].

Finally, identification of novel therapeutic targets is needed for those cases that recur and/or metastasize despite optimal therapy or display histologic progression to aggressive forms (ie, poorly differentiated thyroid carcinoma [PDTC] and anaplastic carcinoma [AC]). While several exciting targets, such as mutated BRAF protein [23,24] and increased RET protein expression due to *RET/PTC* rearrangement [25,26], are being pursued in clinical trials, molecular profiling promises to deliver other signaling pathways that could be inhibited with targeted therapeutics.

In this article, the most relevant genomic work on thyroid tumors performed to date is reviewed along with some general comments about the potential impact of genomic biology on thyroid pathology and the management of patients with thyroid nodules and cancer.

Genomic technology and biology

Description of the available genomic technologies is beyond the scope of this article; nonetheless, a few introductory comments about genomic biology are warranted. Readers interested in learning about genomic technologies are directed to numerous technical review articles [27–35]. The application of DNA microarrays in pathology research has also been recently reviewed [36].

The successful development of genomic technologies would not have been possible without the complete determination of the sequence of the human genome [37,38]. This landmark accomplishment, together with technical advances in chip-based genomic technologies [39] and cancer bioinformatics [40–44], have come together to catalyze a transformation of the way laboratory-based molecular biology research is performed. Once the domain of biologists working alone or in small teams, genomic science is a large team effort that requires a broad spectrum of expertise to be successful. Despite the effort and cost of assembling these genomic teams, the benefits are clearly worth the investment as *genomicists* are now discovering things that just 10 years ago were almost unimaginable, such as a direct comparison of the genomes of 12 species of *Drosophila* [45,46]. The impact on medicine should be equally large with some predicting a future in which individuals will have their genome routinely sequenced as part of the delivery of optimal health care via personalized medicine [47,48].

Gene expression studies with a focus on tumor biology and pathogenesis

The study by Huang and colleagues [49] was one of the first to use DNA microarrays to examine gene expression in a small cohort (n = 8) of papillary carcinomas (PCs) compared with case-matched normal thyroid samples. A robust set of 226 differentially expressed genes was derived using a combination of fold change and paired *t* tests. Among the genes whose expression was decreased in the PCs were several genes specifically related to thyroid function (eg, *TPO*), providing evidence that PC, while considered a well-differentiated tumor, is less differentiated than normal thyroid. The overexpressed gene list included many genes previously associated with PC, such as *FN1* and the *MET* oncogene. In addition, many genes not previously associated with PC were identified such as *CITED1*. Interestingly, a predominance of genes related to cell adhesion were also identified, consistent with the morphologic observation that PCs are generally invasive tumors that frequently metastasize to regional lymph nodes and to distant sites such as lung and bone. Despite the small cohort size, this significant study revealed a consistent gene expression profile that provided insight into the biology of PC and also identified several potential pathologic markers.

Some studies have combined morphologic and genotypic data with gene expression profiling data to define expression profiles that correlate with specific mutations. For example, using a cohort of 51 PCs and analyzing their gene expression profiles together with their morphologies (classical type, follicular variant, and tall cell variant) and mutations, distinct gene expression profiles were defined for PCs with *RAS, BRAF,* and *RET/PTC* mutations [50]. Correlations were uncovered between gene expression and morphology, and between gene expression and mutation, but mutation was more highly correlated to gene expression than morphology. One tumor without a detectable mutation was predicted based on its expression profile to have a *RET/PTC* mutation and was shown to contain such a rearrangement that was subsequently discovered to be a novel rearrangement between *RET* and *HOOK3* [51]. This study revealed that mutational status is the main source of gene expression in PC, suggesting that these mutations are dominant events in these tumors.

Several studies have specifically focused on FCs that contain a balanced translocation between the *PAX8* and *PPARG* genes [52–54]. First described by Kroll and colleagues [55] in 2000, this translocation, together with the well-recognized *RET/PTC* rearrangements, distinguished thyroid carcinoma as an epithelial tumor possessing recurrent chromosomal rearrangements well before their discovery in prostate carcinoma [56]. Some have questioned why DNA microarray studies on similar thyroid tumors yield little overlap in their lists of differentially expressed genes. However, the studies by Lacroix and colleagues [53] and Giordano and colleagues [52] identified a highly overlapping set of genes that were preferentially expressed in FCs with this translocation. Given that *PPARG* encodes a transcription factor, it was interesting to uncover via bioinformatics that many of the differentially expressed genes were known PPARγ targets, suggesting that the PAX8-PPARγ fusion protein retains some of the transcriptional activity of wild-type PPARγ. Transient transfection experiments confirmed this finding. These studies have implications for the pathogenesis of this type of FC, suggesting that the fusion gene may function as an oncogene analogous to other fusion genes present in leukemia and soft tissue tumors [57]. This view is supported by several recent studies that show that this fusion leads to increased cell growth and decreased thyroid differentiation [58,59]. Although much work remains to be done in this area, such as developing transgenic mouse models of FC with the *PAX8-PPARg* translocation, these studies clearly demonstrate how genomic gene expression data can be used to generate mechanistic hypotheses and further our understanding of thyroid tumor pathogenesis.

DNA microarray studies have also focused on specific signaling pathways in an attempt to better understand the role of the pathway in a particular diseased state. One such study examined the cAMP signaling pathway in autonomous functioning follicular adenomas [60]. Using cultured primary thyrocytes stimulated with TSH, they showed more similarity in gene expression between the cultured cells and autonomous adenomas compared with PC. Furthermore, several genes that operate as negative regulators of signal transduction were expressed at lower levels in the adenomas compared with the TSH-stimulated cultures. These results indicate a loss of negative feedback control in autonomous adenomas and suggest they may be the result of activation of cAMP signaling together with suppression of negative feedback mechanisms.

A recent study by Vasko and colleagues [61] examined the difference between gene expression in the central and invasive areas of seven PCs. While this is a subtle comparison and therefore a difficult experimental design, many differentially expressed genes, some of which are related to epithelial-to-mesenchymal transition (EMT), were identified. EMT is the process whereby tumor cells dedifferentiate from an epithelial phenotype to a mesenchymal phenotype via loss of cell-to-cell contact and cytoskeletal remodeling, resulting in a migratory phenotype [62]. As a result, EMT is thought to be crucial to tumor metastasis [63,64]. The EMT result was extended and validated by examining by immunohistochemistry a larger set of PCs for vimentin expression, thought to be one of the defining features of EMT [65]. This study provides support for the idea that the invasive front of PC is biologically distinct from the central portion of the tumor and that EMT plays a role in defining the PC phenotype, a suggestion consistent with their observed invasive nature.

The association between thyroid carcinoma and radiation exposure was well documented before 1986 [66–78]. After the Chernobyl accident that year, the subsequent dramatic increase in the incidence of thyroid cancer in children in exposed countries provided unequivocal confirmation of this association [79–81] and an opportunity to study the effects of ionizing radiation on thyroid cancer [82]. Using transcriptional profiling, Detours and colleagues [83] compared gene expression in 12 PCs from the Chernobyl Tissue Bank (CTB) and 14 PCs from French patients with no history of exposure to ionizing radiation and, despite an absence of correlation between global gene expression and radiation, uncovered a distinct set of genes related to radiation susceptibility, although previous work from the same group failed to do so [84]. Using supervised analyses with multiple classification procedures, they found 256 differentially expressed genes between the 2 PC cohorts. These genes were enriched for genes related to H_2O_2 response and homologous recombination. While this study did identify some gene expression differences in radiation-associated and non–radiation-associated PCs, the study design was less than ideal due to different proportions of *BRAF* and *RET/PTC* mutations among the two groups, a known source of gene expression variation in PC [50]. A larger study better controlled for mutation would be needed to fully resolve whether radiation-associated PCs are biologically different from other PCs.

Gene expression studies with a focus on tumor classification and diagnosis

Given the difficulties associated with the diagnosis of some thyroid tumors, especially follicular-patterned tumors, it is not surprising that numerous studies have focused on using gene expression derived from genomic studies with the intent to develop a novel diagnostic approach. While none of these have yet been sufficiently validated to justify clinical implementation, it is nonetheless worthwhile to closely examine a selection of these studies as a proxy of what is possible and to clarify what remains to be accomplished.

To date, there have been at least 15 studies published in the English literature that have primarily focused on using genomic data for thyroid tumor diagnosis and classification [50,85–98]. Some studies have focused on the simple separation of benign and malignant nodules, an approach that would be useful if successfully implemented preoperatively using samples derived from fine-needle aspirations (FNAs). Other studies have compared specific tumor types, such as PC and FC. Still other studies have examined tumors within a specific diagnostic category with different mutations. The overall clinical applicability of using gene expression profiling has been reviewed [99], with an optimistic prediction of implementation of preoperative molecular profiling in the next few years.

The type of statistical methodology varies widely among these studies. Many investigators have used hierarchical clustering (HC) as the sole classification tool, although HC has been deemed by many statisticians as not sufficiently rigorous for tumor classification [100]. Other studies have used such methods as principal components analysis, multidimensional scaling, linear discrimination analysis, singular value decomposition, leave-one-out cross validation, and machine learning such as support vector machines. Description of these methods and when and how they should be applied is beyond the scope of this article. Interested readers are referred to these reviews [31,101–105].

Review of all of the diagnostically oriented studies is beyond the scope of this article. However, a few studies are discussed to highlight the potential and limitations of this approach. Mazzanti and colleagues [95] profiled 71 thyroid tumors (classical PC, FVPC, FA, and hyperplastic nodules [HN]) using cDNA microarrays. Principal component analysis revealed an overall organization of tumors based on diagnosis, a finding that provides support for the quality of the microarray data. By comparing the benign tumors (FA plus HN) to the PCs, a set of 47 genes was derived and used to construct a diagnostic predictor model that accurately predicted the diagnosis of the tumors using a leave-one-out cross-validation method. Despite a lack of genotyping data for common PC mutations and the lack of FC samples, this study was one of the first to highlight the potential of gene expression profiles as a diagnostic tool for thyroid tumors.

Several studies have focused on the difficult separation of FA and FC. Barden and colleagues [86] generated gene expression profiles for a small cohort of 17 FAs and FCs and derived a set of 105 differentially expressed genes. Five tumors, a relatively small testing set, were correctly classified using hierarchical clustering. Similarly, Weber and colleagues [96] used a slightly larger set of 24 FAs and FCs to derive a set of 80 genes that were differentially expressed between the groups. From this group, a set of three genes was selected and then evaluated as a gene-expression classifier using an independent set of 31 tumors. The results were very promising, with a sensitivity of 100%, specificity of 94.7%, and an accuracy of 96.7%, and await independent validation by other groups.

Gene-expression profiles have also been used for mutation prediction. By first defining mutation-specific profiles for PCs with *RAS, BRAF,* and *RET/PTC* mutations, it was then possible to accurately predict the mutational status of 40 PCs by leave-one-out cross validation using as few as one gene per mutation class [50]. Not unexpectedly, the gene whose expression was most correlated with *RET/PTC* rearrangement was *RET*.

A recent study [89] using spotted cDNA microarray specifically addressed the issue of diagnostically difficult follicular-patterned tumors; those sometimes classified as having "uncertain malignant potential." This term, along with others, has been proposed for these tumors [106], although it has not been widely accepted due to their noncommittal nature. Nonetheless, this study appropriately focused on tumors with uncertain or intermediate histologic features. Comparing gene expression in 10 of these tumors (designated

T-UM) to tumors with clear-cut histologic diagnoses (PC, FVPC, FTC, and FTA), the T-UMs were classified into benign and malignant groups. This study, although it tested a relatively small group of T-UMs, provides support for the goal of developing objective pathologic parameters for follicular-patterned thyroid tumors.

The ultimate goal of much of this diagnostic work is to improve the accuracy of preoperative thyroid FNA. Using 22 FNA specimens of thyroid nodules and a hierarchical clustering–based classifier derived from 25 genes, Lubitz and colleagues [94] showed that diagnosis prediction of FNA samples was feasible and accurate in most cases. Despite the small validation size and lack of a robust statistical classifier, this study illustrates the potential of gene-expression profiling to improve the preoperative diagnosis of thyroid tumors.

Meta-analyses

Given the large numbers of microarray studies performed using thyroid tumors, a meta-analysis of 21 published gene-expression studies was performed on 10 different expression platforms [91]. Because of the diversity of methodologies used by the studies, it was impossible to merge all of the raw data. Therefore, the analysts examined the overlap between studies of reported differentially expressed genes. Many diagnostic comparisons were performed, but a large "cancer versus noncancer" analysis revealed a list of 107 genes that included well-recognized genes such as *MET*, *TIMP1*, *FN1*, *TPO*, *CITED1*, and *KRT19*, as well as less recognized genes such as *EPS8*, *PROS1*, and *CRABP1*. Interestingly, the same group performed a true meta-analysis by merging the raw image files from those fewer studies that employed a common platform (Affymetrix GeneChips) and compared the results to the larger meta-review. Forty-three of the 107 genes identified initially were identified by both methods. This was an encouraging result, but it was clear that reprocessing the microarray data in a consistent manner would improve the results.

A similar meta-analysis was performed by Eszlinger and colleagues [87]. Using several expression datasets corresponding to PC, autonomously functioning thyroid nodules, and cold thyroid nodules, they verified a support vector machine-based PC classifier. Collectively, these two meta-analyses demonstrate the value of this approach, despite the technical hurdles of combining microarray datasets, especially when large, single-institutional datasets are not available.

Gene expression studies with a focus on identification of therapeutic targets

Although nearly all microarray studies can be used to identify differentially expressed genes whose protein products could serve as therapeutic targets, several studies have focused on this aspect together with identification

of prognostic markers. Combining multiple molecular approaches, Wreesmann and colleagues [107] identified *MUC1* as an independent prognostic
factor for PC and suggested that it could serve as a therapeutic target. Using
a mouse model of PC that develops pulmonary metastases with high frequency, Zou and colleagues [108] found increased expression of *S100A4*
and suggested that this protein could serve as a therapeutic target. This
work was extended to human tumors [109]. A recently reported cDNA expression study using PCs from Middle Eastern countries confirmed high
MET expression in this tumor [110], an established molecular target present
in several tumor types [111].

Correlation between gene expression and tumor morphology

One of the most consistent observations in the studies reviewed herein
(and also present in microarray studies of other tumors in which I have participated) is the correlation between global gene expression in a tumor and
its histopathology. This is completely logical, as the morphology of a given
tumor reflects the integration of all the genetic changes present in the tumor
cell DNA sequence together with those epigenetic changes present in DNA
and histones (for a review on epigenetics, see Egger and colleagues [112]).
Many, but not all, of these genetic and epigenetic changes are manifested
through changes in transcription that are readily measurable by DNA microarrays. Thus, in my opinion, any molecular information about a tumor
that directly contradicts what a pathologist can derive from its morphology
should be treated with a healthy dose of suspicion. Accordingly, the view
among most pathologists is that microscopy will remain the mainstay of tumor classification [113] and that molecular pathology will enhance rather
than replace morphology [114].

MicroRNA studies

MicroRNAs (miRNA) are a recently described class of small, noncoding
RNA molecules that act as regulators during development and differentiation [115]. Chip-based profiling has permitted simultaneous investigation
of numerous miRNAs in a variety of human tumor types [116–121], and
a few studies have specifically profiled miRNAs in thyroid tumors [122–
125]. The first such study by He and colleagues [125], using miRNA microarrays and nine tumor-normal matched PCs, found several overexpressed
miRNA genes out of 460 miRNA genes. A set of five overexpressed miRNA
genes was able to accurately distinguish PC and normal thyroid, a finding
with diagnostic potential. Interestingly, one miRNA (miR-221) was overexpressed in normal tissue adjacent to PC, suggesting that this may be an early
event in PC pathogenesis, although this finding requires validation.
Combining gene-expression data with the miRNA profiles and using bioinformatics, 19 putative target genes, including *KIT,* were identified.

Consistent with this hypothesis, *KIT* expression was decreased in the majority of tumors with high expression of miR-221, -222, and -146b. Similarly, miR-221 and miR-222 were confirmed to be highly expressed in resected PCs, FNA samples of PCs, and thyroid cancer cell lines in an independent study [124]. Functional studies of miR-221 suggest a role for overexpression of this microRNA in thyroid carcinogenesis. Two miRNAs, miR-197 and miR-346, were also identified as being overexpressed in FC, and both are thought to play a role in the development of FC [123]. Recently, an miRNA profile specific to AC was reported [122]. Collectively, these studies strongly suggest a vital role for specific miRNAs as key factors in the development and progression of thyroid cancer.

Chromosomal studies

Despite the common mutations associated with thyroid cancer, such as those of the *RET/RAS/BRAF* signaling pathway, it is broadly recognized that cancer is a multistep process and therefore these tumors should possess many other genetics and epigenetic changes [126]. As a result, there is a need to systematically examine the thyroid cancer genome for recurrent changes, similar to what is being done for more common cancers (see Weir and colleagues [127] for an example on lung adenocarcinoma).

Many studies on thyroid cancer have used comparative genomic hybridization (CGH) [128–152]. First described by Kallioniemi and colleagues in 1992 [153], CGH is a technique that can be used to systematically examine the cancer genome to identify large, recurrent genomic alterations such as DNA copy number gains and losses. The initial form of CGH uses metaphase DNA and suffers from low mapping resolution. Array CGH (aCGH) provides a higher mapping resolution and has been used in a several cancer studies [154].

Collectively, the reported chromosomal gains and losses are substantial, yet difficult to fully characterize in a meaningful way. One of the most interesting CGH studies demonstrated that thyroid carcinoma associated with radiation exposure harbored two- to fourfold higher levels of recurrent chromosomal gains [155], consistent with the view that DNA damage secondary to ionizing radiation leads to chromosomal copy number alterations.

A recent aCGH study of PCs used DNA from laser capture microdissected tumors to catalog recurrent chromosomal gains and losses [149]. This study uncovered a higher frequency of gains and losses than previously reported, a finding attributed to higher mapping resolution of aCGH and the enrichment of tumor DNA due to microdissection. While these results are exciting, the study cohort was relatively small (eight tumors and three cell lines). Therefore, these findings need to be validated with more tumors and other technologies such as whole genome mapping DNA microarrays that can identify focal chromosomal copy number changes in cancer [127].

Remaining challenges

Despite the significant advances outlined in this article, there are several areas in which little genomic work has been reported, but in which genomic approaches have the potential to further advance the field of thyroid cancer. Two such areas are discussed in the following sections.

Genomic definition of poorly differentiated carcinoma

Poorly differentiated thyroid cancer (PDTC) is a controversial entity that lacks a consensus regarding definition and diagnostic criteria. It is agreed that PDTC represents an intermediate form between differentiated (papillary and follicular) carcinomas and anaplastic (undifferentiated) carcinoma [156]. As an intermediate form of thyroid carcinoma, the PDTC diagnostic category contains two boundaries, one with differentiated carcinomas and another with undifferentiated carcinomas. As a result, the potential for diagnostic disagreement is considerable despite work in this area [157], and the development of an objective set of diagnostic criteria would be helpful. Some have argued that tumor pattern alone is not sufficient to define PDTC [158]. The genetics changes associated with progression from differentiated to PDTC and ATC have been reviewed [159]. It is clear that the current histologic and molecular studies have not produced a definition sufficient for reliable sorting of thyroid tumors into well-differentiated, poorly differentiated, and undifferentiated categories. Transcriptional profiling, if applied to a large enough cohort of thyroid tumors of all of histopathologic types, has the potential to objectively define these diagnostic categories. However, a well-funded, multi-institutional effort would be needed to accomplish this goal.

Analysis of thyroid cancer progression

Related to the above discussion on PDTC, genomic biology could be used to expand our understanding of thyroid cancer progression, beginning with differentiated forms and ending at undifferentiated carcinoma, similar to what has been done for prostate carcinoma [160–162]. This will be challenging but highly beneficial, as thyroid mortality is often related to histologic progression to aggressive forms. A better understanding of this multistep process will permit the identification of molecular targets that will form the basis for combination therapies that will needed for the treatment of these aggressive cancers.

Medullary thyroid carcinoma

Relative to the amount of genomic research performed on follicular cell thyroid tumors, there has been little done on medullary thyroid carcinoma (MTC). This reflects both the rarer nature of MTC and the advanced state of knowledge regarding the genetics of *RET* mutations in MTC. Nonetheless, the available genomic studies on MTC are reviewed as follows.

By generating gene-expression profiles of benign pheochromocytomas and MTC from patients with multiple endocrine neoplasia (MEN) type 2A and 2B that harbor specific *RET* mutations, Jain and colleagues [163] defined distinct expression profiles between extracellular (MEN2A) and intracellular (MEN2B) *RET* mutations. Genes related to EMT were preferentially expressed in MEN2B-associated MTCs. Interestingly, high levels of CHM1, a protein that is expressed in chondrocytes of growth plates and thought to regulate growth of bone and cartilage [164], were present in MEN2B-associated MTCs and correlated to the presence of skeletal abnormalities similar to those found in Marfan syndrome. These observations again demonstrate how genomic studies can provide clues to the pathogenesis of disease, and that gene expression profiles of thyroid tumors reflect their underlying mutational status.

Applying CGH to a cohort of MTCs, Marsh and colleagues [165] uncovered copy number imbalances including large deletions of 1p, 3q, 4, 9q, 13q, and 22q and an amplification of chromosome 19. Similar to CGH studies of nonmedullary carcinoma, the observed copy number changes likely correspond to gains and loss of oncogenes and tumor suppressor genes, respectively. However, the regions of interest were large and housed many genes, thereby making identification of those genes contributing to carcinogenesis difficult.

A recent genome association study elucidated potential sources of intrafamilial and interfamilial phenotypic variability observed related to age of onset and tumor histology [166]. By examining 417 single-nucleotide polymorphisms (SNPs) of 69 genes related to RET signaling in two large MTC cohort cases and two large control cohorts, 7 low-penetrance genes associated with sporadic MTC risk were identified. One such SNP, located in the promoter of *CDKN2B*, was shown to alter the binding of the transcription factor HNF1, thereby providing a possible mechanistic explanation for this observation. This study extends our knowledge of sporadic MTC beyond the mutational status of *RET* and provides insight into how several genes involved in RET signaling can subtly impact the phenotype of this disease.

Molecular profiling and its potential impact on thyroid pathology and management of patients with thyroid nodules and cancer

As discussed previously, the morphology of a given tumor, including thyroid tumors, is thought to reflect the integration of its underlying genetic and epigenetic changes. Many of these changes are manifested through changes in gene transcription and thus can be easily identified and measured by transcriptomic profiling. The power of these genomic techniques is clearly demonstrated in the studies presented herein. However, what remains to be seen is whether genomic information can transform the practice of thyroid pathology (including cytology), the management of patients with thyroid nodules, and the management of thyroid cancer patients. Given the work performed to date, it is reasonable to be optimistic that molecular profiling in various forms to be determined will be successful in all of these matters. Specifically, one can envision that molecular profiling, probably in the form of quantitative reverse transcriptase–polymerase chain reaction (RT-PCR) on a subset of highly informative molecules, will be applied to cytology FNA specimens to deliver accurate diagnoses that will extend beyond the information provided by routine cytologic evaluation. Some promising preliminary work has already been done in this area [167–169]. The end result of this will be improved selection of (1) those patients who require surgical intervention and (2) those patients whose nodules can safely be monitored. This will drive down the incidence of thyroidectomies for benign disease and correspondingly increase the yield of thyroid cancer at surgery.

Furthermore, the benefits of molecular profiling will not be restricted to preoperative evaluation of thyroid nodules. After resection of a carcinoma, molecular profiling promises to provide much more information about the behavior of a given tumor and should also provide guidance on selecting the optimal therapy. For example, molecular profiling should be able to identify those well-differentiated tumors that are at high risk for recurrence and metastasis. This will permit more conservative treatment for patients with tumors predicted to have low-risk disease, and conversely permit more aggressive therapy for patients with high-risk tumors. Gene expression–based risk assessment and stratification is being done for more common carcinomas and some types of leukemia (for examples, see Refs. [170–174]) and should also work for thyroid carcinomas. Similarly, prediction of response to therapy holds the greatest promise for molecular profiling. Much work has been done in this area on other tumor types [175–180] and it is reasonable to expect this to be true for predicting response to RAI for well-differentiated thyroid cancer.

In summary, research in genomics and molecular profiling has advanced our understanding of thyroid tumor biology. Translation of this knowledge to pathology practice and the thyroid clinic will lead to advances in the care of patients with thyroid nodules and thyroid cancer.

Acknowledgments

I thank my many colleagues at the University of Michigan with whom I have had the pleasure of collaborating on numerous genomic studies, especially Rork Kuick for his outstanding and ongoing statistical and bioinformatics support. I also thank Sara Williams for excellent administrative support.

References

[1] Hirokawa M, Carney JA, Goellner JR, et al. Observer variation of encapsulated follicular lesions of the thyroid gland. Am J Surg Pathol 2002;26(11):1508–14.

[2] Franc B, de la Salmoniere P, Lange F, et al. Interobserver and intraobserver reproducibility in the histopathology of follicular thyroid carcinoma. Hum Pathol 2003;34(11): 1092–100.

[3] Lloyd RV, Erickson LA, Casey MB, et al. Observer variation in the diagnosis of follicular variant of papillary thyroid carcinoma. Am J Surg Pathol 2004;28(10):1336–40.

[4] Sapio MR, Posca D, Raggioli A, et al. Detection of RET/PTC, TRK and BRAF mutations in preoperative diagnosis of thyroid nodules with indeterminate cytological findings. Clin Endocrinol (Oxf) 2007;66(5):678–83.

[5] Pizzolanti G, Russo L, Richiusa P, et al. Fine-needle aspiration molecular analysis for the diagnosis of papillary thyroid carcinoma through BRAF(V600E) mutation and RET/PTC rearrangement. Thyroid 2007;17(11):1109–15.

[6] Kumagai A, Namba H, Akanov Z, et al. Clinical implications of pre-operative rapid BRAF analysis for papillary thyroid cancer. Endocr J 2007;54(3):399–405.

[7] Trovisco V, Soares P, Sobrinho-Simoes M. B-RAF mutations in the etiopathogenesis, diagnosis, and prognosis of thyroid carcinomas. Hum Pathol 2006;37(7):781–6.

[8] Sapio MR, Posca D, Troncone G, et al. Detection of BRAF mutation in thyroid papillary carcinomas by mutant allele-specific PCR amplification (MASA). Eur J Endocrinol 2006; 154(2):341–8.

[9] Rowe LR, Bentz BG, Bentz JS. Utility of BRAF V600E mutation detection in cytologically indeterminate thyroid nodules. Cytojournal 2006;3:10.

[10] Jin L, Sebo TJ, Nakamura N, et al. BRAF mutation analysis in fine needle aspiration (FNA) cytology of the thyroid. Diagn Mol Pathol 2006;15(3):136–43.

[11] Chung KW, Yang SK, Lee GK, et al. Detection of BRAFV600E mutation on fine needle aspiration specimens of thyroid nodule refines cyto-pathology diagnosis, especially in BRAF600E mutation-prevalent area. Clin Endocrinol (Oxf) 2006;65(5):660–6.

[12] Xing M, Tufano RP, Tufaro AP, et al. Detection of BRAF mutation on fine needle aspiration biopsy specimens: a new diagnostic tool for papillary thyroid cancer. J Clin Endocrinol Metab 2004;89(6):2867–72.

[13] Jonklaas J. Role of radioactive iodine for adjuvant therapy and treatment of metastases. J Natl Compr Canc Netw 2007;5(6):631–40.

[14] Shaha AR. Advances in the management of thyroid cancer. Int J Surg 2005;3(3):213–20.

[15] Mizukami Y, Michigishi T, Nonomura A, et al. Distant metastases in differentiated thyroid carcinomas: a clinical and pathologic study. Hum Pathol 1990;21(3):283–90.

[16] Mazzaferri EL. Management of low-risk differentiated thyroid cancer. Endocr Pract 2007; 13(5):498–512.

[17] Hamming JF, Van de Velde CJ, Goslings BM, et al. Prognosis and morbidity after total thyroidectomy for papillary, follicular and medullary thyroid cancer. Eur J Cancer Clin Oncol 1989;25(9):1317–23.

[18] DeGroot LJ, Kaplan EL, Shukla MS, et al. Morbidity and mortality in follicular thyroid cancer. J Clin Endocrinol Metab 1995;80(10):2946–53.

[19] Witt RL, McNamara AM. Prognostic factors in mortality and morbidity in patients with differentiated thyroid cancer. Ear Nose Throat J 2002;81(12):856–63.

[20] Kingma G, van den Bergen HA, de Vries JE. Prognostic scoring systems in differentiated thyroid carcinoma: which is the best? Neth J Surg 1991;43(3):63–6.

[21] Sawka AM, Thephamongkhol K, Brouwers M, et al. Clinical review 170: a systematic review and metaanalysis of the effectiveness of radioactive iodine remnant ablation for well-differentiated thyroid cancer. J Clin Endocrinol Metab 2004;89(8):3668–76.

[22] Weber F, Eng C. Gene-expression profiling in differentiated thyroid cancer—a viable strategy for the practice of genomic medicine? Future Oncol 2005;1(4):497–510.

[23] Mitsiades CS, Negri J, McMullan C, et al. Targeting BRAFV600E in thyroid carcinoma: therapeutic implications. Mol Cancer Ther 2007;6(3):1070–8.

[24] Salvatore G, De Falco V, Salerno P, et al. BRAF is a therapeutic target in aggressive thyroid carcinoma. Clin Cancer Res 2006;12(5):1623–9.

[25] Kim DW, Jo YS, Jung HS, et al. An orally administered multitarget tyrosine kinase inhibitor, SU11248, is a novel potent inhibitor of thyroid oncogenic RET/papillary thyroid cancer kinases. J Clin Endocrinol Metab 2006;91(10):4070–6.

[26] Lanzi C, Cassinelli G, Cuccuru G, et al. RET/PTC oncoproteins: molecular targets of new drugs. Tumori 2003;89(5):520–2.

[27] Brentani RR, Carraro DM, Verjovski-Almeida S, et al. Gene expression arrays in cancer research: methods and applications. Crit Rev Oncol Hematol 2005;54(2):95–105.

[28] Carter NP. Methods and strategies for analyzing copy number variation using DNA microarrays. Nat Genet 2007;39(7 Suppl):S16–21.

[29] Draghici S, Khatri P, Eklund AC, et al. Reliability and reproducibility issues in DNA microarray measurements. Trends Genet 2006;22(2):101–9.

[30] Hoheisel JD. Microarray technology: beyond transcript profiling and genotype analysis. Nat Rev Genet 2006;7(3):200–10.

[31] Lee NH, Saeed AI. Microarrays: an overview. Methods Mol Biol 2007;353:265–300.

[32] Mandruzzato S. Technological platforms for microarray gene expression profiling. Adv Exp Med Biol 2007;593:12–8.

[33] Mockler TC, Chan S, Sundaresan A, et al. Applications of DNA tiling arrays for whole-genome analysis. Genomics 2005;85(1):1–15.

[34] Petersen DW, Kawasaki ES. Manufacturing of microarrays. Adv Exp Med Biol 2007;593: 1–11.

[35] Stoughton RB. Applications of DNA microarrays in biology. Annu Rev Biochem 2005;74: 53–82.

[36] Pollack JR. A perspective on DNA microarrays in pathology research and practice. Am J Pathol 2007;171(2):375–85.

[37] Venter JC, Adams MD, Myers EW, et al. The sequence of the human genome. Science 2001; 291(5507):1304–51.

[38] Lander ES, Linton LM, Birren B, et al. Initial sequencing and analysis of the human genome. Nature 2001;409(6822):860–921.

[39] Schena M, Shalon D, Davis RW, et al. Quantitative monitoring of gene expression patterns with a complementary DNA microarray. Science 1995;270(5235):467–70.

[40] Hanauer DA, Rhodes DR, Sinha-Kumar C, et al. Bioinformatics approaches in the study of cancer. Curr Mol Med 2007;7(1):133–41.

[41] Hanai T, Hamada H, Okamoto M. Application of bioinformatics for DNA microarray data to bioscience, bioengineering and medical fields. J Biosci Bioeng 2006;101(5): 377–84.

[42] Szallasi Z. Bioinformatics. Gene expression patterns and cancer. Nat Biotechnol 1998; 16(13):1292–3.

[43] Coleman WB. Cancer bioinformatics: addressing the challenges of integrated postgenomic cancer research. Cancer Invest 2004;22(1):161–3.

[44] Roberts ML, Kottaridis SD. Interpreting microarray data: towards the complete bioinformatics toolkit for cancer. Cancer Genomics Proteomics 2007;4(4):301–8.

[45] Clark AG, Eisen MB, Smith DR, et al. Evolution of genes and genomes on the *Drosophila* phylogeny. Nature 2007;450(7167):203–18.

[46] Stark A, Lin MF, Kheradpour P, et al. Discovery of functional elements in 12 *Drosophila* genomes using evolutionary signatures. Nature 2007;450(7167):219–32.

[47] Hutchison CA 3rd. DNA sequencing: bench to bedside and beyond. Nucleic Acids Res 2007;35(18):6227–37.

[48] Wolinsky H. The thousand-dollar genome. Genetic brinkmanship or personalized medicine? EMBO Rep 2007;8(10):900–3.

[49] Huang Y, Prasad M, Lemon WJ, et al. Gene expression in papillary thyroid carcinoma reveals highly consistent profiles. Proc Natl Acad Sci U S A 2001;98(26):15044–9.

[50] Giordano TJ, Kuick R, Thomas DG, et al. Molecular classification of papillary thyroid carcinoma: distinct BRAF, RAS, and RET/PTC mutation-specific gene expression profiles discovered by DNA microarray analysis. Oncogene 2005;24(44):6646–56.

[51] Ciampi R, Giordano TJ, Wikenheiser-Brokamp K, et al. HOOK3-RET: a novel type of RET/PTC rearrangement in papillary thyroid carcinoma. Endocr Relat Cancer 2007; 14(2):445–52.

[52] Giordano TJ, Au AY, Kuick R, et al. Delineation, functional validation, and bioinformatic evaluation of gene expression in thyroid follicular carcinomas with the PAX8-PPARG translocation. Clin Cancer Res 2006;12(7 Pt 1):1983–93.

[53] Lacroix L, Lazar V, Michiels S, et al. Follicular thyroid tumors with the PAX8-PPARgamma1 rearrangement display characteristic genetic alterations. Am J Pathol 2005; 167(1):223–31.

[54] Lui WO, Foukakis T, Liden J, et al. Expression profiling reveals a distinct transcription signature in follicular thyroid carcinomas with a PAX8-PPAR(gamma) fusion oncogene. Oncogene 2005;24(8):1467–76.

[55] Kroll TG, Sarraf P, Pecciarini L, et al. PAX8-PPARgamma1 fusion oncogene in human thyroid carcinoma [corrected]. Science 2000;289(5483):1357–60.

[56] Tomlins SA, Rhodes DR, Perner S, et al. Recurrent fusion of TMPRSS2 and ETS transcription factor genes in prostate cancer. Science 2005;310(5748):644–8.

[57] Reddi HV, McIver B, Grebe SK, et al. The paired box-8/peroxisome proliferator-activated receptor-gamma oncogene in thyroid tumorigenesis. Endocrinology 2007;148(3):932–5.

[58] Espadinha C, Cavaco BM, Leite V. PAX8PPARgamma stimulates cell viability and modulates expression of thyroid-specific genes in a human thyroid cell line. Thyroid 2007;17(6): 497–509.

[59] Au AY, McBride C, Wilhelm KG Jr, et al. PAX8-peroxisome proliferator-activated receptor gamma (PPARgamma) disrupts normal PAX8 or PPARgamma transcriptional function and stimulates follicular thyroid cell growth. Endocrinology 2006;147(1): 367–76.

[60] van Staveren WC, Solis DW, Delys L, et al. Gene expression in human thyrocytes and autonomous adenomas reveals suppression of negative feedbacks in tumorigenesis. Proc Natl Acad Sci U S A 2006;103(2):413–8.

[61] Vasko V, Espinosa AV, Scouten W, et al. Gene expression and functional evidence of epithelial-to-mesenchymal transition in papillary thyroid carcinoma invasion. Proc Natl Acad Sci U S A 2007;104(8):2803–8.

[62] Thiery JP, Sleeman JP. Complex networks orchestrate epithelial-mesenchymal transitions. Nat Rev Mol Cell Biol 2006;7(2):131–42.

[63] Thiery JP. Epithelial-mesenchymal transitions in tumour progression. Nat Rev Cancer 2002;2(6):442–54.

[64] Thiery JP, Chopin D. Epithelial cell plasticity in development and tumor progression. Cancer Metastasis Rev 1999;18(1):31–42.

[65] Kokkinos MI, Wafai R, Wong MK, et al. Vimentin and epithelial-mesenchymal transition in human breast cancer—observations in vitro and in vivo. Cells Tissues Organs 2007; 185(1–3):191–203.

[66] Makarewicz CR. Radiation and thyroid cancer. JAMA 1984;251(10):1280.

[67] Dolphin GW. Radiation exposure and thyroid cancer. Br J Radiol 1972;45(538):795.

[68] Roudebush CP, Asteris GT. Radiation-associated thyroid cancer. J Indiana State Med Assoc 1978;71(8):780–2.

[69] Roudebush CP, Asteris GT, DeGroot LJ. Natural history of radiation-associated thyroid cancer. Arch Intern Med 1978;138(11):1631–4.

[70] Sonenberg M, Leeper RB. Radiation-induced cancer of the thyroid. Clin Bull 1978;8(1): 29–33.

[71] Curtin CT, McHeffy B, Kolarsick AJ. Thyroid and breast cancer following childhood radiation. Cancer 1977;40(6):2911–3.

[72] Williamson ME. Thyroid cancer following exposure to ionizing radiation. J Am Osteopath Assoc 1977;76(11):98–101.

[73] Greenspan FS. Radiation exposure and thyroid cancer. JAMA 1977;237(19):2089–91.

[74] DeGroot LJ. Radiation and thyroid cancer. Proc Inst Med Chic 1976;31(4):95–6.

[75] Asteris GT, DeGroot LJ. Thyroid cancer: relationship to radiation exposure and to pregnancy. J Reprod Med 1976;17(4):209–16.

[76] Debra DW Jr. Radiation and thyroid cancer. New concerns. J Med Assoc Ga 1975;64(10): 395–6.

[77] Dolphin GW. Thyroid cancer: radiation carcinogenesis. Recent Results Cancer Res 1980; 73:23–30.

[78] Duffy BJ Jr. Can radiation cause thyroid cancer. J Clin Endocrinol Metab 1957;17(11): 1383–8.

[79] Ivanov VK, Gorski AI, Tsyb AF, et al. Radiation-epidemiological studies of thyroid cancer incidence among children and adolescents in the Bryansk oblast of Russia after the Chernobyl accident (1991-2001 follow-up period). Radiat Environ Biophys 2006;45(1):9–16.

[80] Kopecky KJ, Stepanenko V, Rivkind N, et al. Childhood thyroid cancer, radiation dose from Chernobyl, and dose uncertainties in Bryansk Oblast, Russia: a population-based case-control study. Radiat Res 2006;166(2):367–74.

[81] Minenko VF, Ulanovsky AV, Drozdovitch VV, et al. Individual thyroid dose estimates for a case-control study of Chernobyl-related thyroid cancer among children of Belarus—part II. Contributions from long-lived radionuclides and external radiation. Health Phys 2006; 90(4):312–27.

[82] Nikiforov YE. Radiation-induced thyroid cancer: what we have learned from Chernobyl. Endocr Pathol 2006;17(4):307–17.

[83] Detours V, Delys L, Libert F, et al. Genome-wide gene expression profiling suggests distinct radiation susceptibilities in sporadic and post-Chernobyl papillary thyroid cancers. Br J Cancer 2007;97(6):818–25.

[84] Detours V, Wattel S, Venet D, et al. Absence of a specific radiation signature in post-Chernobyl thyroid cancers. Br J Cancer 2005;92(8):1545–52.

[85] Aldred MA, Huang Y, Liyanarachchi S, et al. Papillary and follicular thyroid carcinomas show distinctly different microarray expression profiles and can be distinguished by a minimum of five genes. J Clin Oncol 2004;22(17):3531–9.

[86] Barden CB, Shister KW, Zhu B, et al. Classification of follicular thyroid tumors by molecular signature: results of gene profiling. Clin Cancer Res 2003;9(5):1792–800.

[87] Eszlinger M, Wiench M, Jarzab B, et al. Meta- and reanalysis of gene expression profiles of hot and cold thyroid nodules and papillary thyroid carcinoma for gene groups. J Clin Endocrinol Metab 2006;91(5):1934–42.

[88] Finley DJ, Zhu B, Barden CB, et al. Discrimination of benign and malignant thyroid nodules by molecular profiling. Ann Surg 2004;240(3):425–36 [discussion: 436–7].

[89] Fontaine JF, Mirebeau-Prunier D, Franc B, et al. Microarray analysis refines classification of non-medullary thyroid tumours of uncertain malignancy. Oncogene 2007; [epub ahead of print].

[90] Fujarewicz K, Jarzab M, Eszlinger M, et al. A multi-gene approach to differentiate papillary thyroid carcinoma from benign lesions: gene selection using support vector machines with bootstrapping. Endocr Relat Cancer 2007;14(3):809–26.

[91] Griffith OL, Melck A, Jones SJ, et al. Meta-analysis and meta-review of thyroid cancer gene expression profiling studies identifies important diagnostic biomarkers. J Clin Oncol 2006; 24(31):5043–51.

[92] Jarzab B, Wiench M, Fujarewicz K, et al. Gene expression profile of papillary thyroid cancer: sources of variability and diagnostic implications. Cancer Res 2005;65(4): 1587–97.

[93] Lubitz CC, Gallagher LA, Finley DJ, et al. Molecular analysis of minimally invasive follicular carcinomas by gene profiling. Surgery 2005;138(6):1042–8 [discussion: 1048–49].

[94] Lubitz CC, Ugras SK, Kazam JJ, et al. Microarray analysis of thyroid nodule fine-needle aspirates accurately classifies benign and malignant lesions. J Mol Diagn 2006;8(4):490–8, [quiz: 528].

[95] Mazzanti C, Zeiger MA, Costouros NG, et al. Using gene expression profiling to differentiate benign versus malignant thyroid tumors. Cancer Res 2004;64(8):2898–903.

[96] Weber F, Shen L, Aldred MA, et al. Genetic classification of benign and malignant thyroid follicular neoplasia based on a three-gene combination. J Clin Endocrinol Metab 2005; 90(5):2512–21.

[97] Yano Y, Uematsu N, Yashiro T, et al. Gene expression profiling identifies platelet-derived growth factor as a diagnostic molecular marker for papillary thyroid carcinoma. Clin Cancer Res 2004;10(6):2035–43.

[98] Yukinawa N, Oba S, Kato K, et al. A multi-class predictor based on a probabilistic model: application to gene expression profiling-based diagnosis of thyroid tumors. BMC Genomics 2006;7:190.

[99] Lubitz CC, Fahey TJ 3rd. Gene expression profiling of thyroid tumors—clinical applicability. Nat Clin Pract Endocrinol Metab 2006;2(9):472–3.

[100] Simon R, Radmacher MD, Dobbin K, et al. Pitfalls in the use of DNA microarray data for diagnostic and prognostic classification. J Natl Cancer Inst 2003;95(1):14–8.

[101] Belacel N, Wang Q, Cuperlovic-Culf M. Clustering methods for microarray gene expression data. OMICS 2006;10(4):507–31.

[102] Breitling R. Biological microarray interpretation: the rules of engagement. Biochim Biophys Acta 2006;1759(7):319–27.

[103] Dupuy A, Simon RM. Critical review of published microarray studies for cancer outcome and guidelines on statistical analysis and reporting. J Natl Cancer Inst 2007;99(2):147–57.

[104] Ness SA. Basic microarray analysis: strategies for successful experiments. Methods Mol Biol 2006;316:13–33.

[105] Weeraratna AT, Taub DD. Microarray data analysis: an overview of design, methodology, and analysis. Methods Mol Biol 2007;377:1–16.

[106] Williams ED. Guest editorial: two proposals regarding the terminology of thyroid tumors. Int J Surg Pathol 2000;8(3):181–3.

[107] Wreesmann VB, Sieczka EM, Socci ND, et al. Genome-wide profiling of papillary thyroid cancer identifies MUC1 as an independent prognostic marker. Cancer Res 2004;64(11): 3780–9.

[108] Zou M, Famulski KS, Parhar RS, et al. Microarray analysis of metastasis-associated gene expression profiling in a murine model of thyroid carcinoma pulmonary metastasis: identification of S100A4 (Mts1) gene overexpression as a poor prognostic marker for thyroid carcinoma. J Clin Endocrinol Metab 2004;89(12):6146–54.

[109] Zou M, Al-Baradie RS, Al-Hindi H, et al. S100A4 (Mts1) gene overexpression is associated with invasion and metastasis of papillary thyroid carcinoma. Br J Cancer 2005;93(11): 1277–84.

[110] Siraj AK, Bavi P, Abubaker J, et al. Genome-wide expression analysis of Middle Eastern papillary thyroid cancer reveals c-MET as a novel target for cancer therapy. J Pathol 2007;213(2):190–9.

[111] Christensen JG, Burrows J, Salgia R. c-Met as a target for human cancer and characterization of inhibitors for therapeutic intervention. Cancer Lett 2005;225(1):1–26.

[112] Egger G, Liang G, Aparicio A, et al. Epigenetics in human disease and prospects for epigenetic therapy. Nature 2004;429(6990):457–63.

[113] Rosai J. Why microscopy will remain a cornerstone of surgical pathology. Lab Invest 2007; 87(5):403–8.

[114] Giordano TJ. Molecular profiling and personalized predictive pathology: challenge to the academic surgical pathology community. Am J Surg Pathol 2006;30(3):402–4.

[115] Miska EA. How microRNAs control cell division, differentiation and death. Curr Opin Genet Dev 2005;15(5):563–8.

[116] Lu J, Getz G, Miska EA, et al. MicroRNA expression profiles classify human cancers. Nature 2005;435(7043):834–8.

[117] Yanaihara N, Caplen N, Bowman E, et al. Unique microRNA molecular profiles in lung cancer diagnosis and prognosis. Cancer Cell 2006;9(3):189–98.

[118] Blower PE, Verducci JS, Lin S, et al. MicroRNA expression profiles for the NCI-60 cancer cell panel. Mol Cancer Ther 2007;6(5):1483–91.

[119] Lui WO, Pourmand N, Patterson BK, et al. Patterns of known and novel small RNAs in human cervical cancer. Cancer Res 2007;67(13):6031–43.

[120] Zanette DL, Rivadavia F, Molfetta GA, et al. miRNA expression profiles in chronic lymphocytic and acute lymphocytic leukemia. Braz J Med Biol Res 2007;40(11):1435–40.

[121] Zhang B, Pan X, Cobb GP, et al. microRNAs as oncogenes and tumor suppressors. Dev Biol 2007;302(1):1–12.

[122] Visone R, Pallante P, Vecchione A, et al. Specific microRNAs are downregulated in human thyroid anaplastic carcinomas. Oncogene 2007;26(54):7590–5.

[123] Weber F, Teresi RE, Broelsch CE, et al. A limited set of human MicroRNA is deregulated in follicular thyroid carcinoma. J Clin Endocrinol Metab 2006;91(9):3584–91.

[124] Pallante P, Visone R, Ferracin M, et al. MicroRNA deregulation in human thyroid papillary carcinomas. Endocr Relat Cancer 2006;13(2):497–508.

[125] He H, Jazdzewski K, Li W, et al. The role of microRNA genes in papillary thyroid carcinoma. Proc Natl Acad Sci U S A 2005;102(52):19075–80.

[126] Kondo T, Ezzat S, Asa SL. Pathogenetic mechanisms in thyroid follicular-cell neoplasia. Nat Rev Cancer 2006;6(4):292–306.

[127] Weir BA, Woo MS, Getz G, et al. Characterizing the cancer genome in lung adenocarcinoma. Nature 2007;450(7171):893–8.

[128] Chen X, Knauf JA, Gonsky R, et al. From amplification to gene in thyroid cancer: a high-resolution mapped bacterial-artificial-chromosome resource for cancer chromosome aberrations guides gene discovery after comparative genome hybridization. Am J Hum Genet 1998;63(2):625–37.

[129] Hemmer S, Wasenius VM, Knuutila S, et al. Comparison of benign and malignant follicular thyroid tumours by comparative genomic hybridization. Br J Cancer 1998;78(8):1012–7.

[130] Frisk T, Kytola S, Wallin G, et al. Low frequency of numerical chromosomal aberrations in follicular thyroid tumors detected by comparative genomic hybridization. Genes Chromosomes Cancer 1999;25(4):349–53.

[131] Hemmer S, Wasenius VM, Knuutila S, et al. DNA copy number changes in thyroid carcinoma. Am J Pathol 1999;154(5):1539–47.

[132] Komoike Y, Tamaki Y, Sakita I, et al. Comparative genomic hybridization defines frequent loss on 16p in human anaplastic thyroid carcinoma. Int J Oncol 1999;14(6):1157–62.

[133] Tallini G, Hsueh A, Liu S, et al. Frequent chromosomal DNA unbalance in thyroid oncocytic (Hurthle cell) neoplasms detected by comparative genomic hybridization. Lab Invest 1999;79(5):547–55.

[134] Singh B, Lim D, Cigudosa JC, et al. Screening for genetic aberrations in papillary thyroid cancer by using comparative genomic hybridization. Surgery 2000;128(6):888–93 [discussion: 893–4].

[135] Wilkens L, Benten D, Tchinda J, et al. Aberrations of chromosomes 5 and 8 as recurrent cytogenetic events in anaplastic carcinoma of the thyroid as detected by fluorescence in situ hybridisation and comparative genomic hybridisation. Virchows Arch 2000;436(4):312–8.

[136] Kjellman P, Lagercrantz S, Hoog A, et al. Gain of 1q and loss of 9q21.3-q32 are associated with a less favorable prognosis in papillary thyroid carcinoma. Genes Chromosomes Cancer 2001;32(1):43–9.

[137] Bauer AJ, Cavalli LR, Rone JD, et al. Evaluation of adult papillary thyroid carcinomas by comparative genomic hybridization and microsatellite instability analysis. Cancer Genet Cytogenet 2002;135(2):182–6.

[138] Corso C, Ulucan H, Parry EM, et al. Comparative analysis of two thyroid tumor cell lines by fluorescence in situ hybridization and comparative genomic hybridization. Cancer Genet Cytogenet 2002;137(2):108–18.

[139] Wreesmann VB, Ghossein RA, Patel SG, et al. Genome-wide appraisal of thyroid cancer progression. Am J Pathol 2002;161(5):1549–56.

[140] Brunaud L, Zarnegar R, Wada N, et al. Chromosomal aberrations by comparative genomic hybridization in thyroid tumors in patients with familial nonmedullary thyroid cancer. Thyroid 2003;13(7):621–9.

[141] Dettori T, Frau DV, Lai ML, et al. Aneuploidy in oncocytic lesions of the thyroid gland: diffuse accumulation of mitochondria within the cell is associated with trisomy 7 and progressive numerical chromosomal alterations. Genes Chromosomes Cancer 2003;38(1): 22–31.

[142] Miura D, Wada N, Chin K, et al. Anaplastic thyroid cancer: cytogenetic patterns by comparative genomic hybridization. Thyroid 2003;13(3):283–90.

[143] Roque L, Rodrigues R, Pinto A, et al. Chromosome imbalances in thyroid follicular neoplasms: a comparison between follicular adenomas and carcinomas. Genes Chromosomes Cancer 2003;36(3):292–302.

[144] Richter H, Braselmann H, Hieber L, et al. Chromosomal imbalances in post-Chernobyl thyroid tumors. Thyroid 2004;14(12):1061–4.

[145] Rodrigues RF, Roque L, Rosa-Santos J, et al. Chromosomal imbalances associated with anaplastic transformation of follicular thyroid carcinomas. Br J Cancer 2004;90(2): 492–6.

[146] Wreesmann VB, Ghossein RA, Hezel M, et al. Follicular variant of papillary thyroid carcinoma: genome-wide appraisal of a controversial entity. Genes Chromosomes Cancer 2004;40(4):355–64.

[147] Castro P, Eknaes M, Teixeira MR, et al. Adenomas and follicular carcinomas of the thyroid display two major patterns of chromosomal changes. J Pathol 2005;206(3):305–11.

[148] Foukakis T, Thoppe SR, Lagercrantz S, et al. Molecular cytogenetic characterization of primary cultures and established cell lines from non-medullary thyroid tumors. Int J Oncol 2005;26(1):141–9.

[149] Finn S, Smyth P, O'Regan E, et al. Low-level genomic instability is a feature of papillary thyroid carcinoma: an array comparative genomic hybridization study of laser capture microdissected papillary thyroid carcinoma tumors and clonal cell lines. Arch Pathol Lab Med 2007;131(1):65–73.

[150] Lee JJ, Foukakis T, Hashemi J, et al. Molecular cytogenetic profiles of novel and established human anaplastic thyroid carcinoma models. Thyroid 2007;17(4): 289–301.

[151] Rodrigues R, Roque L, Espadinha C, et al. Comparative genomic hybridization, BRAF, RAS, RET, and oligo-array analysis in aneuploid papillary thyroid carcinomas. Oncol Rep 2007;18(4):917–26.

[152] Stoler DL, Nowak NJ, Matsui S, et al. Comparative genomic instabilities of thyroid and colon cancers. Arch Otolaryngol Head Neck Surg 2007;133(5):457–63.

[153] Kallioniemi A, Kallioniemi OP, Sudar D, et al. Comparative genomic hybridization for molecular cytogenetic analysis of solid tumors. Science 1992;258(5083):818–21.

[154] Pinkel D, Albertson DG. Array comparative genomic hybridization and its applications in cancer. Nat Genet 2005;(37 Suppl):S11–7.

[155] Kimmel RR, Zhao LP, Nguyen D, et al. Microarray comparative genomic hybridization reveals genome-wide patterns of DNA gains and losses in post-Chernobyl thyroid cancer. Radiat Res 2006;166(3):519–31.

[156] Rosai J. Poorly differentiated thyroid carcinoma: introduction to the issue, its landmarks, and clinical impact. Endocr Pathol 2004;15(4):293–6.

[157] Sakamoto A. Definition of poorly differentiated carcinoma of the thyroid: the Japanese experience. Endocr Pathol 2004;15(4):307–11.

[158] Albores-Saavedra J, Carrick K. Where to set the threshold between well differentiated and poorly differentiated follicular carcinomas of the thyroid. Endocr Pathol 2004;15(4): 297–305.

[159] Nikiforov YE. Genetic alterations involved in the transition from well-differentiated to poorly differentiated and anaplastic thyroid carcinomas. Endocr Pathol 2004;15(4): 319–27.

[160] Kim JH, Dhanasekaran SM, Mehra R, et al. Integrative analysis of genomic aberrations associated with prostate cancer progression. Cancer Res 2007;67(17):8229–39.

[161] Tomlins SA, Mehra R, Rhodes DR, et al. Integrative molecular concept modeling of prostate cancer progression. Nat Genet 2007;39(1):41–51.

[162] Varambally S, Yu J, Laxman B, et al. Integrative genomic and proteomic analysis of prostate cancer reveals signatures of metastatic progression. Cancer Cell 2005;8(5):393–406.

[163] Jain S, Watson MA, DeBenedetti MK, et al. Expression profiles provide insights into early malignant potential and skeletal abnormalities in multiple endocrine neoplasia type 2B syndrome tumors. Cancer Res 2004;64(11):3907–13.

[164] Nakamichi Y, Shukunami C, Yamada T, et al. Chondromodulin I is a bone remodeling factor. Mol Cell Biol 2003;23(2):636–44.

[165] Marsh DJ, Theodosopoulos G, Martin-Schulte K, et al. Genome-wide copy number imbalances identified in familial and sporadic medullary thyroid carcinoma. J Clin Endocrinol Metab 2003;88(4):1866–72.

[166] Ruiz-Llorente S, Montero-Conde C, Milne RL, et al. Association study of 69 genes in the RET pathway identifies low-penetrance loci in sporadic medullary thyroid carcinoma. Cancer Res 2007;67(19):9561–7.

[167] Denning KM, Smyth PC, Cahill SF, et al. A molecular expression signature distinguishing follicular lesions in thyroid carcinoma using preamplification RT-PCR in archival samples. Mod Pathol 2007;20(10):1095–102.

[168] Foukakis T, Gusnanto A, Au AY, et al. A PCR-based expression signature of malignancy in follicular thyroid tumors. Endocr Relat Cancer 2007;14(2):381–91.

[169] Rosen J, He M, Umbricht C, et al. A six-gene model for differentiating benign from malignant thyroid tumors on the basis of gene expression. Surgery 2005;138(6):1050–6 [discussion: 1056–7].

[170] Lu Y, Lemon W, Liu PY, et al. A gene expression signature predicts survival of patients with stage I non-small cell lung cancer. PLoS Med 2006;3(12):2229–43.

[171] Furlow B. Gene-expression profiles predict secondary leukaemia risk. Lancet Oncol 2006; 7(4):287.

[172] Desmedt C, Piette F, Loi S, et al. Strong time dependence of the 76-gene prognostic signature for node-negative breast cancer patients in the TRANSBIG multicenter independent validation series. Clin Cancer Res 2007;13(11):3207–14.

[173] Wang Y, Klijn JG, Zhang Y, et al. Gene-expression profiles to predict distant metastasis of lymph-node-negative primary breast cancer. Lancet 2005;365(9460):671–9.

[174] Spentzos D, Levine DA, Ramoni MF, et al. Gene expression signature with independent prognostic significance in epithelial ovarian cancer. J Clin Oncol 2004;22(23):4700–10.

[175] Parissenti AM, Hembruff SL, Villeneuve DJ, et al. Gene expression profiles as biomarkers for the prediction of chemotherapy drug response in human tumour cells. Anticancer Drugs 2007;18(5):499–523.

[176] Kim IJ, Lim SB, Kang HC, et al. Microarray gene expression profiling for predicting complete response to preoperative chemoradiotherapy in patients with advanced rectal cancer. Dis Colon Rectum 2007;50(9):1342–53.

[177] Jensen EH, McLoughlin JM, Yeatman TJ. Microarrays in gastrointestinal cancer: is personalized prediction of response to chemotherapy at hand? Curr Opin Oncol 2006;18(4):374–80.

[178] Takata R, Katagiri T, Kanehira M, et al. Predicting response to methotrexate, vinblastine, doxorubicin, and cisplatin neoadjuvant chemotherapy for bladder cancers through genome-wide gene expression profiling. Clin Cancer Res 2005;11(7):2625–36.

[179] Selvanayagam ZE, Cheung TH, Wei N, et al. Prediction of chemotherapeutic response in ovarian cancer with DNA microarray expression profiling. Cancer Genet Cytogenet 2004;154(1):63–6.

[180] Mariadason JM, Arango D, Shi Q, et al. Gene expression profiling-based prediction of response of colon carcinoma cells to 5-fluorouracil and camptothecin. Cancer Res 2003; 63(24):8791–812.

ELSEVIER
SAUNDERS

Endocrinol Metab Clin N Am
37 (2008) 333–362

ENDOCRINOLOGY
AND METABOLISM
CLINICS
OF NORTH AMERICA

Intragenic Mutations in Thyroid Cancer

Manuel Sobrinho-Simões, MD, PhD[a,b,c],
Valdemar Máximo, PhD[a,b],
Ana Sofia Rocha, PhD[a], Vitor Trovisco, PhD[a],
Patricia Castro, PhD[a], Ana Preto, PhD[a,d],
Jorge Lima, PhD[a], Paula Soares, PhD[a,b],*

[a]Institute of Molecular Pathology and Immunology of the University of Porto, Rua Roberto
Frias s/n, 4200-465 Porto, Portugal
[b]Department of Pathology, University of Porto, Al. Prof. Hernãni Monteiro,
4200-319 Porto, Portugal
[c]Department of Anatomic Pathology, Hospital São João, Al. Prof. Hernãni Monteiro,
4200-319 Porto, Portugal
[d]Department of Biology, University of Minho, Campus de Gualtar, 4710-057 Braga, Portugal

The close genotype-phenotype relationship that characterizes thyroid oncology stimulated the authors to address this article by using a mixed, genetic and phenotypic approach.

Within the group of well differentiated carcinomas, RET/PTC1 and the BRAF^{V600E} mutation tend to concentrate in cases of conventional papillary carcinoma (PTC); RET/PTC3 and, perhaps, BRAF$^{VK600-1E}$ appear to be associated with the solid variant of PTC; N-RAS^{Q61R} and BRAF^{K601E} mutations tend to concentrate in cases of the follicular variant of PTC (FVPTC), while a PAX8-peroxisome proliferator-activated receptor $-\gamma$ (PPARγ) rearrangement is found in benign and malignant tumors displaying a prominent follicular growth pattern (follicular thyroid adenoma or FTA, follicular thyroid carcinoma or FTC, and FVPTC). The same holds true regarding Hürthle cell tumors (HCT) and anaplastic thyroid carcinomas (ATC), which also present quite characteristic genetic alterations.

This work was supported by a grant from The Late David and Esther Bernstein Halpern Fund and by the Portuguese Foundation for Science and Technology (Fundação para a Ciência e Tecnologia), through the project funding (POCI/FEDER, project POCTI/SAU-OBS/56175/2004).

* Corresponding author. Institute of Molecular Pathology and Immunology of the University of Porto, Rua Roberto Frias s/n, 4200-465 Porto, Portugal.

E-mail address: psoares@ipatimup.pt (P. Soares).

The authors' decision regarding the organization of the article is reflected in the headings of the sections, some of which are centered on the alterations of specific genes (eg, BRAF, PAX8-PPARγ), while in others the genetic alterations have been linked with pathologic entities (eg, HCT and poorly differentiated thyroid carcinoma [PDTC], and ATC). In one section the authors address, together with the genetic alterations, cytogenetic and DNA content issues (RAS mutations and aneuploidy).

To achieve a good articulation with the other articles in this issue, the authors do not discuss RET mutations, nor RET and NTRK1 rearrangements; the article also does not address in depth the alterations of the genes of PTEN/PI3K/AKT pathway, nor the genetic and epigenetic alterations of cell-cell and cell-matrix adhesion proteins and growth factors.

For the sake of completeness the authors decided to include two short sections, one on the genes mutated in hyperfunctioning tumors despite their benign nature in most cases, and another on the alterations in succinate dehydrogenase (SDH) genes in C-cell lesions.

Thyroid stimulating hormone receptor and guanine-nucleotide-binding proteins of the stimulatory family mutations in hyperfunctioning tumors

The majority of the thyroid tumors are benign lesions that can be detected in more than 50% of adults subjected to routine thyroid echography [1]. Thyroid nodules are the most common thyroid benign tumors, and can be classified according to their scintigraphic characteristics as "hot," "cold," or "warm." The etiology of hot nodules (also known as autonomous functioning nodules) is well characterized, whereas the etiopathogenesis of cold nodules is less well understood [1].

Thyroid stimulating hormone (TSH) and iodine are the two major physiologic regulators that control the function and size of the thyroid: TSH positively, iodide negatively. After binding to its membrane receptor (TSHr), TSH activates guanine-nucleotide-binding proteins of the stimulatory family (Gs) to stimulate the adenylate cyclase (AC)-cAMP pathway and phospholipase C, ultimately inducing growth and function of thyroid cells [2].

The cyclic adenosine monophosphate (cAMP) cascade in the thyroid corresponds to the canonic model of the β-adrenergic receptor cascade. These receptors are classic seven-transmembrane receptors controlling transducing guanosine triphosphate (GTP)-binding proteins. Activated G proteins belong to the Gs class and activate adenylyl cyclase. Alpha-sGTP directly binds to and activates adenylyl cyclase. The cAMP generated by adenylyl cyclase binds to the regulatory subunit of protein kinase A (PKA) and releases this now-active unit. The activated, released catalytic unit of PKA phosphorylates serines and threonines in the set of proteins that it recognizes. These phosphorylations, through more or less complicated cascades, lead to the increased thyrocyte proliferation and function. Besides PKA, cAMP activates in the thyroid the exchange protein directly activated by cAMP (EPAC), which activates the small G protein RAP. The Ca2+-inositol 1,4,5-triphosphate cascade also corresponds, in the thyroid, to the canonic model of the muscarinic or α1-adrenergic receptor-activated cascades. This is activated in the human thyrocyte by TSH.

Some growth factors and hormones act on their target cells by receptors that contain a single transmembrane segment. They interact with the extracellular domain and activate the intracellular domain, which phosphorylates proteins on their tyrosines. The first step in activation is interprotein tyrosine phosphorylation, followed by binding of various protein substrates on tyrosine phosphates containing segments of the receptor. Such binding, through SRC homology domains (SH2), leads to direct activation or to phosphorylation of these proteins on their tyrosines and to membrane localization. In turn, these cause sequential activation of the RAS and RAF proto-oncogenes, mitogen-activated protein (MAP) kinase kinase, MAP kinase, and so on. This cascade is associated with thyrocyte proliferation and loss of function and differentiation.

Mutational events in hot or hyperfunctioning thyroid nodules

In 1989, Dumont and colleagues [3] raised the possibility that overactivity of the cAMP system, caused by molecular defects in the TSH cascade, could account for a fraction of thyroid benign tumors. Soon after, mutations of Gs somatotrophs were described [4], and similar mutations (also called Gsp mutations) were found in some toxic FTA (Table 1) [5–7]. The mutated residues (Arg201, Glu227) are homologous to those found mutated in the RAS proto-oncogenes: that is, the mutations decrease the endogenous GTPase activity of the G protein, resulting in a constitutively active molecule.

Constitutive activation of TSH receptor as the result of point mutations was then identified by Parma and colleagues [8] to be the cause of most hyperfunctioning nodules. These mutations generally involve the extracellular loops of the transmembrane domain and the transmembrane segments, and are proven to induce hyperfunction by transfection studies [9]. Most aminoacidic substitutions found in toxic FTA or toxic thyroid hyperplasia share some characteristics: they increase the constitutive activity of the receptor toward stimulation of adenylyl-cyclase and do not display constitutive activity toward the inositolphosphate/diacylglycerol [9]. The prevalence of TSHr mutations in hyperfunctioning adenomas varies from 20% to 82% in patients with similar iodine supply. This discrepancy may reflect the different sensitivities of the methods used for mutation screening; furthermore, while some investigators studied the entire TSHr gene, others have concentrated their studies in the analysis of TSHr mutational hotspot (exon 10). Similarly, the Gs gene mutation frequency ranges from 8% to 75% [10]. Fifty percent of the mutation-negative cases show a monoclonal origin when tested for X chromosome inactivation, suggesting a mutation in a gene other than those described above [11,12]. Because the phenotype of thyroid autonomy is

Table 1
Summary of the results published on mutation analysis on thyroid hot and cold nodules

Reference	Histology	TSHr	Gs	RAS
Parma and colleagues [8]	Hyperfunctioning adenomas	3/11	No data (nd)	nd
Takeshita and colleagues [211]	Solitary adenomas	1/38	1/38	nd
Tanaka and colleagues [212]	Thyroid hot adenomas	3/10	2/10	nd
Derwahl and colleagues [213]	Hot nodules	27/33	2/33	nd
Parma and colleagues [214]	Hot nodules	27/38	2/38	nd
Vassart and colleagues [215]	Hot nodules	15/31	0/31	nd
Führer and colleagues [216,217]	Hot nodules	13/27	nd	nd
Khron and colleagues [12]	Hot nodules	14/20	0/20	nd
Tonacchera and colleagues [218]	Hot follicular adenomas	12/15	1/15	nd
Tonacchera and colleagues [13]	Cold adenomas (two with features of malignancy)	0/15	0/15	
Khron and colleagues [219]	Hot nodules	19/47	nd	0/47
	Cold nodules	0/41		1/41
Russo and colleagues [220]	Carcinomas	3/14	nd	1/14+
Spambalg and colleagues [21]	Follicular carcinomas	2/20	0/20	nd
	Papillary carcinoma	0/8	0/8	
	Hürthle cell carcinoma	0/1	0/1	
	Anaplastic carcinoma	0/1	0/1	
Russo and colleagues [221]	Insular thyroid carcinoma	1/1	0	0
Bourasseau and colleagues [222]	Hot carcinomas	0/4	0/4	nd
	Cold carcinomas	0/4	0/4	
Führer and colleagues [223]	Toxic Follicular carcinoma	2/2	nd	nd
	Non-functional lung metastases	0/2		
Niepomniszcze and colleagues [23]	Follicular carcinoma	1/1	0/1	1/1

associated with constitutive cAMP activation, it is likely that further candidate genes will be located on this signaling cascade.

Mutational events in cold thyroid nodules

In contrast to hyperfunctioning nodules, cold nodules are believed to have their origin in mutations of genes linked with dedifferentiation. At variance with most series that reported the absence of mutations in TSHr and Gs [13–15], mutations in Gs protein were detected in 27% of nonfunctioning adenomas in one series, an observation which has not been reproduced in any subsequent study [13–15]. Mutations in other cAMP effectors, such as EPAC and its downstream target RAP1, have not been detected in 10 thyroid cold nodules [16]. These findings were further confirmed by Castro and colleagues [17].

The lack of mutations in the cAMP differentiation pathway led to the screening of genes belonging to transformational pathways, such as the mitogen activated protein kinase (MAPK) pathway. Activating mutations in the RAS proto-oncogenes pathway have been detected in 20% of thyroid adenomas [18,19], with frequencies similar to those found in FTC and FVPTC (see below).

Another difference between cold and hot nodules is the predominant monoclonality of the first, as compared with the latter, suggesting a different process of nodule development (reviewed in [10]) (see Table 1).

TSHr and Gs gene mutations in thyroid carcinomas

The involvement of constitutive activation of the cAMP cascade in carcinomas has not yet been firmly established. Based on available data, TSHr and Gs gene mutations are not involved in carcinogenesis, except maybe in a small proportion of cases [20,21]. Other family members of G proteins activated by TSHr were also screened for the presence of mutations, but none were found [22].

In thyroid carcinomas with high basal adenylate cyclase activity and a poor response to TSH, mutations in TSHr and Gs were reported in 12% of FTC and in 13% of PTC [14,15]. Niepomniszcze and colleagues [23] described a case of a FTC presenting as a hot nodule; mutation analysis revealed point mutations in both TSHr and K-RAS, leading the investigators to suggest that RAS mutation would be the driver mutation to transformation, because hot nodules only rarely progress to carcinoma [24]. Gozu and colleagues [25] described a TSHr mutation in a PTC presenting as a hot nodule, and a similar observation was made by Camacho and colleagues [26] in a FTC. However, the role of TSHr mutations in transformation was not established, as the presence of mutations in oncogenes associated to either PTC or FTC was not screened in any of the studies. Finally, Russo and colleagues [27] described an autonomously functioning Hürthle cell carcinoma with a TSHr mutation and absence of either a RAS or TP53 mutation [27].

From the data available in the literature, it seems that activation of the cAMP pathway is not a major player in cell transformation. Most hyperfunctioning tumors harbor both TSHr mutations and proto-oncogene mutations; this coexistence suggests that carcinomas arise from the activity of classical oncogenes, such as RAS and RET/PTC, and that the TSHr and Gs mutations confer hyperfunctioning features to the neoplasms.

Mutations in RAS and other genes and aneuploidy

Three human RAS genes (N, H, and K-RAS) are frequently involved in human tumorigenesis. RAS mutations produce constitutively active RAS proteins, which are key intracellular signal transducers that can activate several downstream pathways, namely the classical RAF-MEK-ERK pathway (for a review, see [28,29]).

RAS genes mutations are particularly prevalent in FTA and FTC and, less frequently, in PTC (for a review, see [1,30]). Their prevalence in PTC varies widely from series to series, being relatively rare (0%–16%) in conventional PTC [30–33] and much more frequent (greater than 25%) in the FVPTC [17,34–36]. The mutations associated with thyroid tumors involve predominantly codon 61 of N-RAS and, to a less extent, of H-RAS [17,30,34,35].

Giaretti and colleagues [37–39] showed that activating mutations of K-RAS were involved in the control of chromosome stability in aneuploidy in colorectal tumors. Fagin [40] advanced that a similar mechanism, also involving RAS, might cause aneuploidy in follicular thyroid tumors.

The ploidy of thyroid tumors and tumor-like lesions has been extensively studied by many groups [41–45]. It is known that FTA and FTC are often aneuploid, whereas PTC are usually diploid or near-diploid, and these differences would fit with the assumption that RAS mutations play a role in the aneuploidization process [41–48]. This assumption has not been confirmed, however, in studies focusing in differences of DNA content in each type of lesion (see below). The reported aneuploidy frequencies in the different types of thyroid lesions vary in the available series. In goiters, the frequency of aneuploidy ranges from 10% to 22% [45,49–51], in FTA from 18% to 52% [41,45,47,49,52], and in FTC from 15% to 65% [41,45,49,52,53]. A close relationship between aneuplody and RAS mutations was not found in any tumor type. In FTA, the aneuploidy seems to be closely related to a specific morphologic pattern: the fetal-like pattern [45,54].

In thyroid tumors, there is no correlation between the presence of an abnormal DNA content and malignancy, because benign lesions often show an aneuploid phenotype, whereas malignant tumors may be diploid [41,43–45,49]. In thyroid oncology, the correlation between aneuploidy and prognosis is not as clear as in other tumor models, but several studies demonstrated that the presence of aneuploidy is an adverse prognostic factor in thyroid carcinomas [55,56].

The evaluation of the DNA content in thyroid tumors has been complemented with cytogenetic studies, including Giemsa-banding, comparative genome hybridization (CGH), and fluorescence in situ hybridization [57–59]. Follicular tumors (FTA and FTC) frequently show copy sequence alterations [44,54,60–62]. Gains affecting chromosomes 5, 7, 12, 17, 19, and 20 are typically seen in both tumor types [54,57], and gain of chromosome 7 appears to be the most common alteration [44,54,57,60–62]. Gain of whole chromosome 7 is the most frequent change in follicular tumors [44,57, 60–62], particularly in tumors displaying a fetal-like growth pattern [54]. Loss of chromosome arm 15q is frequent in FTA, and appears to represent a major difference between FTA and FTC [57].

Loss of 22q has been reported in several cytogenetic studies of thyroid lesions, being more prevalent in widely invasive FTC [43,44]. Some investigators also found loss of 22q in FTA [57] and in PTC [63].

Taking into consideration the available cytogenetic data, the existence of two main pathways for thyroid follicular carcinogenesis have been advanced: one is characterized by gross aneuploidy and a fetal-like growth pattern, displaying chromosomal gains; the other occurs in lesions with a classic follicular growth pattern and a diploid or near-diploid DNA content, displaying frequent chromosomal losses [54,64].

The genetic defects (if any) that are facilitating the aneuploidization of thyroid tumors are still unknown. Ouyang and colleagues [65] searched for mutations in the mitotic checkpoint genes (BUB1 and BUBR1), and found that these genes are not mutated in the thyroid cell lines investigated.

Kim and colleagues [66] demonstrated a strong relationship between the expression of the pituitary tumor transforming gene (also known as securin), which is a mitotic checkpoint protein that inhibits sister chromatid separation during mitosis, and the degree of genetic instability in thyroid cancers.

The advanced relationship between RAS activation and chromosomal instability [40] has received some indirect support, by the finding of a significant association between H-RAS 81T $\rightarrow$ C polymorphism, together with increased amount of p21 (which is the active form of RAS), and the occurrence of aneuploidy in thyroid follicular tumors [67]. The reason underlying such an association has not been clarified yet.

PAX8-PPARγ rearrangements

The genes involved in the translocation t(2;3)(q13;p25) that is relatively frequent in follicular tumors were identified in FTC [68]. This rearrangement creates a fusion gene, encompassing the promoter proximal 5′ coding sequence of the thyroid-specific transcription factor PAX8 gene and most of the coding sequence of the PPARγ gene [68]. Kroll and colleagues [68] claimed the PAX8-PPARγ rearrangement was specific of FTC because it was not detected in any of the 20 FTAs, nor in any of the 10 hyperplastic nodules and 10 PTC included in their series [68].

Later studies showed that the PAX8-PPARγ rearrangement was not specific of FTC because it was also detected in FTA [69,70], as well as in PTC, with a prominent follicular growth pattern [17,59].

Although the PAX8-PPARγ rearrangement was only identified recently, specific rearrangements involving the PPARγ locus had been reported previously in follicular tumors. Roque and colleagues [71] reported a clonal t(2;3)(q13;p25) in a FTC and its bone metastasis. A similar clonal rearrangement had been detected previously by Sozzi and colleagues [72] t(2;3)(q12~q13;p24~p25) in two FTA. Other reports describing tumors with chromosome alterations involving 3p25 had also been published, such as those on t(1;3)(p13;p25) [73] and t(3;7)(p25;q34) [74] in FTC.

The oncogenic function and mechanisms of action of PAX8-PPARγ fusion protein are not yet fully understood. Kroll and colleagues [68] demonstrated that the PAX8-PPARγ fusion protein does not stimulate thiazolidinedione-induced transcription and that the fusion protein can inhibit the wild-type PPARγ transcriptional activation [68]. Powell and colleagues [75] showed that the PAX8-PPARγ fusion protein have oncogenic properties, leading to increased cell cycle transition, reduced apoptosis and loss of contact inhibition, and matrix-independent growth. These effects appear to be mediated, at least in part, by wild type PPARγ inhibition [75], confirming the results obtained previously [68]. Studies using PPARγ agonists showed that in their presence thyroid cancer cells redifferentiate and proliferate less [76], thus supporting the idea that loss of PPARγ function would have opposite effects.

At variance with the aforementioned evidence, an up-regulation of the expression of several known or suspected PPARγ target genes was detected in FTC with PAX8-PPARγ rearrangement, such as angiopoietin-like 4 and aquaporin 7 [77]. This result contradicts the assumption that the chimeric protein acts through a dominant negative effect on the wild type PPARγ, and shows that the oncogenic mechanisms of PAX8-PPARγ rearrangement remains to be fully clarified.

The clinical importance of the rearrangement also remains disputable. Nikiforova and colleagues [33] found an association of PAX-PPARγ rearrangement with the younger age of FTA and FTC patients and overtly invasive features of the FTC. In the authors' series, the younger age of the patients with tumors displaying the rearrangement has been confirmed, but there were not enough invasive cases to evaluate the relationship with prominent vascular invasiveness [17]. In two other series it was reported that patients with PPARγ-negative tumors have less well-differentiated tumors and are more likely to have metastatic disease [78,79].

BRAF mutations

Activating oncogenic mutations of the BRAF gene are the most frequent genetic events detected in PTC (36%–83%) [80–82]. BRAF is a pivotal member of the RAF-MEK-ERK signaling pathway, of which active normal and oncogenic RAS, RET (RET/PTC), and NTRK1 (the other prominent PTC proto-oncogenes) are known elicitors. Alterations in these genes nearly do not overlap and account for about 70% of all PTC cases, and for that reason it is assumed that underlying PTC development is the linear activation of the RET/PTC(NTRK1)-RAS-BRAF-MEK-ERK signaling pathway [80,81,83,84], a concept further reinforced by in vitro experiments demonstrating the BRAF-dependent activation of the ERK signaling pathway by RET/PTC [85,86].

BRAF mutations are not randomly distributed by PTC histotypes: the hotspot BRAF^{V600E} closely clusters to PTC cases of predominant papillary architecture, irrespective of the histologic variant being conventional PTC (C-PTC), tall cell PTC, oncocytic PTC, or papillary microcarcinoma and is rare in cases of predominant follicular architecture [83,84,87–90]. In the FVPTC, another activating BRAF mutation (BRAF^{K601E}) has been detected in about 7% of cases [88,89]. Moreover, the in-frame deletion BRAF$^{VK600-1E}$ was detected by the authors' group in a case of solid variant of PTC [91]; it is unknown, however, whether this or other rare BRAF alterations show any histotype clustering [17,92–94].

Observations in PTCs arising within struma ovarii confirmed the phenotype-marker nature of BRAF mutations: C-PTC lesions harbored the BRAF^{V600E} mutation, whereas FVPTC presented BRAF^{K601E} and the rare deletion BRAF$^{TV599-600M}$ [95,96]. A higher in vitro kinase activity of BRAF^{V600E} in comparison to BRAF^{K601E} [97], and higher mitogenicity of RET/PTC3 in comparison to RET/PTC1 [98] have been reported, but it remains to be understood how these and other functional differences may contribute to different phenotypes.

Etiopathogenically, BRAF mutations are possibly early or even initiating events in PTC, as they are frequently detected in papillary microcarcinoma (20%–52%) [88,89,99,100]. These mutations have been found even in minute incidental cases (17%) [101]. The assumption that BRAF mutations serve as causative events in PTC has been supported by the development of invasive PTC-like lesions in thyroid-targeted BRAF^{V600E} transgenic mice [102], and by the requirement of mutant BRAF protein to the induction [85,86] and maintenance [103] of tumoral features (eg, growth and survival) in in vitro thyroid cell models. Furthermore, BRAF^{V600E}-harboring papillary microcarcinomas [88,89] and the BRAF^{V600E}-transgenic mice thyroid lesions predominantly display a papillary pattern [102], thus reinforcing the mentioned genotype-phenotype association.

BRAF mutations have been related to a more aggressive clinical behavior of PTC, as several studies have associated their presence with parameters regarded as indicators of poor prognosis: older age at diagnosis [36,87,88,104], male gender [105,106], extra-thyroid invasion [36,87,107,108], lymph node metastization [82,106–108], higher tumor staging [36,87,108,109], and recurrence [106,108]. Despite these reports, the prognostic meaning of BRAF mutations is controversial, not only because some groups did not find the aforementioned associations [84,99,100,110–112], but also because most studies did not take into account the close association of the BRAF^{V600E} mutation with the PTC histotypes, which are usually associated with higher levels of extrathyroid extension, lymph node metastases, and recurrence [36,88–90,108,113]. The histologic bias is well demonstrated in the study by Xing and colleagues [108], who found that the association of BRAF mutations to extrathyroid extension, lymph node metastization, and higher tumor staging detected in univariate analysis, were lost after the adjustment of the analysis for PTC histotype. Hence, it remains to be confirmed whether or not, within the cases with papillary histotypes, BRAF mutations are significantly associated with poor prognosis [88,90,106,108].

A study that came to sustain the advanced aggressive character of BRAF mutations in PTCs was the report by Oler and colleagues [92] on the increase of BRAF mutations in PTC metastases in comparison to the primary lesions: while five of eight C-PTC primary lesions harbored BRAF^{V600E}, all eight metastases were BRAF-mutated, three of them bearing the in-frame deletion BRAF$^{VK600-1E}$. It was suggested that these data implied that lymph node metastization of PTC could be promoted by, or even require, the acquisition of BRAF mutation [92]. However, similar studies by other investigators [114–116] did not confirm such increase of BRAF mutations in PTC metastases and, therefore, the involvement of BRAF mutations in general—and of the BRAF$^{VK600-1E}$ in particular—in PTC metastization also remains controversial issue.

The frequency of BRAF mutations and their hotspot incidence (almost all 1799T-A, BRAF^{V600E}) turn its detection into a putative useful molecular marker for the preoperative diagnosis of difficult PTC cases. In fact, the reliable detection of BRAF mutations (as well as of RET/PTC) in thyroid fine-needle aspirates has been consistently reported [111,117–121]. Nonetheless, the value of such application may be lessened by the rarity of BRAF^{V600E} in the FVPTC, which is the histotype that raises more difficult diagnostic problems, namely regarding the distinction between FTC and FTA [122].

A well-known etiologic factor in PTC is ionizing radiation, as shown by the large increase of PTC incidence in children after the nuclear accident of Chernobyl [123]. In this setting RET/PTC are highly prevalent and, conversely, BRAF point mutations are rare [124–127], thus indicating that radiation mainly induces double-strand DNA breaks (followed by illegitimate recombination) [128]. This assumption has been reinforced by the finding of activating rearrangement of the BRAF gene (AKAP9-BRAF) in some post-Chernobyl childhood cases [129]. The rearrangement derives from the paracentric inversion of 7q and leads to the fusion of the N-terminal region of AKAP9 with BRAF kinase domain. It ultimately leads to the expression of the active BRAF kinase domain [129] by the disposal of its autoinhibitory N-terminal region, as in the viral oncogenic homolog v-RAF [130–132]. Aside from the series of Ciampi and colleagues [129], BRAF rearrangement has not been reported by other groups in sporadic or radiation-induced PTC.

BRAF mutations are very rare both in Chernobyl cases and in sporadic childhood PTC cases [88,126,127,133,134], and appear to be associated to older age at diagnosis [36,87,88,104]. Consequently, the rarity of BRAF mutations in post-Chernobyl cases may be either because of their irrelevance in a strong radiation background or simply because of their reduced tumorigenic potential, leading to longer latency periods [88]. In a recent study of PTC cases of atom bomb survivors by Takahashi and colleagues [135], BRAF point mutations were associated both to lower radiation doses, a finding that concurs with the former hypothesis, and to longer latency periods, which also supports the latter.

There are several drugs that efficiently inhibit BRAF or its downstream effectors, remarkably MEK1/2, that are at clinical trial with promising results [136]. BAY43-9006 (also known as sorafenib), for instance, seems promising as it efficiently impairs the growth of thyroid carcinoma-derived cell lines, harboring BRAF mutations or not [137,138]. Similarly, two other RAF kinase inhibitors, NVP-AAL881-NX and NVP-LBT613-AG-8, were shown to inhibit proliferation and survival of thyroid carcinoma-derived cell lines [139]. Additionally, BRAF^{V600E}, but not BRAF^{WT}, was shown to require the HSP90 chaperone for its stability, envisioning the usage of HSP90 inhibitors for thyroid cancer (and melanoma and colon cancer) treatment [140,141].

Mutations in oxidative phosphorylation and Krebs cycle genes in Hürthle cell tumors

Although it is difficult or even impossible to evaluate critically the huge amount of data on record, it seems that the HCT do not differ substantially from their non-Hürthle cell counterparts, regarding the prevalence of aneuploidy, trisomy of chromosomes 5, 7, and 12, and mutations of oncogenes and oncosuppressor genes (RET/PTC and NTRK1 rearrangements, RAS, TP53, and BRAF mutations) (for a thorough review, see Refs. [89,142,143]). HCT do differ, however, from their non-Hürthle cell counterparts regarding the prevalence of mitochondrial protein alterations encoded by genes of both mitochondrial DNA (mtDNA) and nuclear DNA (nDNA) [142,144,145].

A specific mtDNA alteration—a large deletion encompassing 4977 bp of mtDNA—known as the mtDNA common deletion (CD), is often found in oncocytic thyroid tumors and was proposed as a hallmark of these tumors, also known as Hürthle cell tumors [144,146,147]. This deletion removes seven oxidative phosphorylation (OXPHOS) genes (ATPase6, ATPase8, COIII, ND3, ND4L, ND4, and ND5) and five tRNAs (glycine, arginine, histidine, serine, and leucine), thus resulting in severe impairment of the OXPHOS system.

The mtDNA CD was found in every thyroid tumor with oncocytic features, irrespective of the histologic subtype (PTC, FTC, and FTA) [144]. The mtDNA CD has also been detected in nononcocytic thyroid tumors, but with a significantly lower frequency (18.8% of PTC, 0% of FTC, and 33.3% of FTA) [144]. The relative amount of deleted mtDNA molecules within each tumor was also assessed and was found to be significantly higher ($P = .0001$) in oncocytic thyroid tumors than in nononcocytic thyroid tumors [144]. The highest value of the mtDNA CD detected in Hürthle cell tumors was 16% of the total mtDNA amount, suggesting that above that level the neoplastic cells were not viable [144].

Traditionally, the association between mtDNA CD and oncocytic phenotype has been explained through a positive feedback mechanism: the severe impairment of the OXPHOS system (as a consequence of the mtDNA CD) would engage and activate nuclear genes that control mitochondrial number, resulting in an increase in the mitochondrial mass [148–150].

MtDNA mutations are also frequently detected in benign and malignant HCT [144,145,151]. They occur both in the "C" tract of the D-loop region and in all of the 13 genes that encode OXPHOS proteins, being more frequent in Complex I genes than in the genes of the other Complexes [144,145,151]. Occasionally, mutations in some tRNAs have also been detected [144]. The OXPHOS gene mutations include frameshift and point mutations (both silent and missense mutations). Disruptive mutations (either frameshift or nonsense) tended to be concentrated in Complex I genes, without any apparent concentration in a single gene [144,145,151].

MtDNA variants affecting genes of Complex V (ATPase6 and ATPase8) were much more frequent in HCT than in their non-Hürthle cell counterparts, and were more frequently detected in malignant tumors than in adenomas [144,145]. These findings do not indicate that these mtDNA variants are associated with an increased risk for tumor development, but they suggest that, in case the patient harboring such variants will develop a thyroid tumor, it is more likely that the tumor will have oncocytic features and be malignant [144].

Gasparre and colleagues [145] found that the only breast tumor of their series that presented a disruptive somatic mtDNA mutation (also located in a Complex I gene) was a mitochondrion-rich tumor, thus reinforcing the association of disruptive mtDNA Complex I mutations with the occurrence of the oncocytic phenotype of thyroid tumors. In line with this rationale when addressing the association of the mtDNA CD with oncocytic features— severe impairment of the OXPHOS system because the mtDNA CD would lead to a positive feedback in the nucleus, resulting in accumulating dysfunctional mitochondria—the disruptive Complex I mutations (and in the genes of other mitochondrial respiratory chain complexes) found in a subset of oncocytic thyroid tumors may also result in OXPHOS system impairment and, subsequently, to accumulation of abnormal mitochondria [144,145].

The familial forms of benign and malignant HCT may be caused by a germline mutation in GRIM-19, a dual-function nuclear gene involved in mitochondrial metabolism and cell death [152–154]. GRIM-19 has been mapped to chromosome 19p13.2 [153] and is the human homolog of the bovine subunit of the mitochondrial NADH:ubiquinone oxireductase complex (Complex I) of the mitochondrial respiratory chain [155]. Down-regulation of GRIM-19 has been shown to confer a growth advantage on cells and to reduce the likelihood that they will enter apoptosis [152].

Recently, somatic missense mutations of GRIM-19 were detected in one Hürthle cell FTC and two Hürthle cell PTC, and a germline mutation was detected in a Hürthle cell PTC arising in a thyroid with multiple Hürthle cell benign nodules and familial history of HCT [156]; no mutations were detected in any of the 20 cases of non-Hürthle follicular and papillary carcinomas, nor in any of the 96 blood donor samples [156]. The GRIM-19 mutations detected are the first nuclear gene mutations specific to Hürthle cell tumors reported to date [156].

In one of the sporadic Hürthle cell PTC positive for GRIM-19 mutations, the authors have also detected a RET/PTC-1 rearrangement, suggesting that GRIM-19 mutation may serve as a predisposing alteration for the occurrence of tumors with oncocytic transformation, and that other alterations, such as RET/PTC rearrangement or BRAF mutation, may be necessary for the acquisition of the malignant phenotype.

The presence of abundant (and abnormal) mitochondria in the cytoplasm of the neoplastic cells may be seen throughout the entire tumor (primary oncocytic transformation), indicating that the carcinogenic hit has occurred in cells with pre-existing mitochondrial alterations, or in part of the tumor ("secondary" oncocytic transformation), indicating that the mitochondrial abnormalities have occurred after tumor initiation [142,150]. For a complete review on Hürthle cell tumors, see Lima and colleagues [157].

Mutations in SDH genes in medullary carcinoma and C-cell hyperplasia

Mutations in the genes encoding mitochondrial succinate dehydrogenase subunits B, C and D (SDHB, SDHC and SDHD, also called SDH genes) have been identified from 2000 on in hereditary and sporadic paragangliomas and pheochromocytomas [158,159]. The authors have identified one MEN2-like family in which all the affected individuals presented an alteration (H50R) in exon 2 of the SDHD gene [160]. Screening of exons 8 to 16 of the RET gene revealed an alteration in exon 13 (Y791N), which was present in three individuals of the family but did not segregate with the disease. These findings, together with the aforementioned role of SDHD mutations in other endocrine lesions, support the assumption that the SDHD H50R alteration is the probable cause of this inherited C-cell hyperplasia [160].

In addition to the MEN2-like family, the authors have also searched for germline mutations in SDH genes in apparently sporadic medullary thyroid carcinomas (MTCs) without germline RET mutations. The authors have identified five different germline SDHB (two) and SDHD (three) alterations in 6 out of 20 (30%) patients (Jorge Lima and colleagues, unpublished data, 2007). One patient harbored a double alteration in SDHB (A6A and ISV2-36 G>T) and five patients were found to have missense coding alterations in SDHD: three harbored the H50R alteration, one the G12S alteration, and the remaining patient presented both the G12S and the S68S alterations in exon 3 (Jorge Lima and colleagues, unpublished data, 2007). No alterations were disclosed in SDHC. Although the aforementioned SDH alterations were also present in the normal, healthy population, there was a trend for an over-representation of the H50R alteration in patients with MTC ($P = .08$). Moreover, patients with germline SDHD alterations had a (not significantly) lower mean age at diagnosis (46 years) than the patients without germline SDHD alterations (51 years).

Two other articles have searched for germline SDHB and SDHD mutations in patients with MTC. Montani and colleagues [161] have screened for SDHB and SDHD germline mutations in a series of MTC subjects, and found an accumulation of alterations (S163P in SDHB as well as G12S and H50R in SDHD) among MTC subjects (17.1% harbored an alteration in SDHB or in SDHD), when compared with a control population (1.2% with SDHB or SDHD mutations). Cascon and colleagues [162] searched for SDHD mutations in two families with hereditary non-RET C-cell hyperplasia and in sporadic MTC. They found no alterations related to the inherited C-cell hyperplasia, as well as no evidence that the presence of the H50R is strongly associated with the risk of sporadic MTC [162]; however, the presence of the H50R alteration was associated with a significantly lower ($P = .02$) age at diagnosis in sporadic MTC [162].

Recently, it was reported an association of mtDNA transversion mutations (the majority being located in Complex I genes) with familial MTC/MEN2 syndrome, thus reinforcing the putative role played by mitochondrial alterations in this setting [160–163]. Further studies are necessary to confirm whether or not mtDNA alterations and alterations in nuclear genes encoding mitochondrial proteins (eg, SDHD) may predispose to C-cell hyperplasia and modulate the occurrence of MTC.

Mutations in TP53 and other genes in poorly differentiated and anaplastic carcinomas

TP53 mutations

Well-differentiated thyroid carcinomas (WDTC) represent an excellent example of that minority of human cancer types that appear not to require mutational inactivation of TP53. Protein expression and gene mutation analysis of TP53 in WDTC showed that TP53 mutation is a rare event in these carcinomas. Putting together the results obtained by several studies, which looked for TP53 mutations, 98% of the WDTC (PTC and FCT) analyzed have a normal TP53 [164–168].

In thyroid tumors, TP53 gene inactivation seems to play an important role in the progression from differentiated to anaplastic carcinoma, occurring together with an increase in cellular proliferation [169–171]. It seems that this transition occurs, in WDTC in general and PTC in particular, in a quite abrupt way at variance with a stepwise process in other tumor models [172]. Several investigators who studied the expression and mutations of TP53 in PTC coexisting with ATC, found TP53 expression and mutation only in the undifferentiated counterparts [167,173,174]. Mutations in TP53 seem to be restricted to more advanced forms of carcinoma, mainly PDTC (approximately 28%) and ATC (approximately 64%) (Table 2). Virtually, all the mutations reported are located in the known hotspots (exons 5–9), codon 273 being the one that is more often affected [164,165,167,173].

It is possible that progression and dedifferentiation in thyroid lesions in vivo results, as proposed by Wynford-Thomas [175], from a two-step mechanism, explained by the need for the differentiation switch (epithelial-mesenchymal transition) and the TP53 mutation to arise independently in the same cell before any selective advantage is obtained [175,176]. Taking into consideration the data on the progression of WDTC to less differentiated and undifferentiated forms of thyroid cancer, together with the high frequency of TP53 inactivation, gross genetic alterations, and aneuploidy, it is likely that in the more advanced steps of progression, inactivation of TP53 ("suppressor pathway") represents the most frequent mechanism of genomic instability in thyroid cancer. This is in accordance with the sequential increase in chromosomal complexity observed in CGH studies from WDTC to PDTC and ATC [58,177–179].

Table 2
Summary of the results published on mutation analysis of TP53 in poorly differentiated thyroid carcinoma and anaplastic thyroid carcinoma

Reference	Methods	PDTC	ATC
Ito and colleagues [167]	PCR-RFLP, SQ	–	6/7 (86%)
Donghi and colleagues [164]	PCR, SSCP	2/8 (25%)	5/7 (71%)
Fagin and colleagues [165]	PCR, SSCP	–	5/6 (86%)
Zou and colleagues [169]	PCR, SSCP	–	1/5 (20%)
Dobashi and colleagues [224]	PCR, SQ	2/6 (33%)	4/6 (66%)
Ho and colleagues [225]	PCR, SQ	5/29 (17%)	–
Takeuchi and colleagues [226]	PCR, SSCP	14/46 (38%)	–
Wang and colleagues [189]	PCR	–	9/16 (56%)

Abbreviations: PCR, polymerase chain reaction; RFLP, restriction fragment length polymorphism; SQ, sequencing; SSCP, single strand conformation polymorphism.

P53 can trigger cell-cycle growth arrest or the apoptotic pathway in response to DNA damage [180,181]. Furthermore, P53 is a positive regulator of BAX expression and a negative regulator of BCL-2 expression [180,181]. High levels of BCL-2 protein favor cell survival, whereas high levels of wild-type P53 lead to an increase in BAX and a decrease in BCL-2, pushing toward apoptotic cell death. A positive correlation between apoptotic index and P53 expression was found in WDTC [180,182], suggesting that (over) expression of nonmutated P53 could be inducing cell death. An inverse correlation between BCL-2 and P53 expression was observed in ATC [171,180,182]. The characterization of P53 and BCL-2 expression may be expected to give an indication of the ability for survival or death [181].

The frequency of TP53 mutations in ATC in the different series lies between 20% and 86% [164,165,167,169]. Even considering the different sensitivities of the different methodologies, it is tempting to advance that at least in a minority of cases, alterations in genes other than TP53 can lead to a similar end stage of tumor development. WNT pathway and CDK/CDKI molecules, which were found altered in thyroid cell lines and primary tumors, appear to be good candidates for such an alternative role with regard to mutated TP53-like alterations [183,184].

RAS mutations

RAS genes, notably N-RAS, are consistently found mutated in less differentiated thyroid tumors. The prevalence of RAS mutations ranges between 18% and 63% in PDTC, and between 4% and 60% in ATC (Table 3) [174,185–188].

RAS mutations were shown to be associated with aggressive tumor phenotypes and poor prognosis [188]. It was also shown that PDTC cases with mutated N-RAS are significantly associated with the appearance of hematogenous (particularly bone) metastases [185,186].

Because of the association found between RAS mutations and guarded prognosis in PDTC and ATC, and because of the activation of N-RAS oncogenes in WDTC, Wang and colleagues [189] proposed that particular

Table 3
Summary of the results published on mutation analysis of RAS in poorly differentiated thyroid carcinoma and anaplastic thyroid carcinoma

Reference	Methods	PDTC	ATC
Manenti and colleagues [186]	PCR	3/11 (27%),	1/5 (20%)
Capella and colleagues [227]	PCR, RFLP	–	5/13 (38%)
Pilotti and colleagues [228]	PCR, SSCP	5/8 (63%)	–
Basolo and colleagues [185]	PCR, SQ	8/44 (18%)	15/29 (52%)
Garcia-Rostan and colleagues [188]	PCR, SQ	16/29 (55%)	3/5 (60%)
Fukushima and colleagues [229]	PCR, SQ	–	28%
Quiros and colleagues [174]	PCR, SQ	–	1/8 (13%)
Wang and colleagues [189]	PCR	–	5/16 (31%)

attention should be paid to WDTC, particularly FTC, harboring RAS mutation [189,190].

Mutations in WNT pathway genes

Elements of the WNT pathway, particularly CTNNB1 (the gene encoding β-catenin), were also found to be mutated in PDTC and ATC [183]. The first studies by Garcia-Rostan and colleagues [183] reported a frequency of CTNNB1 mutations of 25% in PDTC and 65.5% in ATC [183]. The activating mutations cluster in exon 3, at the phosphorylation sites for ubiquitination and degradation of β-catenin, and are associated with aberrant nuclear immunoreactivity, suggesting WNT pathway activation [183,191]. CTNNB1 mutations were restricted to these two histotypes and significantly associated with poor prognosis, independent of conventional prognostic indicators for thyroid cancer, but not for tumor differentiation [191]. The results from Kim and colleagues [192], demonstrating that the transient overexpression of WNT1 or β-catenin in FRTL-5 cells decreased thyroperoxidase (TPO) mRNA and suppressed TPO-promoter activity, corroborates a putative role of β-catenin activation in loss of differentiation of thyroid cells [192].

At variance with the aforementioned results, Rocha and colleagues [193] did not find mutations in CTNNB1 nor in the CDH1 gene (encoding E-cadherin) in a series of PDTC, but verified alteration in the expression at the protein level, concluding that loss of E-cadherin rather than CTNNB1 mutation is the crucial event in determining the differentiation "level" of thyroid carcinoma [193]. The quite different percentages of CTNNB1 mutations reported in different series of PDTC [183,191,193,194] probably reflect the heterogeneity of tumors that are included under the umbrella category of PDTC [195].

Kurihara and colleagues [194] investigated the status of the components and target genes of the WNT signaling pathway in 22 ATC from Japanese patients, and found nuclear and cytoplasmic positive staining of β-catenin in 40.9% of the 22 ATC samples, whereas CTNNB1 gene mutations were only observed in 4.5% of the cases. Mutations in adenomatous polyposis coli (APC) and Axin were detected in 9% and 81.8% of the ATC samples, respectively, in the same series [194]. To the best of the authors' knowledge, no other investigators have described mutations in APC or the Axin gene in PDTC and undifferentiated thyroid cancer. APC mutations have also been detected in a variant of WDTC that some authors consider to be PTC-related [196]; this particular subset of thyroid tumor (the so-called cribiform morular variant of WDTC) occurs both in the context of familial forms of adenomatous polyposis, and in a sporadic setting as the result of somatic mutation of APC and CTNNB1 [196,197].

BRAF mutations

Regarding the prevalence of BRAF mutations in PDTC and ATC, there exists also some contradictory evidence. The BRAF^{V600E} mutation has been

screened in PDTC by Nikiforova and colleagues [87], who found the mutation in 2 out of 16 cases (13%); the two positive cases had a PTC component
in which the BRAF^{V600E} was also detected. The authors' group did not detect BRAF mutations (V600E or K600E) in a series of PDTC that were selected in a biased way, because it was decided to exclude PTC with foci of
solid growth pattern, PTC with an insular component, and insular, trabecular and solid PDTC with nuclei of the PTC type [198,199]. These criteria
have surely contributed to reducing the heterogeneity of tumors classified
as PDTC [195,200] and may explain the absence of BRAF mutations in
any of the cases of PDTC of the authors' series [198]. Such an absence of
BRAF mutations supports the assumption that these PDTC fit the original
description of insular carcinoma [201] and insular-like carcinoma (solid or
trabecular carcinoma) without PTC nuclei [202]; the authors' data fit with
the assumption that these PDTC are more closely related to FTC than to
PTC [198]. These findings confirm data previously obtained by electron microscopy, morphometry, and lectin histochemistry in a group of PDTC selected according to the same criteria used in this study [195]. On the other
hand, the data obtained by Nikiforova and colleagues [87] indicate that
PTC-derived PDTC may display BRAF mutations.

In ATC, there are also quite different results on the prevalence of BRAF
mutations from series to series (0% to 50%) [87,109,187,198]. Overall, and
considering only the largest series, the mutation is present in about 25%
to 35% of the cases of ATC [87,109,187]. The frequent detection of BRAF-
mutated ATCs together with a BRAF-mutated PTC component suggests,
as with the findings in PDTC, that they may be derived from BRAF-
mutated PTC. Takano and colleagues [203] showed recently that 33.3%
of ATC accompanying PTC showed BRAF^{V600E} mutation in both components. The investigators raise the possibility that BRAF^{V600E} mutations can
be implicated in the progression from WDTC, namely PTC, to more undifferentiated and advanced thyroid tumors, although this issue remains controversial (see above) [203]. Regardless of the putative prognostic meaning
of BRAF mutations in WDTC, it is clear that BRAF mutation does not prevent the evolution to ATC in contrast to the evolution of tumors with RET/
PTC [204]. Both in primary tumors and in thyroid cell lines was the coexistence of BRAF and TP53 mutations in the same cells shown, supporting the
assumption that BRAF-mutated PTC can evolve to ATCs via a superim-
posed TP53 mutation [174].

PI3K mutations

The occurrence of genetic alterations in the phosphatidylinositol 3-kinase
(PI3K)/AKT pathway in thyroid tumors was evaluated in WDTC and ATC
[205]. Activating PI3K mutations located within the kinase domain were
found in 23% of ATC and at lower prevalence in WDTC [206]. In cases
showing coexisting differentiated carcinoma, the mutations were restricted

to the ATC component [206]. Hou and colleagues [190] investigated the overall occurrence and relationship of genetic alterations in the PI3K/AKT pathway in thyroid tumors, having found genetic alterations along this pathway (RAS, PI3K, and PTEN) in 58% of ATC; however PI3K alterations were detected only in 12% of the cases. Coexistence of genetic alterations in the pathway was increasingly seen with progression from differentiated tumors to undifferentiated ATC. Hou and colleagues suggested that progression of WDTC to ATC may be facilitated by the coexistence of PI3K/AKT pathway-related genetic alterations. More recently, Wang and colleagues [189] did not find PI3K mutations in a series of 16 ATC [189]. According to Liu and colleagues [207], gene amplification instead of mutation seems to be a frequent mechanism of PI3K deregulation in thyroid tumors; this mechanism was found by these investigators in 42% of ATC, although they claimed one cannot exclude the contribution of aneuploidy to the high copy number of alleles of the PIK3CA gene often observed in ATC [207].

The disclosure of alterations in PI3K/AKT pathway in ATC led to the suggestion that this pathway should be explored as a therapeutic target for thyroid cancers, particularly PDTC and ATC, that correspond to the subset of thyroid tumors more refractory to conventional therapeutic approaches.

RET/PTC and PAX8-PPARγ in poorly differentiated thyroid carcinoma and anaplastic thyroid carcinoma

Thyroid specific rearrangements found in WDTC (RET/PTC in PTC and PAX8-PPARγ in FTC and FVPTC) are only rarely reported in PDTC or ATC [69,204,208,209], despite the frequent occurrence of foci of WDTC in PDTC and ATC. This suggests that tumors harboring these rearrangements do not usually evolve toward undifferentiated carcinomas, thus reinforcing the assumption that most rearranged PTC and FTC do not tend to progress toward more advanced steps of neoplastic development.

Nakashima and colleagues [210] reported RET amplification in six cases of ATC, showing the ATC cases with stronger P53 immunoreactivity, higher RET amplification-positive cells. Since RET amplification was correlated with P53 accumulation, it was advanced that RET amplification might also result from the high level of genomic instability [210].

References

[1] Kondo T, Ezzat S, Asa SL. Pathogenetic mechanisms in thyroid follicular-cell neoplasia. Nat Rev Cancer 2006;6(4):292–306.

[2] Corvilain B, Laurent E, Lecomte M, et al. Role of the cyclic adenosine 3′,5′-monophosphate and the phosphatidylinositol-Ca2+ cascades in mediating the effects of thyrotropin and iodide on hormone synthesis and secretion in human thyroid slices. J Clin Endocrinol Metab 1994;79(1):152–9.

[3] Dumont JE, Jauniaux JC, Roger PP. The cyclic AMP-mediated stimulation of cell proliferation. Trends Biochem Sci 1989;14(2):67–71.

[4] Landis CA, Masters SB, Spada A, et al. GTPase inhibiting mutations activate the alpha chain of Gs and stimulate adenylyl cyclase in human pituitary tumours. Nature 1989;340(6236):692–6.

[5] Lyons J, Landis CA, Harsh G, et al. Two G protein oncogenes in human endocrine tumors. Science 1990;249(4969):655–9.

[6] Suarez HG, du Villard JA, Caillou B, et al. Gsp mutations in human thyroid tumours. Oncogene 1991;6(4):677–9.

[7] O'Sullivan C, Barton CM, Staddon SL, et al. Activating point mutations of the gsp oncogene in human thyroid adenomas. Mol Carcinog 1991;4(5):345–9.

[8] Parma J, Duprez L, Van Sande J, et al. Somatic mutations in the thyrotropin receptor gene cause hyperfunctioning thyroid adenomas. Nature 1993;365(6447):649–51.

[9] Parma J, Van Sande J, Swillens S, et al. Somatic mutations causing constitutive activity of the thyrotropin receptor are the major cause of hyperfunctioning thyroid adenomas: identification of additional mutations activating both the cyclic adenosine 3′,5′-monophosphate and inositol phosphate-Ca2+ cascades. Mol Endocrinol 1995;9(6):725–33.

[10] Krohn K, Paschke R. Somatic mutations in thyroid nodular disease. Mol Genet Metab 2002;75(3):202–8.

[11] Trulzsch B, Krohn K, Wonerow P, et al. Detection of thyroid-stimulating hormone receptor and Gsalpha mutations: in 75 toxic thyroid nodules by denaturing gradient gel electrophoresis. J Mol Med 2001;78(12):684–91.

[12] Krohn K, Führer D, Holzapfel HP, et al. Clonal origin of toxic thyroid nodules with constitutively activating thyrotropin receptor mutations. J Clin Endocrinol Metab 1998;83(1): 130–4.

[13] Tonacchera M, Vitti P, Agretti P, et al. Functioning and nonfunctioning thyroid adenomas involve different molecular pathogenetic mechanisms. J Clin Endocrinol Metab 1999; 84(11):4155–8.

[14] Farid NR, Shi Y, Zou M. Molecular basis of thyroid cancer. Endocr Rev 1994;15(2): 202–32.

[15] Said S, Schlumberger M, Suarez HG. Oncogenes and anti-oncogenes in human epithelial thyroid tumors. J Endocrinol Invest 1994;17(5):371–9.

[16] Vanvooren V, Allgeier A, Nguyen M, et al. Mutation analysis of the Epac-Rap1 signaling pathway in cold thyroid follicular adenomas. Eur J Endocrinol 2001;144(6):605–10.

[17] Castro P, Rebocho AP, Soares RJ, et al. PAX8-PPARgamma rearrangement is frequently detected in the follicular variant of papillary thyroid carcinoma. J Clin Endocrinol Metab 2006;91(1):213–20.

[18] Motoi N, Sakamoto A, Yamochi T, et al. Role of Ras mutation in the progression of thyroid carcinoma of follicular epithelial origin. Pathol Res Pract 2000;196(1):1–7.

[19] Esapa CT, Johnson SJ, Kendall-Taylor P, et al. Prevalence of Ras mutations in thyroid neoplasia. Clin Endocrinol (Oxf) 1999;50(4):529–35.

[20] Cetani F, Tonacchera M, Pinchera A, et al. Genetic analysis of the TSH receptor gene in differentiated human thyroid carcinomas. J Endocrinol Invest 1999;22(4):273–8.

[21] Spambalg D, Sharifi N, Elisei R, et al. Structural studies of the thyrotropin receptor and Gs alpha in human thyroid cancers: low prevalence of mutations predicts infrequent involvement in malignant transformation. J Clin Endocrinol Metab 1996;81(11):3898–901.

[22] Ringel MD, Saji M, Schwindinger WF, et al. Absence of activating mutations of the genes encoding the alpha-subunits of G11 and Gq in thyroid neoplasia. J Clin Endocrinol Metab 1998;83(2):554–9.

[23] Niepomniszcze H, Suarez H, Pitoia F, et al. Follicular carcinoma presenting as autonomous functioning thyroid nodule and containing an activating mutation of the TSH receptor (T620I) and a mutation of the Ki-RAS (G12C) genes. Thyroid 2006;16(5):497–503.

[24] Dremier S, Coppee F, Delange F, et al. Clinical Review 84: Thyroid autonomy: mechanism and clinical effects. J Clin Endocrinol Metab 1996;81(12):4187–93.

[25] Gozu H, Avsar M, Bircan R, et al. Does a Leu 512 Arg thyrotropin receptor mutation cause an autonomously functioning papillary carcinoma? Thyroid 2004;14(11):975–80.

[26] Camacho P, Gordon D, Chiefari E, et al. A Phe 486 thyrotropin receptor mutation in an autonomously functioning follicular carcinoma that was causing hyperthyroidism. Thyroid 2000;10(11):1009–12.

[27] Russo D, Wong MG, Costante G, et al. A Val 677 activating mutation of the thyrotropin receptor in a Hürthle cell thyroid carcinoma associated with thyrotoxicosis. Thyroid 1999; 9(1):13–7.

[28] Bos JL. Ras oncogenes in human cancer: a review. Cancer Res 1989;49(17):4682–9.

[29] Peyssonnaux C, Eychene A. The Raf/MEK/ERK pathway: new concepts of activation. Biol Cell 2001;93(1–2):53–62.

[30] Vasko V, Ferrand M, Di Cristofaro J, et al. Specific pattern of RAS oncogene mutations in follicular thyroid tumors. J Clin Endocrinol Metab 2003;88(6):2745–52.

[31] Lazzereschi D, Mincione G, Coppa A, et al. Oncogenes and antioncogenes involved in human thyroid carcinogenesis. J Exp Clin Cancer Res 1997;16(3):325–32.

[32] Sugg SL, Ezzat S, Zheng L, et al. Oncogene profile of papillary thyroid carcinoma. Surgery 1999;125(1):46–52.

[33] Nikiforova MN, Lynch RA, Biddinger PW, et al. RAS point mutations and PAX8-PPAR gamma rearrangement in thyroid tumors: evidence for distinct molecular pathways in thyroid follicular carcinoma. J Clin Endocrinol Metab 2003;88(5):2318–26.

[34] Zhu Z, Gandhi M, Nikiforova MN, et al. Molecular profile and clinical-pathologic features of the follicular variant of papillary thyroid carcinoma. An unusually high prevalence of ras mutations. Am J Clin Pathol 2003;120(1):71–7.

[35] Di Cristofaro J, Marcy M, Vasko V, et al. Molecular genetic study comparing follicular variant versus classic papillary thyroid carcinomas: association of N-ras mutation in codon 61 with follicular variant. Hum Pathol 2006;37(7):824–30.

[36] Adeniran AJ, Zhu Z, Gandhi M, et al. Correlation between genetic alterations and microscopic features, clinical manifestations, and prognostic characteristics of thyroid papillary carcinomas. Am J Surg Pathol 2006;30(2):216–22.

[37] Giaretti W, Molinu S, Ceccarelli J, et al. Chromosomal instability, aneuploidy, and gene mutations in human sporadic colorectal adenomas. Cell Oncol 2004;26(5–6):301–5.

[38] Giaretti W, Pujic N, Rapallo A, et al. K-ras-2 G-C and G-T transversions correlate with DNA aneuploidy in colorectal adenomas. Gastroenterology 1995;108(4):1040–7.

[39] Giaretti W, Rapallo A, Geido E, et al. Specific K-ras2 mutations in human sporadic colorectal adenomas are associated with DNA near-diploid aneuploidy and inhibition of proliferation. Am J Pathol 1998;153(4):1201–9.

[40] Fagin JA. Minireview: Branded from the start—distinct oncogenic initiating events may determine tumor fate in the thyroid. Mol Endocrinol 2002;16(5):903–11.

[41] Johannessen JV, Sobrinho-Simões M, Lindmo T, et al. The diagnostic value of flow cytometric DNA measurements in selected disorders of the human thyroid. Am J Clin Pathol 1982;77(1):20–5.

[42] Belge G, Thode B, Rippe V, et al. A characteristic sequence of trisomies starting with trisomy 7 in benign thyroid tumors. Hum Genet 1994;94(2):198–202.

[43] Hemmer S, Wasenius VM, Knuutila S, et al. Comparison of benign and malignant follicular thyroid tumours by comparative genomic hybridization. Br J Cancer 1998;78(8):1012–7.

[44] Barril N, Carvalho-Sales AB, Tajara EH. Interphase cytogenetic analysis of normal tissue of thyroid gland by fluorescence in situ hybridization. Cancer Genet Cytogenet 1999;114(2): 162–4.

[45] Castro P, Sansonetty F, Soares P, et al. Fetal adenomas and minimally invasive follicular carcinomas of the thyroid frequently display a triploid or near triploid DNA pattern. Virchows Arch 2001;438(4):336–42.

[46] Cusick EL, Ewen SW, Krukowski ZH, et al. DNA aneuploidy in follicular thyroid neoplasia. Br J Surg 1991;78(1):94–6.

[47] Schelfhout LJ, Cornelisse CJ, Goslings BM, et al. Frequency and degree of aneuploidy in benign and malignant thyroid neoplasms. Int J Cancer 1990;45(1):16–20.

[48] Stern Y, Segal K, Medalia O, et al. DNA ploidy in papillary carcinoma of the thyroid gland in children and adolescents. Int J Pediatr Otorhinolaryngol 1998;46(1–2):67–70.

[49] Hostetter AL, Hrafnkelsson J, Wingren SO, et al. A comparative study of DNA cytometry methods for benign and malignant thyroid tissue. Am J Clin Pathol 1988;89(6):760–3.

[50] Soares P, Sobrinho-Simões M. Recent advances in cytometry, cytogenetics and molecular genetics of thyroid tumours and tumour-like lesions. Pathol Res Pract 1995;191(4):304–17.

[51] Francia G, Azzolina L, Mantovani T, et al. Heterogeneity of nuclear DNA pattern and its relationship with cell cycle activity parameters in multinodular goitre. Clin Endocrinol (Oxf) 1997;46(6):649–54.

[52] Christov K. Flow cytometric DNA measurements in human thyroid tumors. Virchows Arch B Cell Pathol Incl Mol Pathol 1986;51(3):255–63.

[53] Schurmann G, Mattfeldt T, Feichter G, et al. Stereology, flow cytometry, and immunohistochemistry of follicular neoplasms of the thyroid gland. Hum Pathol 1991;22(2): 179–84.

[54] Castro P, Eknaes M, Teixeira MR, et al. Adenomas and follicular carcinomas of the thyroid display two major patterns of chromosomal changes. J Pathol 2005;206(3):305–11.

[55] Joensuu H, Klemi PJ. DNA aneuploidy in adenomas of endocrine organs. Am J Pathol 1988;132(1):145–51.

[56] Sturgis CD, Caraway NP, Johnston DA, et al. Image analysis of papillary thyroid carcinoma fine-needle aspirates: significant association between aneuploidy and death from disease. Cancer 1999;87(3):155–60.

[57] Roque L, Rodrigues R, Pinto A, et al. Chromosome imbalances in thyroid follicular neoplasms: a comparison between follicular adenomas and carcinomas. Genes Chromosomes Cancer 2003;36(3):292–302.

[58] Rodrigues RF, Roque L, Rosa-Santos J, et al. Chromosomal imbalances associated with anaplastic transformation of follicular thyroid carcinomas. Br J Cancer 2004;90(2):492–6.

[59] Castro P, Roque L, Magalhaes J, et al. A subset of the follicular variant of papillary thyroid carcinoma harbors the PAX8-PPARgamma translocation. Int J Surg Pathol 2005;13(3): 235–8.

[60] van den Berg E, Oosterhuis JW, de Jong B, et al. Cytogenetics of thyroid follicular adenomas. Cancer Genet Cytogenet 1990;44(2):217–22.

[61] Criado B, Barros A, Suijkerbuijk RF, et al. Detection of numerical alterations for chromosomes 7 and 12 in benign thyroid lesions by in situ hybridization. Histological implications. Am J Pathol 1995;147(1):136–44.

[62] Belge G, Roque L, Soares J, et al. Cytogenetic investigations of 340 thyroid hyperplasias and adenomas revealing correlations between cytogenetic findings and histology. Cancer Genet Cytogenet 1998;101(1):42–8.

[63] Roque L, Nunes VM, Ribeiro C, et al. Karyotypic characterization of papillary thyroid carcinomas. Cancer 2001;92(10):2529–38.

[64] Sobrinho-Simões M, Preto A, Rocha AS, et al. Molecular pathology of well-differentiated thyroid carcinomas. Virchows Arch 2005;447(5):787–93.

[65] Ouyang B, Knauf JA, Ain K, et al. Mechanisms of aneuploidy in thyroid cancer cell lines and tissues: evidence for mitotic checkpoint dysfunction without mutations in BUB1 and BUBR1. Clin Endocrinol (Oxf) 2002;56(3):341–50.

[66] Kim D, Pemberton H, Stratford AL, et al. Pituitary tumour transforming gene (PTTG) induces genetic instability in thyroid cells. Oncogene 2005;24(30):4861–6.

[67] Castro P, Soares P, Gusmao L, et al. H-RAS 81 polymorphism is significantly associated with aneuploidy in follicular tumors of the thyroid. Oncogene 2006;25(33):4620–7.

[68] Kroll TG, Sarraf P, Pecciarini L, et al. PAX8-PPARgamma1 fusion oncogene in human thyroid carcinoma [corrected]. Science 2000;289(5483):1357–60.

[69] Marques AR, Espadinha C, Catarino AL, et al. Expression of PAX8-PPAR gamma 1 rearrangements in both follicular thyroid carcinomas and adenomas. J Clin Endocrinol Metab 2002;87(8):3947–52.

[70] Cheung L, Messina M, Gill A, et al. Detection of the PAX8-PPAR gamma fusion oncogene in both follicular thyroid carcinomas and adenomas. J Clin Endocrinol Metab 2003;88(1):354–7.

[71] Roque L, Castedo S, Clode A, et al. Deletion of 3p25–>pter in a primary follicular thyroid carcinoma and its metastasis. Genes Chromosomes Cancer 1993;8(3):199–203.

[72] Sozzi G, Miozzo M, Cariani TC, et al. A t(2;3)(q12-13;p24-25) in follicular thyroid adenomas. Cancer Genet Cytogenet 1992;64(1):38–41.

[73] Jenkins RB, Hay ID, Herath JF, et al. Frequent occurrence of cytogenetic abnormalities in sporadic nonmedullary thyroid carcinoma. Cancer 1990;66(6):1213–20.

[74] Lui WO, Kytola S, Anfalk L, et al. Balanced translocation (3;7)(p25;q34): another mechanism of tumorigenesis in follicular thyroid carcinoma? Cancer Genet Cytogenet 2000; 119(2):109–12.

[75] Gregory Powell J, Wang X, Allard BL, et al. The PAX8/PPARgamma fusion oncoprotein transforms immortalized human thyrocytes through a mechanism probably involving wild-type PPARgamma inhibition. Oncogene 2004;23(20):3634–41.

[76] Park JW, Zarnegar R, Kanauchi H, et al. Troglitazone, the peroxisome proliferator-activated receptor-gamma agonist, induces antiproliferation and redifferentiation in human thyroid cancer cell lines. Thyroid 2005;15(3):222–31.

[77] Lacroix L, Lazar V, Michiels S, et al. Follicular thyroid tumors with the PAX8-PPAR-gamma1 rearrangement display characteristic genetic alterations. Am J Pathol 2005; 167(1):223–31.

[78] Marques AR, Espadinha C, Frias MJ, et al. Underexpression of peroxisome proliferator-activated receptor (PPAR)gamma in PAX8/PPARgamma-negative thyroid tumours. Br J Cancer 2004;91(4):732–8.

[79] Sahin M, Allard BL, Yates M, et al. PPARgamma staining as a surrogate for PAX8/PPAR-gamma fusion oncogene expression in follicular neoplasms: clinicopathological correlation and histopathological diagnostic value. J Clin Endocrinol Metab 2005;90(1):463–8.

[80] Kimura ET, Nikiforova MN, Zhu Z, et al. High Prevalence of BRAF Mutations in Thyroid Cancer: Genetic Evidence for Constitutive Activation of the RET/PTC-RAS-BRAF Signaling Pathway in Papillary Thyroid Carcinoma. Cancer Res 2003;63(7):1454–7.

[81] Soares P, Trovisco V, Rocha AS, et al. BRAF mutations and RET/PTC rearrangements are alternative events in the etiopathogenesis of PTC. Oncogene 2003;22(29):4578–80.

[82] Kim KH, Kang DW, Kim SH, et al. Mutations of the BRAF gene in papillary thyroid carcinoma in a Korean population. Yonsei Med J 2004;45(5):818–21.

[83] Frattini M, Ferrario C, Bressan P, et al. Alternative mutations of BRAF, RET and NTRK1 are associated with similar but distinct gene expression patterns in papillary thyroid cancer. Oncogene 2004;23(44):7436–40.

[84] Puxeddu E, Moretti S, Elisei R, et al. BRAF^{V599E} Mutation Is the Leading Genetic Event in Adult Sporadic Papillary Thyroid Carcinomas. J Clin Endocrinol Metab 2004;89(5): 2414–20.

[85] Mitsutake N, Miyagishi M, Mitsutake S, et al. BRAF mediates RET/PTC-induced MAPK activation in thyroid cells: functional support for requirement of the RET/PTC-RAS-BRAF pathway in papillary thyroid carcinogenesis. Endocrinology 2006;147(2):1014–9.

[86] Melillo RM, Castellone MD, Guarino V, et al. The RET/PTC-RAS-BRAF linear signaling cascade mediates the motile and mitogenic phenotype of thyroid cancer cells. J Clin Invest 2005;115(4):1068–81.

[87] Nikiforova MN, Kimura ET, Gandhi M, et al. BRAF Mutations in thyroid tumors are restricted to papillary carcinomas and anaplastic or poorly differentiated carcinomas arising from papillary carcinomas. J Clin Endocrinol Metab 2003;88(11):5399–404.

[88] Trovisco V, Soares P, Preto A, et al. Type and prevalence of BRAF mutations are closely associated with papillary thyroid carcinoma histotype and patients' age but not with tumour aggressiveness. Virchows Arch 2005;446(6):589–95.

[89] Trovisco V, Vieira DCI, Soares P, et al. BRAF mutations are associated with some histological types of papillary thyroid carcinoma. J Pathol 2004;202(2):247–51.

[90] Fugazzola L, Mannavola D, Cirello V, et al. BRAF mutations in an Italian cohort of thyroid cancers. Clin Endocrinol (Oxf) 2004;61(2):239–43.

[91] Trovisco V, Soares P, Soares R, et al. A new BRAF gene mutation detected in a case of a solid variant of papillary thyroid carcinoma. Hum Pathol 2005;36(6):694–7.

[92] Oler G, Ebina KN, Michaluart P Jr, et al. Investigation of BRAF mutation in a series of papillary thyroid carcinoma and matched-lymph node metastasis reveals a new mutation in metastasis. Clin Endocrinol (Oxf) 2005;62(4):509–11.

[93] Carta C, Moretti S, Passeri L, et al. Genotyping of an Italian papillary thyroid carcinoma cohort revealed high prevalence of BRAF mutations, absence of RAS mutations and allowed the detection of a new mutation of BRAF oncoprotein (BRAF(V599lns). Clin Endocrinol (Oxf) 2006;64(1):105–9.

[94] Hou P, Liu D, Xing M. Functional characterization of the T1799-1801del and A1799-1816ins BRAF mutations in papillary thyroid cancer. Cell Cycle 2007;6(3):377–9.

[95] Flavin R, Smyth P, Crotty P, et al. BRAF T1799A mutation occurring in a case of malignant struma ovarii. Int J Surg Pathol 2007;15(2):116–20.

[96] Schmidt J, Derr V, Heinrich MC, et al. BRAF in papillary thyroid carcinoma of ovary (Struma Ovarii). Am J Surg Pathol 2007;31(9):1337–43.

[97] Wan PT, Garnett MJ, Roe SM, et al. Mechanism of activation of the RAF-ERK signaling pathway by oncogenic mutations of B-RAF. Cell 2004;116(6):855–67.

[98] Basolo F, Giannini R, Monaco C, et al. Potent mitogenicity of the RET/PTC3 oncogene correlates with its prevalence in tall-cell variant of papillary thyroid carcinoma. Am J Pathol 2002;160(1):247–54.

[99] Sedliarou I, Saenko V, Lantsov D, et al. The BRAFT1796A transversion is a prevalent mutational event in human thyroid microcarcinoma. Int J Oncol 2004;25(6):1729–35.

[100] Kim TY, Kim WB, Song JY, et al. The BRAF mutation is not associated with poor prognostic factors in Korean patients with conventional papillary thyroid microcarcinoma. Clin Endocrinol (Oxf) 2005;63(5):588–93.

[101] Ugolini C, Giannini R, Lupi C, et al. Presence of BRAF V600E in Very Early Stages of Papillary Thyroid Carcinoma. Thyroid 2007;17(5):381–8.

[102] Knauf JA, Ma X, Smith EP, et al. Targeted expression of BRAFV600E in thyroid cells of transgenic mice results in papillary thyroid cancers that undergo dedifferentiation. Cancer Res 2005;65(10):4238–45.

[103] Liu D, Liu Z, Condouris S, et al. BRAF V600E maintains proliferation, transformation, and tumorigenicity of BRAF-mutant papillary thyroid cancer cells. J Clin Endocrinol Metab 2007;92(6):2264–71.

[104] Fugazzola L, Puxeddu E, Avenia N, et al. Correlation between B-RAFV600E mutation and clinico-pathologic parameters in papillary thyroid carcinoma: data from a multicentric Italian study and review of the literature. Endocr Relat Cancer 2006;13(2):455–64.

[105] Xu X, Quiros RM, Gattuso P, et al. High Prevalence of BRAF Gene Mutation in Papillary Thyroid Carcinomas and Thyroid Tumor Cell Lines. Cancer Res 2003;63(15):4561–7.

[106] Kim TY, Kim WB, Rhee YS, et al. The BRAF mutation is useful for prediction of clinical recurrence in low-risk patients with conventional papillary thyroid carcinoma. Clin Endocrinol (Oxf) 2006;65(3):364–8.

[107] Jin L, Sebo TJ, Nakamura N, et al. BRAF mutation analysis in fine needle aspiration (FNA) cytology of the thyroid. Diagn Mol Pathol 2006;15(3):136–43.

[108] Xing M, Westra WH, Tufano RP, et al. BRAF mutation predicts a poorer clinical prognosis for papillary thyroid cancer. J Clin Endocrinol Metab 2005;90(12):6373–9.

[109] Namba H, Nakashima M, Hayashi T, et al. Clinical Implication of Hot Spot BRAF Mutation, V599E, in Papillary Thyroid Cancers. J Clin Endocrinol Metab 2003;88(9):4393–7.

[110] Liu RT, Chen YJ, Chou FF, et al. No correlation between BRAFV600E mutation and clinicopathological features of papillary thyroid carcinomas in Taiwan. Clin Endocrinol (Oxf) 2005;63(4):461–6.

[111] Chung KW, Yang SK, Lee GK, et al. Detection of BRAFV600E mutation on fine needle aspiration specimens of thyroid nodule refines cyto-pathology diagnosis, especially in BRAF600E mutation-prevalent area. Clin Endocrinol (Oxf) 2006;65(5):660–6.

[112] Sapio MR, Posca D, Troncone G, et al. Detection of BRAF mutation in thyroid papillary carcinomas by mutant allele-specific PCR amplification (MASA). Eur J Endocrinol 2006; 154(2):341–8.

[113] Trovisco V, Soares P, Sobrinho-Simões M. B-RAF mutations in the etiopathogenesis, diagnosis, and prognosis of thyroid carcinomas. Hum Pathol 2006;37(7):781–6.

[114] Vasko V, Hu S, Wu G, et al. High prevalence and possible de novo formation of BRAF mutation in metastasized papillary thyroid cancer in lymph nodes. J Clin Endocrinol Metab 2005;90(9):5265–9.

[115] Kim J, Giuliano AE, Turner RR, et al. Lymphatic mapping establishes the role of BRAF gene mutation in papillary thyroid carcinoma. Ann Surg 2006;244(5):799–804.

[116] Trovisco V, Couto JP, Cameselle-Teijeiro J, et al. Aquisition of BRAF gene mutations is not a requirement for nodal metastization of PTC. Clin Endocrinology, in press.

[117] Cohen Y, Rosenbaum E, Clark DP, et al. Mutational analysis of BRAF in fine needle aspiration biopsies of the thyroid: a potential application for the preoperative assessment of thyroid nodules. Clin Cancer Res 2004;10(8):2761–5.

[118] Xing M, Tufano RP, Tufaro AP, et al. Detection of BRAF mutation on fine needle aspiration biopsy specimens: a new diagnostic tool for papillary thyroid cancer. J Clin Endocrinol Metab 2004;89(6):2867–72.

[119] Hayashida N, Namba H, Kumagai A, et al. A rapid and simple detection method for the BRAF(T1796A) mutation in fine-needle aspirated thyroid carcinoma cells. Thyroid 2004; 14(11):910–5.

[120] Salvatore G, Giannini R, Faviana P, et al. Analysis of BRAF point mutation and RET/ PTC rearrangement refines the fine-needle aspiration diagnosis of papillary thyroid carcinoma. J Clin Endocrinol Metab 2004;89(10):5175–80.

[121] Domingues R, Mendonca E, Sobrinho L, et al. Searching for RET/PTC rearrangements and BRAF V599E mutation in thyroid aspirates might contribute to establish a preoperative diagnosis of papillary thyroid carcinoma. Cytopathology 2005;16(1):27–31.

[122] Baloch ZW, Gupta PK, Yu GH, et al. Follicular variant of papillary carcinoma. Cytologic and histologic correlation. Am J Clin Pathol 1999;111(2):216–22.

[123] Williams D. Cancer after nuclear fallout: lessons from the Chernobyl accident. Nat Rev Cancer 2002;2(7):543–9.

[124] Nikiforov YE, Rowland JM, Bove KE, et al. Distinct pattern of ret oncogene rearrangements in morphological variants of radiation-induced and sporadic thyroid papillary carcinomas in children. Cancer Res 1997;57(9):1690–4.

[125] Nikiforova MN, Ciampi R, Salvatore G, et al. Low prevalence of BRAF mutations in radiation-induced thyroid tumors in contrast to sporadic papillary carcinomas. Cancer Lett 2004;209(1):1–6.

[126] Lima J, Trovisco V, Soares P, et al. BRAF Mutations Are Not a Major Event in Post-Chernobyl Childhood Thyroid Carcinomas. J Clin Endocrinol Metab 2004;89(9): 4267–71.

[127] Kumagai A, Namba H, Saenko VA, et al. Low Frequency of BRAFT1796A Mutations in Childhood Thyroid Carcinomas. J Clin Endocrinol Metab 2004;89(9):4280–4.

[128] Caudill CM, Zhu Z, Ciampi R, et al. Dose-dependent generation of RET/PTC in human thyroid cells after in vitro exposure to gamma-radiation: a model of carcinogenic chromosomal rearrangement induced by ionizing radiation. J Clin Endocrinol Metab 2005;90(4): 2364–9.

[129] Ciampi R, Knauf JA, Kerler R, et al. Oncogenic AKAP9-BRAF fusion is a novel mechanism of MAPK pathway activation in thyroid cancer. J Clin Invest 2005;115(1):94–101.

[130] Chong H, Guan KL. Regulation of Raf through phosphorylation and N terminus-C terminus interaction. J Biol Chem 2003;278(38):36269–76.

[131] Tran NH, Frost JA. Phosphorylation of Raf-1 by p21-activated kinase 1 and Src regulates Raf-1 autoinhibition. J Biol Chem 2003;278(13):11221–6.

[132] Tran NH, Wu X, Frost JA. B-Raf and Raf-1 are regulated by distinct autoregulatory mechanisms. J Biol Chem 2005;280(16):16244–53.

[133] Penko K, Livezey J, Fenton C, et al. BRAF mutations are uncommon in papillary thyroid cancer of young patients. Thyroid 2005;15(4):320–5.

[134] Powell N, Jeremiah S, Morishita M, et al. Frequency of BRAF T1796A mutation in papillary thyroid carcinoma relates to age of patient at diagnosis and not to radiation exposure. J Pathol 2005;205(5):558–64.

[135] Takahashi K, Eguchi H, Arihiro K, et al. The presence of BRAF point mutation in adult papillary thyroid carcinomas from atomic bomb survivors correlates with radiation dose. Mol Carcinog 2007;46(3):242–8.

[136] Thompson N, Lyons J. Recent progress in targeting the Raf/MEK/ERK pathway with inhibitors in cancer drug discovery. Curr Opin Pharmacol 2005;5(4):350–6.

[137] Salvatore G, De Falco V, Salerno P, et al. BRAF is a therapeutic target in aggressive thyroid carcinoma. Clin Cancer Res 2006;12(5):1623–9.

[138] Preto and colleagues, submitted.

[139] Ouyang B, Knauf JA, Smith EP, et al. Inhibitors of Raf kinase activity block growth of thyroid cancer cells with RET/PTC or BRAF mutations in vitro and in vivo. Clin Cancer Res 2006;12(6):1785–93.

[140] da Rocha Dias S, Friedlos F, Light Y, et al. Activated B-RAF is an Hsp90 client protein that is targeted by the anticancer drug 17-allylamino-17-demethoxygeldanamycin. Cancer Res 2005;65(23):10686–91.

[141] Grbovic OM, Basso AD, Sawai A, et al. V600E B-Raf requires the Hsp90 chaperone for stability and is degraded in response to Hsp90 inhibitors. Proc Natl Acad Sci USA 2006; 103(1):57–62.

[142] Máximo V, Sobrinho-Simões M. Hurthle cell tumours of the thyroid. A review with emphasis on mitochondrial abnormalities with clinical relevance. Virchows Arch 2000;437(2): 107–15.

[143] Cheung CC, Ezzat S, Ramyar L, et al. Molecular basis off Hürthle cell papillary thyroid carcinoma. J Clin Endocrinol Metab 2000;85(2):878–82.

[144] Máximo V, Soares P, Lima J, et al. Mitochondrial DNA somatic mutations (point mutations and large deletions) and mitochondrial DNA variants in human thyroid pathology: a study with emphasis on Hürthle cell tumors. Am J Pathol 2002;160(5):1857–65.

[145] Gasparre G, Porcelli AM, Bonora E, et al. Disruptive mitochondrial DNA mutations in complex I subunits are markers of oncocytic phenotype in thyroid tumors. Proc Natl Acad Sci USA 2007;104(21):9001–6.

[146] Máximo V, Soares P, Rocha AS, et al. The common deletion of mitochondrial DNA is found in goiters and thyroid tumors with and without oxyphil cell change. Ultrastruct Pathol 1998;22(3):271–3.

[147] Máximo V, Sobrinho-Simões M. Mitochondrial DNA 'common' deletion in Hürthle cell lesions of the thyroid. J Pathol 2000;192(4):561–2.

[148] Attardi G, Yoneda M, Chomyn A. Complementation and segregation behavior of disease-causing mitochondrial DNA mutations in cellular model systems. Biochim Biophys Acta 1995;1271(1):241–8.

[149] Heddi A, Faure-Vigny H, Wallace DC, et al. Coordinate expression of nuclear and mitochondrial genes involved in energy production in carcinoma and oncocytoma. Biochim Biophys Acta 1996;1316(3):203–9.

[150] Sobrinho-Simões M, Máximo V, Castro IV, et al. Hürthle (oncocytic) cell tumors of thyroid: etiopathogenesis, diagnosis and clinical significance. Int J Surg Pathol 2005;13(1):29–35.

[151] Yeh JJ, Lunetta KL, Van Orsouw NJ, et al. Somatic mitochondrial DNA (mtDNA) mutations in papillary thyroid carcinomas and differential mtDNA sequence variants in cases with thyroid tumours. Oncogene 2000;19(16):2060–6.

[152] Angell JE, Lindner DJ, Shapiro PS, et al. Identification of GRIM-19, a novel cell death-regulatory gene induced by the interferon-beta and retinoic acid combination, using a genetic approach. J Biol Chem 2000;275(43):33416–26.

[153] Chidambaram NV, Angell JE, Ling W, et al. Chromosomal localization of human GRIM-19, a novel IFN-beta and retinoic acid-activated regulator of cell death. J Interferon Cytokine Res 2000;20(7):661–5.

[154] Lufei C, Ma J, Huang G, et al. GRIM-19, a death-regulatory gene product, suppresses Stat3 activity via functional interaction. EMBO J 2003;22(6):1325–35.

[155] Fearnley IM, Carroll J, Shannon RJ, et al. GRIM-19, a cell death regulatory gene product, is a subunit of bovine mitochondrial NADH:ubiquinone oxidoreductase (complex I). J Biol Chem 2001;276(42):38345–8.

[156] Máximo V, Botelho T, Capela J, et al. Somatic and germline mutation in GRIM-19, a dual function gene involved in mitochondrial metabolism and cell death, is linked to mitochondrion-rich (Hürthle cell) tumours of the thyroid. Br J Cancer 2005;92(10):1982–9.

[157] Lima J, Máximo V, Soares P, et al. Mitochondria and oncocytomas. In: Singh KK, editor. Mitochondria and Cancer. New York: Springer, in press.

[158] Eng C, Kiuru M, Fernandez MJ, et al. A role for mitochondrial enzymes in inherited neoplasia and beyond. Nat Rev Cancer 2003;3(3):193–202.

[159] Gottlieb E, Tomlinson IP. Mitochondrial tumour suppressors: a genetic and biochemical update. Nat Rev Cancer 2005;5(11):857–66.

[160] Lima J, Teixeira-Gomes J, Soares P, et al. Germline succinate dehydrogenase subunit D mutation segregating with familial non-RET C cell hyperplasia. J Clin Endocrinol Metab 2003;88(10):4932–7.

[161] Montani M, Schmitt AM, Schmid S, et al. No mutations but an increased frequency of SDHx polymorphisms in patients with sporadic and familial medullary thyroid carcinoma. Endocr Relat Cancer 2005;12(4):1011–6.

[162] Cascon A, Cebrian A, Pollan M, et al. Succinate dehydrogenase D variants do not constitute a risk factor for developing C cell hyperplasia or sporadic medullary thyroid carcinoma. J Clin Endocrinol Metab 2005;90(4):2127–30.

[163] Abu-Amero KK, Alzahrani AS, Zou M, et al. Association of mitochondrial DNA transversion mutations with familial medullary thyroid carcinoma/multiple endocrine neoplasia type 2 syndrome. Oncogene 2006;25(5):677–84.

[164] Donghi R, Longoni A, Pilotti S, et al. Gene p53 mutations are restricted to poorly differentiated and undifferentiated carcinomas of the thyroid gland. J Clin Invest 1993;91(4):1753–60.

[165] Fagin JA, Matsuo K, Karmakar A, et al. High prevalence of mutations of the p53 gene in poorly differentiated human thyroid carcinomas. J Clin Invest 1993;91(1):179–84.

[166] Wright PA, Lemoine NR, Goretzki PE, et al. Mutation of the p53 gene in a differentiated human thyroid carcinoma cell line, but not in primary thyroid tumours. Oncogene 1991; 6(9):1693–7.

[167] Ito T, Seyama T, Mizuno T, et al. Unique association of p53 mutations with undifferentiated but not with differentiated carcinomas of the thyroid gland. Cancer Res 1992;52(5): 1369–71.

[168] Park KY, Koh JM, Kim YI, et al. Prevalences of Gs alpha, ras, p53 mutations and ret/PTC rearrangement in differentiated thyroid tumours in a Korean population. Clin Endocrinol (Oxf) 1998;49(3):317–23.

[169] Zou M, Shi Y, Farid NR. p53 mutations in all stages of thyroid carcinomas. J Clin Endocrinol Metab 1993;77(4):1054–8.

[170] Soares P, Cameselle-Teijeiro J, Sobrinho-Simões M. Immunohistochemical detection of p53 in differentiated, poorly differentiated and undifferentiated carcinomas of the thyroid. Histopathology 1994;24(3):205–10.

[171] Saltman B, Singh B, Hedvat CV, et al. Patterns of expression of cell cycle/apoptosis genes along the spectrum of thyroid carcinoma progression. Surgery 2006;140(6):899–905 [discussion: 905–6].

[172] Arends JW. Molecular interactions in the Vogelstein model of colorectal carcinoma. J Pathol 2000;190(4):412–6.

[173] Ito T, Seyama T, Mizuno T, et al. Genetic alterations in thyroid tumor progression: association with p53 gene mutations. Jpn J Cancer Res 1993;84(5):526–31.

[174] Quiros RM, Ding HG, Gattuso P, et al. Evidence that one subset of anaplastic thyroid carcinomas are derived from papillary carcinomas due to BRAF and p53 mutations. Cancer 2005;103(11):2261–8.

[175] Wynford-Thomas D. Origin and progression of thyroid epithelial tumours: cellular and molecular mechanisms. Horm Res 1997;47(4–6):145–57.

[176] Wynford-Thomas D, Blaydes J. The influence of cell context on the selection pressure for p53 mutation in human cancer. Carcinogenesis 1998;19(1):29–36.

[177] Miura D, Wada N, Chin K, et al. Anaplastic thyroid cancer: cytogenetic patterns by comparative genomic hybridization. Thyroid 2003;13(3):283–90.

[178] Rodrigues RF, Roque L, Krug T, et al. Poorly differentiated and anaplastic thyroid carcinomas: chromosomal and oligo-array profile of five new cell lines. Br J Cancer 2007;96(8):1237–45.

[179] Wreesmann VB, Ghossein RA, Patel SG, et al. Genome-wide appraisal of thyroid cancer progression. Am J Pathol 2002;161(5):1549–56.

[180] Farid P, Gomb SZ, Peter I, et al. Bcl2, p53 and bax in thyroid tumors and their relation to apoptosis. Neoplasma 2001;48(4):299–301.

[181] Hermann S, Sturm I, Mrozek A, et al. Bax expression in benign and malignant thyroid tumours: dysregulation of wild-type P53 is associated with a high Bax and P21 expression in thyroid carcinoma. Int J Cancer 2001;92(6):805–11.

[182] Moore D, Ohene-Fianko D, Garcia B, et al. Apoptosis in thyroid neoplasms: relationship with p53 and bcl-2 expression. Histopathology 1998;32(1):35–42.

[183] Garcia-Rostan G, Tallini G, Herrero A, et al. Frequent mutation and nuclear localization of beta-catenin in anaplastic thyroid carcinoma. Cancer Res 1999;59(8):1811–5.

[184] Tung WS, Shevlin DW, Bartsch D, et al. Infrequent CDKN2 mutation in human differentiated thyroid cancers. Mol Carcinog 1996;15(1):5–10.

[185] Basolo F, Pisaturo F, Pollina LE, et al. N-ras mutation in poorly differentiated thyroid carcinomas: correlation with bone metastases and inverse correlation to thyroglobulin expression. Thyroid 2000;10(1):19–23.

[186] Manenti G, Pilotti S, Re FC, et al. Selective activation of ras oncogenes in follicular and undifferentiated thyroid carcinomas. Eur J Cancer 1994;30A(7):987–93.

[187] Fukushima T, Suzuki S, Mashiko M, et al. BRAF mutations in papillary carcinomas of the thyroid. Oncogene 2003;22(41):6455–7.

[188] Garcia-Rostan G, Zhao H, Camp RL, et al. Ras mutations are associated with aggressive tumor phenotypes and poor prognosis in thyroid cancer. J Clin Oncol 2003;21(17):3226–35.

[189] Wang Y, Hou P, Yu H, et al. High prevalence and mutual exclusivity of genetic alterations in the phosphatidylinositol-3-kinase/akt pathway in thyroid tumors. J Clin Endocrinol Metab 2007;92(6):2387–90.

[190] Hou P, Liu D, Shan Y, et al. Genetic alterations and their relationship in the phosphatidylinositol 3-kinase/Akt pathway in thyroid cancer. Clin Cancer Res 2007;13(4):1161–70.

[191] Garcia-Rostan G, Camp RL, Herrero A, et al. Beta-catenin dysregulation in thyroid neoplasms: down-regulation, aberrant nuclear expression, and CTNNB1 exon 3 mutations are markers for aggressive tumor phenotypes and poor prognosis. Am J Pathol 2001;158(3):987–96.

[192] Kim WB, Lewis CJ, McCall KD, et al. Overexpression of Wnt-1 in thyrocytes enhances cellular growth but suppresses transcription of the thyroperoxidase gene via different signaling mechanisms. J Endocrinol 2007;193(1):93–106.

[193] Rocha AS, Soares P, Fonseca E, et al. E-cadherin loss rather than beta-catenin alterations is a common feature of poorly differentiated thyroid carcinomas. Histopathology 2003;42(6):580–7.

[194] Kurihara T, Ikeda S, Ishizaki Y, et al. Immunohistochemical and sequencing analyses of the Wnt signaling components in Japanese anaplastic thyroid cancers. Thyroid 2004; 14(12):1020–9.

[195] Sobrinho-Simões M, Sambade C, Fonseca E, et al. Poorly differentiated carcinomas of the thyroid gland: a review of the clinicopathologic features of a series of 28 cases of a heterogeneous, clinically aggressive group of thyroid tumors. Int J Surg Pathol 2002;10(2): 123–31.

[196] Cameselle-Teijeiro J, Ruiz-Ponte C, Loidi L, et al. Somatic but not germline mutation of the APC gene in a case of cribriform-morular variant of papillary thyroid carcinoma. Am J Clin Pathol 2001;115(4):486–93.

[197] Cameselle-Teijeiro J, Chan JK. Cribriform-morular variant of papillary carcinoma: a distinctive variant representing the sporadic counterpart of familial adenomatous polyposis-associated thyroid carcinoma? Mod Pathol 1999;12(4):400–11.

[198] Soares P, Trovisco V, Rocha AS, et al. BRAF mutations typical of papillary thyroid carcinoma are more frequently detected in undifferentiated than in insular and insular-like poorly differentiated carcinomas. Virchows Arch 2004;444(6):572–6.

[199] DeLellis RA, Heitz PU, Eng C, editors. World Health Organization classification of tumours. Pathology and genetics of tumours of endocrine glands. Lyon: IARC Press; 2004.

[200] Ashfaq R, Vuitch F, Delgado R, et al. Papillary and follicular thyroid carcinomas with an insular component. Cancer 1994;73(2):416–23.

[201] Carcangiu ML, Zampi G, Rosai J. Poorly differentiated ("insular") thyroid carcinoma. A reinterpretation of Langhans' "wuchernde Struma". Am J Surg Pathol 1984;8(9):655–68.

[202] Papotti M, Botto Micca F, Favero A, et al. Poorly differentiated thyroid carcinomas with primordial cell component. A group of aggressive lesions sharing insular, trabecular, and solid patterns. Am J Surg Pathol 1993;17(3):291–301.

[203] Takano T, Ito Y, Hirokawa M, et al. BRAF V600E mutation in anaplastic thyroid carcinomas and their accompanying differentiated carcinomas. Br J Cancer 2007;96(10): 1549–53.

[204] Tallini G, Santoro M, Helie M, et al. RET/PTC oncogene activation defines a subset of papillary thyroid carcinomas lacking evidence of progression to poorly differentiated or undifferentiated tumor phenotypes. Clin Cancer Res 1998;4(2):287–94.

[205] Wu G, Mambo E, Guo Z, et al. Uncommon mutation, but common amplifications, of the PIK3CA gene in thyroid tumors. J Clin Endocrinol Metab 2005;90(8):4688–93.

[206] Garcia-Rostan G, Costa AM, Pereira-Castro I, et al. Mutation of the PIK3CA gene in anaplastic thyroid cancer. Cancer Res 2005;65(22):10199–207.

[207] Liu D, Mambo E, Ladenson PW, et al. Letter re: uncommon mutation but common amplifications of the PIK3CA gene in thyroid tumors. J Clin Endocrinol Metab 2005;90(9):5509.

[208] Santoro M, Papotti M, Chiappetta G, et al. RET activation and clinicopathologic features in poorly differentiated thyroid tumors. J Clin Endocrinol Metab 2002;87(1):370–9.

[209] Dwight T, Thoppe SR, Foukakis T, et al. Involvement of the PAX8/peroxisome proliferator-activated receptor gamma rearrangement in follicular thyroid tumors. J Clin Endocrinol Metab 2003;88(9):4440–5.

[210] Nakashima M, Takamura N, Namba H, et al. RET oncogene amplification in thyroid cancer: correlations with radiation-associated and high-grade malignancy. Hum Pathol 2007; 38(4):621–8.

[211] Takeshita A, Nagayama Y, Yokoyama N, et al. Rarity of oncogenic mutations in the thyrotropin receptor of autonomously functioning thyroid nodules in Japan. J Clin Endocrinol Metab 1995;80(9):2607–11.

[212] Tanaka K, Nagayama Y, Takeshita A, et al. Low incidence of the stimulatory G protein alpha-subunit mutations in autonomously functioning thyroid adenomas in Japan. Thyroid 1996;6(3):195–9.

[213] Derwahl M. TSH receptor and Gs-alpha gene mutations in the pathogenesis of toxic thyroid adenomas—a note of caution. J Clin Endocrinol Metab 1996;81(8):2783–5.

[214] Parma J, Duprez L, Van Sande J, et al. Diversity and prevalence of somatic mutations in the thyrotropin receptor and Gs alpha genes as a cause of toxic thyroid adenomas. J Clin Endocrinol Metab 1997;82(8):2695–701.

[215] Vassart G. New pathophysiological mechanisms for hyperthyroidism. Horm Res 1997; 48(Suppl 4):47–50.

[216] Führer D, Holzapfel HP, Wonerow P, et al. Somatic mutations in the thyrotropin receptor gene and not in the Gs alpha protein gene in 31 toxic thyroid nodules. J Clin Endocrinol Metab 1997;82(11):3885–91.

[217] Führer D, Kubisch C, Scheibler U, et al. The extracellular thyrotropin receptor domain is not a major candidate for mutations in toxic thyroid nodules. Thyroid 1998;8(11): 997–1001.

[218] Tonacchera M, Agretti P, Chiovato L, et al. Activating thyrotropin receptor mutations are present in nonadenomatous hyperfunctioning nodules of toxic or autonomous multinodular goiter. J Clin Endocrinol Metab 2000;85(6):2270–4.

[219] Krohn K, Reske A, Ackermann F, et al. Ras mutations are rare in solitary cold and toxic thyroid nodules. Clin Endocrinol (Oxf) 2001;55(2):241–8.

[220] Russo D, Arturi F, Wicker R, et al. Genetic alterations in thyroid hyperfunctioning adenomas. J Clin Endocrinol Metab 1995;80(4):1347–51.

[221] Russo D, Tumino S, Arturi F, et al. Detection of an activating mutation of the thyrotropin receptor in a case of an autonomously hyperfunctioning thyroid insular carcinoma. J Clin Endocrinol Metab 1997;82(3):735–8.

[222] Bourasseau I, Savagner F, Rodien P, et al. No evidence of thyrotropin receptor and Gs(alpha) gene mutation in high iodine uptake thyroid carcinoma. Thyroid 2000;10(9): 761–5.

[223] Führer D, Tannapfel A, Sabri O, et al. Two somatic TSH receptor mutations in a patient with toxic metastasising follicular thyroid carcinoma and non-functional lung metastases. Endocr Relat Cancer 2003;10(4):591–600.

[224] Dobashi Y, Sakamoto A, Sugimura H, et al. Overexpression of p53 as a possible prognostic factor in human thyroid carcinoma. Am J Surg Pathol 1993;17(4):375–81.

[225] Ho YS, Tseng SC, Chin TY, et al. p53 gene mutation in thyroid carcinoma. Cancer Lett 1996;103(1):57–63.

[226] Takeuchi Y, Daa T, Kashima K, et al. Mutations of p53 in thyroid carcinoma with an insular component. Thyroid 1999;9(4):377–81.

[227] Capella G, Matias-Guiu X, Ampudia X, et al. Ras oncogene mutations in thyroid tumors: polymerase chain reaction-restriction-fragment-length polymorphism analysis from paraffin-embedded tissues. Diagn Mol Pathol 1996;5(1):45–52.

[228] Pilotti S, Collini P, Mariani L, et al. Insular carcinoma: a distinct de novo entity among follicular carcinomas of the thyroid gland. Am J Surg Pathol 1997;21(12):1466–73.

[229] Fukushima T, Takenoshita S. Roles of RAS and BRAF mutations in thyroid carcinogenesis. Fukushima J Med Sci 2005;51(2):67–75.

ELSEVIER
SAUNDERS

Endocrinol Metab Clin N Am
37 (2008) 363–374

ENDOCRINOLOGY
AND METABOLISM
CLINICS
OF NORTH AMERICA

Dysregulated RET Signaling in Thyroid Cancer

Maria Domenica Castellone, MD, PhD[a],
Massimo Santoro, MD, PhD[b],*

[a]*Istituto di Endocrinologia ed Oncologia Sperimentale del CNR "G.Salvatore",
Dipartimento di Biologia e Patologia Cellulare e Molecolare, Università di Napoli Federico II,
via S. Pansini 5, 80131 Naples, Italy*
[b]*Dipartimento di Biologia e Patologia Cellulare e Molecolare, Università di Napoli Federico
II, via S. Pansini 5, 80131 Naples, Italy*

The *RET* proto-oncogene, located on chromosome 10q11.2, codes for a transmembrane receptor (RET) that has tyrosine kinase activity. RET is a component of a cell-surface complex that binds glial-derived neurotrophic factor family ligands (GDNF, neurturin, artemin and persephin) in conjunction with a group of coreceptors designated "GDNF-family receptor-α" (GFRα1–4) [1].

As illustrated in Fig. 1, RET features (1) an extracellular portion that includes the cleavable signal peptide, four cadherin-like repeats, and a cysteine-rich domain [2]; (2) a transmembrane portion; and (3) an intracellular portion with the juxtamembrane domain, the tyrosine kinase (RET-TKD) domain split in two subdomains by an insert of 14 amino acids, and a C-terminal tail [3].

Structurally, RET-TKD adopts the typical protein kinase fold consisting of a small N-lobe and a large C-lobe connected by a short linker (see Fig. 1) [3]. In unstimulated conditions, the catalytic domains of most kinases are monomeric and auto-inhibited *in cis* by the C-lobe activation loop (A-loop) that maintains the kinase pocket closed. Ligand binding causes dimerization, rearrangement of the A-loop, and kinase activation [4]. Differently, the RET-TKD is already a dimer in unstimulated conditions. It adopts a *trans*-inhibited head-to-tail inactive dimer conformation in which the substrate-binding site of each monomer is occluded by the contralateral one.

The authors apologize to the many colleagues whose work could not be cited because of space limitations. This study was supported by the Italian Association for Cancer Research.

* Corresponding author.

E-mail address: masantor@unina.it (M. Santoro).

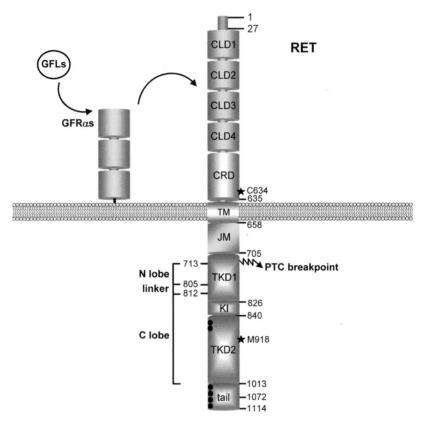

Fig. 1. Schematic drawing of the RET protein. RET is stimulated by complexes of GDNF-family ligands (GFLs) with GPI-anchored GFRα coreceptors. The extracellular RET domain, containing the signal peptide, the four cadherin-like repeats (CLD1-4) and the cysteine-rich domain (CRD), the transmembrane domain (TM), and the intracellular domain with the juxta-membrane region (JM), the core tyrosine kinase domain (TKD), and the C-terminal tail, are shown. The RET TKD is split into two subdomains (TKD1 and 2) by an insert region (KI). As indicated, RET TKD folds in an N-terminal lobe and a C-terminal lobe divided by a short linker. RET is subjected to alternative splicing, which results in two major protein isoforms of 1072 and 1114 amino acids (RET9 and RET51, respectively). RET51 is shown. The position of cysteine 634 (typically mutated in MEN2A) and methionine 918 (mutated in MEN2B) are indicated by stars. The position of the breakpoint occurring in PTC and causing the fusion of the RET TKD (starting at exon 12, residue E713) with heterologous genes (RET/PTC chimeric proteins) is also shown. Black dots mark the position of some critical RET tyrosine phosphorylated sites: Y900 and Y905 in the activation loop and Y1015, Y1062, Y1090, and Y1096 in the carboxyl-terminal tail.

Interaction with GDNF/GFRα probably causes a conformational change that favors the formation of active dimers, thereby relieving the *trans*-inhibition [3].

RET is subjected to alternative splicing, which results in two major protein isoforms of 1072 and 1114 amino acids (RET9 and RET51). RET9 and

RET51 differ in the amino acid region immediately downstream from tyrosine 1062 (Y1062): starting from glycine 1063, RET9 has nine extra residues, whereas RET51 has 51 amino acids including two extraphosphorylation sites, Y1090 and Y1096 [1].

RET function

RET is essential for the development of the sympathetic, parasympathetic, and enteric neurons; male germ cells; and kidney. Knock-out of RET caused renal defects and intestinal agangliosis in genetically modified mice [1]. In humans, germline loss-of-function mutations in RET cause impaired formation of the enteric nervous system and congenital agangliosis of the colon (Hirschsprung's disease; OMIM #142623) [5]. RET also regulates the development of the lymphoid system in the gut, as witnessed by impaired formation of Peyer's patches in case of deficiency of GFRα3 (the receptor for artemin) [6]. Tissue-specific ablation of RET caused adult-onset loss of dopaminergic neurons in the substantia nigra thereby demonstrating that RET exerts essential functions also in the adult [7].

Regarding the thyroid gland, RET is not detectable in normal endoderm-derived thyroid follicular cells. Instead, it is expressed in neural-crest–derived calcitonin-secreting thyroid C cells and is necessary for their development. RET-deficient mice have less calcitonin-immunoreactive cells than do wild-type littermates at birth [8]. GFRα4 (the persephin receptor) is expressed in developing C cells, and newborn GFRα4-deficient mice had reduced thyroid calcitonin levels compared with wild-type littermates [8]. Accordingly, RET signaling up-regulated calcitonin expression in C cell–derived medullary thyroid carcinoma (MTC) cells [9].

RET as an oncogene

RET was isolated in 1985 by Takahashi and coworkers [10] and shown to be activated as a dominant oncogene by a DNA rearrangement (REarranged during Transfection) that probably occurred during the DNA transfection procedure. The first evidence of its involvement in human cancer was obtained in thyroid gland papillary carcinomas [11,12].

Very recently, large-scale genome sequencing revealed a few RET somatic mutations in colon cancer samples [13]. Altered RET expression, rather than structural alterations, has been described in other tumor types, such as neuroblastomas, seminomas, pancreatic and breast carcinomas, myeloid leukemia, and pituitary adenomas. In neuroblastomas, RET is involved in the regulation of the differentiated phenotype [14]. RET is expressed in seminomas, and GDNF-overexpressing mice developed testicular tumors [15]. Pancreatic tumors express RET, and a RET polymorphism (G691S) amplified the proinvasive and proliferative properties of GDNF in pancreatic cancer cells [16]. In breast cancer, *RET* expression coclustered with estrogen receptor and *RET* was induced in E2-treated breast MCF7 cells [17]. *RET* expression in acute myeloid leukemia was typical of samples featuring the t(8;16) (MYST3-CREBBP) rearrangement [18]. Finally, *RET* was expressed in somatotroph-derived pituitary adenomas where it acted as a two-sided tumor regulator: a tumor suppressor (because in the absence of GDNF it functioned as a dependence receptor, was cleaved by caspase-3, and induced cell death) and as an oncogene (because when stimulated, it activated intracellular signaling and promoted cell survival) [19,20].

RET point mutations in medullary thyroid carcinoma

MTC (about 5% of thyroid cancers) is a malignant tumor arising from thyroid C cells. It is inherited in about 25% of cases as a component of the autosomal-dominant multiple endocrine neoplasia type–2 (MEN 2A, MEN 2B, FMTC) syndromes (OMIM #171400) [21]. Point mutations in *RET* are identified in about 98% of familial MTC cases (at the germline level) and in 30% to 50% of the sporadic cases (at the somatic level). These mutations are reviewed elsewhere [22] (see also the COSMIC catalog at www.sanger.ac.uk). Briefly, most MEN 2B patients (95% of cases) carry the M918T mutation in the RET kinase domain (see Fig. 1); in 98% of MEN 2A and 90% of FMTC cases, mutations affect one of few cysteines in the extracellular cysteine-rich domain of RET (see Fig. 1). In sporadic MTC, mutations mainly target M918, V804, and E768 in *RET*. Mutations in other codons or small insertions or deletions are rare. MTC-associated *RET* mutations promote activation of the kinase and oncogenic conversion.

Extracellular cysteine mutants display constitutive kinase activity consequent to the formation of disulfide-bonds [23]; this probably mimics conformational changes induced by ligand binding [24]. Close proximity to the RET transmembrane domain and the correct relative orientation of the cysteines are required for the disulfide-bond to form [23]. Signaling of RET–MEN 2A mutant is not identical to ligand-mediated RET signaling, however, and qualitative differences were identified in the activation of the PI3K/AKT pathway [25].

Instead, mutations targeting the intracellular domain probably modify the structure of the RET-TKD by switching the equilibrium toward the active conformation. Accordingly, the M918T mutation was found to cause a great increase in ATP binding affinity and the formation of a more stable RET-ATP complex [26]. Structurally, some of the intracellular mutations (M918T, P766S, and E768/A919) target positions close to the *trans*-inhibited dimer contact points and may activate RET by destabilizing this inactive dimer conformation [3]. RET(M918T) has been also proposed to have an altered signaling specificity with respect to wild-type RET; recently, it was shown that this particular mutant is already active in the endoplasmic reticulum where it interacts with adapter proteins [27].

RET/PTC rearrangements in papillary thyroid carcinoma

Papillary thyroid carcinoma (PTC) arises from follicular thyroid cells and is the most prevalent thyroid cancer type [28]. In PTC, *RET* is targeted by chromosomal rearrangements that result in the in-frame fusion of part of its intracellular domain (the TKD and the tail, starting at residue E713 through the C-terminus) with the 5'-end of heterologous genes (see Fig. 1). The resulting chimeric sequences are called "RET/PTC." Table 1 lists the known RET/PTC variants, which differ in the RET fusion partner [12,29–40]. Surprisingly, two RET rearrangements, RFP-RET [10] and RET-II (RET/PTC5) [41], which were initially isolated as in vitro artifacts of the DNA transfection procedure, were subsequently found in vivo in PTC patients [33,39].

RET/PTC1 and 3 account for more than 90% of all rearrangements. They result from the fusion of RET to the coiled coil domain containing gene 6 (*CCDC6*, formerly called *H4/D10S170*) or to the nuclear receptor co-activator gene–4 (*NcoA4*, formerly called *RFG/ELE1/ARA70*). *CCDC6* and *NcoA4*, like *RET* itself, map on the long arm of chromosome 10, indicating that a paracentric inversion is the chromosomal aberration that forms RET/PTC1 and 3 (see Table 1). RET/PTC3 is particularly frequent in PTC consequent to the Chernobyl disaster and in PTC in young patients [28,42]. The

Table 1
RET/PTC rearrangements in papillary thyroid cancer

Rearrangement	Name[a]	Other aliases[a]	Chromosome location[a]
RET/PTC1 [12]	*CCDC6 (coiled-coil domain containing 6)*	H4, D10S170	10q21
RET/PTC2 [29]	*PRKAR1A (protein kinase, cAMP-dependent, regulatory, type I, alpha)*	—	17q23
RET/PTC3 [30,31]	*NcoA4 (Nuclear coactivator 4)*	RFG, ELE1, ARA70	10q11
RET/PTC4 [32]	*NcoA4 (Nuclear coactivator 4)*	RFG, ELE1, ARA70	10q11
RET/PTC5 [33]	*GOLGA5 (golgin subfamily a, 5)*	RFG5, RET-II	14q32
RET/PTC6 [34]	*TRIM24 (tripartite motif-containing 24)*	HTIF1, TIFα	7q32–34
RET/PTC7 [34]	*TRIM33 (tripartite motif-containing 33)*	Ectodermin, RFG7, HTIFγ	1p13
RET/PTC8 [35]	*KTN1*	Kinectin 1	14q22.1
RET/PTC9 [36]	*RFG9*	KIAA1468	18q21–22
ELKS–*RET* [37]	*ERC1 (ELKS/RAB6-interacting/ CAST family member 1)*	ELKS, RAB6IP2	12p13.3
PCM1–*RET* [38]	*PCM1 (pericentriolar material 1)*	—	8p21–22
RFP–*RET* [39]	*TRIM27 (tripartite motif-containing 27)*	RFP	6p21
HOOK3–*RET* [40]	*HOOK3 (Homo sapiens hook homolog 3)*	—	8p11.21

[a] Information retrieved from the Entrez Gene database of the National Center for Biotechnology Information.

reader is referred to other articles for a detailed description of the prevalence of RET/PTC rearrangements [28,42].

In vitro and in vivo irradiation induces RET/PTC formation. In thyrocyte nuclei, *RET*, *CCDC6*, and *NcoA4* loci, which are several megabases apart in the linear map of chromosome 10, frequently juxtapose thereby facilitating their nonhomologous recombination on irradiation [43,44].

RET/PTC oncogenes can be causative in thyroid tumorigenesis: (1) RET/PTC expression causes thyrotropin-independent proliferation, impairs the expression of thyroid differentiation markers in rat thyroid follicular cells [45], and induces the irregular nuclear contours that are characteristic of PTC [46]; (2) transgenic mice develop PTC with features very similar to those shown by human PTC [47]; and (3) RET/PTC are found in microscopic PTC foci, thought to be precursors of full-blown PTC, suggesting that they may be early genetic events in PTC development [48].

The mechanism by which RET/PTC rearrangements convert *RET* into a dominantly acting oncogene has been partially clarified. All the translocated amino termini fused to RET are predicted to fold into coiled coils. Fusion with such protein-protein interaction motifs provides RET/PTC kinases with dimerizing interfaces that foster the formation of active dimers [29,49,50]. Moreover, RET/PTC molecules lack the intracellular juxtamembrane domain (see Fig. 1). The juxtamembrane domain forms an integral part of the autoinhibited RET dimer interface. The RET-TKD in the RET/PTC oncoproteins might be favored to adopt the active conformation [3]. Accordingly, the juxtamembrane domain suppressed transforming ability of RET/PTC [51]. Finally, unscheduled RET expression in thyroid follicular cells caused by the fusion to ubiquitously expressed gene partners and delocalization of the rearranged protein to the cytosol probably concur to RET activation.

It is conceivable that RET kinase activation is not the sole consequence of RET/PTC rearrangements and that structural alterations of the *RET* fusion partners may contribute to their oncogenic effects (see Table 1). Perhaps the most convincing support for this hypothesis is provided by *PRKAR1A*, the *RET* fusion partner in the RET/PTC2 rearrangement. *PRKAR1A* encodes the cyclic AMP-dependent protein kinase type I–regulatory subunit [29]. *PRKAR1A* is a bona fide tumor suppressor gene that is mutated in approximately half of Carney complex kindreds. Carney complex predisposes to a variety of tumors including adenomas and papillary and follicular carcinomas of the thyroid [52]. Importantly, *PRKAR1A-null* mice developed thyroid carcinomas [53]. Other RET fusion partners have functions that may be related to tumorigenesis (see Table 1). ERC1 recruits IKBA to the IKK complex, thereby regulating NFkB, a well-known oncogenic transcriptional factor [54,55]. CCDC6 is a proapoptotic factor whose knock-down promoted cell survival [56]. TRIM33 forms a transcriptional complex with the TGFβ signaling intermediates Smad proteins [57,58]. Finally, RFP acts as a transcriptional repressor disabling pRb (retinoblastoma)-mediated differentiation [59,60].

Although thus far RET/PTC rearrangements have been described only in PTC, RET fusion partners may play a role also in cancer types other than PTC. CCDC6 is rearranged to the PDGFRβ RTK in myeloproliferative disorders [61,62] and to the phosphatase PTEN in some PTC cases [63]. In hematologic malignancies, the t(8;9)(p22;p24) translocation caused the fusion of the janus kinase–2 gene with PCM1 [64]. Finally, TRIM24 is rearranged with BRAF in mouse hepatocellular carcinomas [65] and to FGFR1 in a myeloproliferative syndrome [66].

RET signaling

RET signaling has been described in detail elsewhere [67–69]. Briefly, RET signaling depends on the autophosphorylation of several RET tyrosine residues (see Fig. 1) [70]. Tyrosines 900 and 905 (Y900, Y905) map in the kinase A-loop. These tyrosines are essential for RET activation in intact cells [71], although recent biochemical data showed that conformational change of the A-loop is not essential for RET kinase activation [3]. Y905 acts also as a binding site for Grb7/10 adaptors [72]. Moreover, Y905 mediates binding of SH2B1β, a protein that, by obstructing the SHP-1 tyrosine phosphatase, enhances RET phosphorylation [73].

Y1015, a docking site for phospholipase Cγ, is essential for RET function during kidney development probably by *Sprouty* activation [74], and for RET/PTC transforming activity [75]. Y1062 acts as a binding site for several proteins, along with Shc, ShcC, IRS1/2, FRS2, DOK1/4/5, and Enigma, which in turn lead to stimulation of the Ras/MAPK and phosphatidylinositol-3-kinase (PI3K)/AKT pathway [67–69]. RET/PTC also directly phosphorylates phosphoinositide-dependent kinase–1 in the Y9 residue and leads to AKT phosphorylation [76]. Through Y1062, RET mediates also activation of the small GTPase Rap1 [77]. The DOK4 adaptor plays a role in RET-mediated Rap1 activation in pheochromocytoma PC12 cells [78]. Both Rap1 and DOK4 contribute to MAPK activation [77,78]. Y1062 is essential for RET transforming activity [79–81] and for development [74,82,83]. Y1062 ablation induces more severe effects in RET9 than in RET51 monoisomorphic mice, probably because of the redundant activation of the AKT/MAPK pathways through the Y1096 residue, which is not present in RET9 [74].

Serine phosphorylation is crucial also for RET signaling. In particular, S687 in the RET juxtamembrane is phosphorylated by protein kinase and essential for activation of the RAC1 small GTPase/JUN NH(2)-terminal kinase pathway. Mutation in this codon affects the development of the enteric nervous system in transgenic mice [84].

Finally, the activity of RET is controlled at multiple levels by transcription factors that regulate receptor and ligand expression [85–87]; by extracellular signaling factors, such as Rob/Slit [88] and Bmp4 [85,89]; and by intracellular inhibitors of tyrosine kinase activity like *Sprouty* [90,91] or PTEN, whose expression can suppress GDNF/RET-mediated chemotaxis and kidney development [92].

Summary

Since its isolation about 20 years ago, much progress has been made in the understanding of the oncogenic effects exerted by *RET*. The analysis of RET signal transduction has helped to shed considerable light on the Ras/BRAF/MAPK and PI3K/AKT signaling pathways that are crucial for the formation of various thyroid cancer types [93,94]. Genetic testing and prophylactic thyroidectomy are now the gold standard in the treatment of MEN-2 [95]. Recent studies demonstrating that cancers can be removed by directly targeting the disease-causing protein kinase (targeted therapy) suggest that cancer patients in which RET mutations are causative events could benefit from treatment strategies based on the use of kinase inhibitors that intercept RET kinase or downstream signaling [96].

Acknowledgments

The authors gratefully acknowledge Prof. G. Vecchio, Prof. A. Fusco, Prof. R.M. Melillo, Dr F. Carlomagno, and all members of their laboratory for continuous support. They are grateful to Jean Ann Gilder for text editing.

References

[1] Airaksinen MS, Saarma M. The GDNF family: signalling, biological functions and therapeutic value. Nat Rev Neurosci 2002;3(5):383–94.

[2] Anders J, Kjar S, Ibanez CF. Molecular modeling of the extracellular domain of the RET receptor tyrosine kinase reveals multiple cadherin-like domains and a calcium-binding site. J Biol Chem 2001;276(38):35808–17.

[3] Knowles PP, Murray-Rust J, Kjaer S, et al. Structure and chemical inhibition of the RET tyrosine kinase domain. J Biol Chem 2006;281(44):33577–87.

[4] Schlessinger J. Signal transduction: autoinhibition control. Science 2003;300(5620):750–2.

[5] Heanue TA, Pachnis V. Enteric nervous system development and Hirschsprung's disease: advances in genetic and stem cell studies. Nat Rev Neurosci 2007;8(6):466–79.

[6] Veiga-Fernandes H, Coles MC, Foster KE, et al. Tyrosine kinase receptor RET is a key regulator of Peyer's patch organogenesis. Nature 2007;446(7135):547–51.

[7] Kramer ER, Aron L, Ramakers GM, et al. Absence of ret signaling in mice causes progressive and late degeneration of the nigrostriatal system. PLoS Biol 2007;5(3):616–28.

[8] Lindfors PH, Lindahl M, Rossi J, et al. Ablation of persephin receptor glial cell line-derived neurotrophic factor family receptor alpha4 impairs thyroid calcitonin production in young mice. Endocrinology 2006;147(5):2237–44.

[9] Akeno-Stuart N, Croyle M, Knauf JA, et al. The RET kinase inhibitor NVP-AST487 blocks growth and calcitonin gene expression through distinct mechanisms in medullary thyroid cancer cells. Cancer Res 2007;67(14):6956–64.

[10] Takahashi M, Ritz J, Cooper GM. Activation of a novel human transforming gene, ret, by DNA rearrangement. Cell 1985;42(2):581–8.

[11] Fusco A, Grieco M, Santoro M, et al. A new oncogene in human thyroid papillary carcinomas and their lymph-nodal metastases. Nature 1987;328(6126):170–2.

[12] Grieco M, Santoro M, Berlingieri MT, et al. PTC is a novel rearranged form of the ret proto-oncogene and is frequently detected in vivo in human thyroid papillary carcinomas. Cell 1990;60(4):557–63.

[13] Greenman C, Stephens P, Smith R, et al. Patterns of somatic mutation in human cancer genomes. Nature 2007;446(7132):153–8.

[14] Tahira T, Ishizaka Y, Itoh F, et al. Expression of the ret proto-oncogene in human neuroblastoma cell lines and its increase during neuronal differentiation induced by retinoic acid. Oncogene 1991;6(12):2333–8.

[15] Meng X, Lindahl M, Hyvonen ME, et al. Regulation of cell fate decision of undifferentiated spermatogonia by GDNF. Science 2000;287(5457):1489–93.

[16] Sawai H, Okada Y, Kazanjian K, et al. The G691S RET polymorphism increases glial cell line-derived neurotrophic factor-induced pancreatic cancer cell invasion by amplifying mitogen-activated protein kinase signaling. Cancer Res 2005;65(24):11536–44.

[17] Tozlu S, Girault I, Vacher S, et al. Identification of novel genes that co-cluster with estrogen receptor alpha in breast tumor biopsy specimens, using a large-scale real-time reverse transcription-PCR approach. Endocr Relat Cancer 2006;13(4):1109–20.

[18] Camos M, Esteve J, Jares P, et al. Gene expression profiling of acute myeloid leukemia with translocation t(8;16)(p11;p13) and MYST3-CREBBP rearrangement reveals a distinctive signature with a specific pattern of HOX gene expression. Cancer Res 2006;66(14): 6947–54.

[19] Bordeaux MC, Forcet C, Granger L, et al. The RET proto-oncogene induces apoptosis: a novel mechanism for Hirschsprung disease. EMBO J 2000;19(15):4056–63.

[20] Canibano C, Rodriguez NL, Saez C, et al. The dependence receptor Ret induces apoptosis in somatotrophs through a Pit-1/p53 pathway, preventing tumor growth. EMBO J 2007;26(8): 2015–28.

[21] Brandi ML, Gagel RF, Angeli A, et al. Guidelines for diagnosis and therapy of MEN type 1 and type 2. J Clin Endocrinol Metab 2001;86(12):5658–71.

[22] Kouvaraki MA, Shapiro SE, Perrier ND, et al. RET proto-oncogene: a review and update of genotype-phenotype correlations in hereditary medullary thyroid cancer and associated endocrine tumors. Thyroid 2005;15(6):531–44.

[23] Kjaer S, Kurokawa K, Perrinjaquet M, et al. Self-association of the transmembrane domain of RET underlies oncogenic activation by MEN2A mutations. Oncogene 2006;25(53): 7086–95.

[24] Santoro M, Carlomagno F, Romano A, et al. Activation of RET as a dominant transforming gene by germline mutations of MEN2A and MEN2B. Science 1995;267(5196):381–3.

[25] Freche B, Guillaumot P, Charmetant J, et al. Inducible dimerization of RET reveals a specific AKT deregulation in oncogenic signaling. J Biol Chem 2005;280(44):36584–91.

[26] Gujral TS, Singh VK, Jia Z, et al. Molecular mechanisms of RET receptor-mediated oncogenesis in multiple endocrine neoplasia 2B. Cancer Res 2006;66(22):10741–9.

[27] Runeberg-Roos P, Virtanen H, Saarma M. RET(MEN 2B) is active in the endoplasmic reticulum before reaching the cell surface. Oncogene 2007;26(57):7909–15.

[28] Kondo T, Ezzat S, Asa SL. Pathogenetic mechanisms in thyroid follicular-cell neoplasia. Nat Rev Cancer 2006;6(4):292–306.

[29] Bongarzone I, Monzini N, Borrello MG, et al. Molecular characterization of a thyroid tumor-specific transforming sequence formed by the fusion of ret tyrosine kinase and the regulatory subunit RI alpha of cyclic AMP-dependent protein kinase A. Mol Cell Biol 1993; 13(1):358–66.

[30] Bongarzone I, Butti MG, Coronelli S, et al. Frequent activation of ret protooncogene by fusion with a new activating gene in papillary thyroid carcinomas. Cancer Res 1994; 54(11):2979–85.

[31] Santoro M, Dathan NA, Berlingieri MT, et al. Molecular characterization of RET/PTC3; a novel rearranged version of the RETproto-oncogene in a human thyroid papillary carcinoma. Oncogene 1994;9(2):509–16.

[32] Fugazzola L, Pierotti MA, Vigano E, et al. Molecular and biochemical analysis of RET/PTC4, a novel oncogenic rearrangement between RET and ELE1 genes, in a post-Chernobyl papillary thyroid cancer. Oncogene 1996;13(5):1093–7.

[33] Klugbauer S, Demidchik EP, Lengfelder E, et al. Detection of a novel type of RET rearrangement (PTC5) in thyroid carcinomas after Chernobyl and analysis of the involved RET-fused gene RFG5. Cancer Res 1998;58(2):198–203.

[34] Klugbauer S, Rabes HM. The transcription coactivator HTIF1 and a related protein are fused to the RET receptor tyrosine kinase in childhood papillary thyroid carcinomas. Oncogene 1999;18(30):4388–93.

[35] Salassidis K, Bruch J, Zitzelsberger H, et al. Translocation t(10;14)(q11.2:q22.1) fusing the kinetin to the RET gene creates a novel rearranged form (PTC8) of the RET proto-oncogene in radiation-induced childhood papillary thyroid carcinoma. Cancer Res 2000;60(11): 2786–9.

[36] Klugbauer S, Jauch A, Lengfelder E, et al. A novel type of RET rearrangement (PTC8) in childhood papillary thyroid carcinomas and characterization of the involved gene (RFG8). Cancer Res 2000;60(24):7028–32.

[37] Nakata T, Kitamura Y, Shimizu K, et al. Fusion of a novel gene, ELKS, to RET due to translocation t(10;12)(q11;p13) in a papillary thyroid carcinoma. Genes Chromosomes Cancer 1999;25(2):97–103.

[38] Corvi R, Berger N, Balczon R, et al. RET/PCM-1: a novel fusion gene in papillary thyroid carcinoma. Oncogene 2000;19(37):4236–42.

[39] Saenko V, Rogounovitch T, Shimizu-Yoshida Y, et al. Novel tumorigenic rearrangement, Delta rfp/ret, in a papillary thyroid carcinoma from externally irradiated patient. Mutat Res 2003;527(1–2):81–90.

[40] Ciampi R, Giordano TJ, Wikenheiser-Brokamp K, et al. HOOK3-RET: a novel type of RET/PTC rearrangement in papillary thyroid carcinoma. Endocr Relat Cancer 2007; 14(2):445–52.

[41] Ishizaka Y, Tahira T, Ochiai M, et al. Molecular cloning and characterization of human ret-II oncogene. Oncogene Res 1988;3(2):193–7.

[42] Nikiforov YE. RET/PTC rearrangement in thyroid tumors. Endocr Pathol 2002;13(1):3–16.

[43] Nikiforova MN, Stringer JR, Blough R, et al. Proximity of chromosomal loci that participate in radiation-induced rearrangements in human cells. Science 2000;290(5489):138–41.

[44] Gandhi M, Medvedovic M, Stringer JR, et al. Interphase chromosome folding determines spatial proximity of genes participating in carcinogenic RET/PTC rearrangements. Oncogene 2006;25(16):2360–6.

[45] Santoro M, Melillo RM, Grieco M, et al. The TRK and RET tyrosine kinase oncogenes cooperate with ras in the neoplastic transformation of a rat thyroid epithelial cell line. Cell Growth Differ 1993;4(2):77–84.

[46] Fischer AH, Taysavang P, Jhiang SM. Nuclear envelope irregularity is induced by RET/PTC during interphase. Am J Pathol 2003;163(3):1091–100.

[47] Jhiang SM. The RET proto-oncogene in human cancers. Oncogene 2000;19(49):5590–7.

[48] Viglietto G, Chiappetta G, Martinez-Tello FJ, et al. RET/PTC oncogene activation is an early event in thyroid carcinogenesis. Oncogene 1995;11(6):1207–10.

[49] Tong Q, Xing S, Jhiang SM. Leucine zipper-mediated dimerization is essential for the PTC1 oncogenic activity. J Biol Chem 1997;272(14):9043–7.

[50] Monaco C, Visconti R, Barone MV, et al. The RFG oligomerization domain mediates kinase activation and re-localization of the RET/PTC3 oncoprotein to the plasma membrane. Oncogene 2001;20(5):599–608.

[51] Melillo RM, Cirafici AM, De Falco V, et al. The oncogenic activity of RET point mutants for follicular thyroid cells may account for the occurrence of papillary thyroid carcinoma in patients affected by familial medullary thyroid carcinoma. Am J Pathol 2004;165(2): 511–21.

[52] Kirschner LS, Carney JA, Pack SD, et al. Mutations of the gene encoding the protein kinase A type I-alpha regulatory subunit in patients with the Carney complex. Nat Genet 2000; 26(1):89–92.

[53] Kirschner LS, Kusewitt DF, Matyakhina L, et al. A mouse model for the Carney complex tumor syndrome develops neoplasia in cyclic AMP-responsive tissues. Cancer Res 2005; 65(11):4506–14.

[54] Ducut Sigala JL, Bottero V, Young DB, et al. Activation of transcription factor NF-kappaB requires ELKS, an IkappaB kinase regulatory subunit. Science 2004;304(5679):1963–7.

[55] Wu ZH, Shi Y, Tibbetts RS, et al. Molecular linkage between the kinase ATM and NF-kappaB signaling in response to genotoxic stimuli. Science 2006;311(5764):1141–6.

[56] Merolla F, Pentimalli F, Pacelli R, et al. Involvement of H4(D10S170) protein in ATM-dependent response to DNA damage. Oncogene 2007;26(42):6167–75.

[57] Dupont S, Zacchigna L, Cordenonsi M, et al. Germ-layer specification and control of cell growth by Ectodermin, a Smad4 ubiquitin ligase. Cell 2005;121(1):87–99.

[58] He W, Dorn DC, Erdjument-Bromage H, et al. Hematopoiesis controlled by distinct TIF1-gamma and Smad4 branches of the TGFbeta pathway. Cell 2006;125(5):929–41.

[59] Shimono Y, Murakami H, Hasegawa Y, et al. RET finger protein is a transcriptional repressor and interacts with enhancer of polycomb that has dual transcriptional functions. J Biol Chem 2000;275(50):39411–9.

[60] Krutzfeldt M, Ellis M, Weekes DB, et al. Selective ablation of retinoblastoma protein function by the RET finger protein. Mol Cell 2005;18(2):213–24.

[61] Kulkarni S, Heath C, Parker S, et al. Fusion of H4/D10S170 to the platelet-derived growth factor receptor beta in BCR-ABL-negative myeloproliferative disorders with a t(5;10)(q33;q21). Cancer Res 2000;60(13):3592–8.

[62] Schwaller J, Anastasiadou E, Cain D, et al. H4(D10S170), a gene frequently rearranged in papillary thyroid carcinoma, is fused to the platelet-derived growth factor receptor beta gene in atypical chronic myeloid leukemia with t(5;10)(q33;q22). Blood 2001;97(12): 3910–8.

[63] Puxeddu E, Zhao G, Stringer JR, et al. Characterization of novel non-clonal intrachromosomal rearrangements between the H4 and PTEN genes (H4/PTEN) in human thyroid cell lines and papillary thyroid cancer specimens. Mutat Res 2005;570(1):17–32.

[64] Reiter A, Walz C, Watmore A, et al. The t(8;9)(p22;p24) is a recurrent abnormality in chronic and acute leukemia that fuses PCM1 to JAK2. Cancer Res 2005;65(7):2662–7.

[65] Zhong S, Delva L, Rachez C, et al. A RA-dependent, tumour-growth suppressive transcription complex is the target of the PML-RARalpha and T18 oncoproteins. Nat Genet 1999; 23(3):287–95.

[66] Belloni E, Trubia M, Gasparini P, et al. 8p11 myeloproliferative syndrome with a novel t(7;8) translocation leading to fusion of the FGFR1 and TIF1 genes. Genes Chromosomes Cancer 2005;42(3):320–5.

[67] Ichihara M, Murakumo Y, Takahashi M. RET and neuroendocrine tumors. Cancer Lett 2004;204(2):197–211.

[68] Santoro M, Carlomagno F, Melillo RM, et al. Dysfunction of the RET receptor in human cancer. Cell Mol Life Sci 2004;61(23):2954–64.

[69] Arighi E, Borrello MG, Sariola H. RET tyrosine kinase signaling in development and cancer. Cytokine Growth Factor Rev 2005;16(4–5):441–67.

[70] Kawamoto Y, Takeda K, Okuno Y, et al. Identification of RET autophosphorylation sites by mass spectrometry. J Biol Chem 2004;279(14):14213–24.

[71] Iwashita T, Asai N, Murakami H, et al. Identification of tyrosine residues that are essential for transforming activity of the ret proto-oncogene with MEN2A or MEN2B mutation. Oncogene 1996;12(3):481–7.

[72] Pandey A, Liu X, Dixon JE, et al. Direct association between the Ret receptor tyrosine kinase and the Src homology 2-containing adapter protein Grb7. J Biol Chem 1996;271(18): 10607–10.

[73] Donatello S, Fiorino A, Degl'innocenti D, et al. SH2B1beta adaptor is a key enhancer of RET tyrosine kinase signaling. Oncogene 2007;26(45):6546–59.

[74] Jain S, Encinas M, Johnson EM Jr, et al. Critical and distinct roles for key RET tyrosine docking sites in renal development. Genes Dev 2006;20(3):321–33.

[75] Borrello MG, Alberti L, Arighi E, et al. The full oncogenic activity of Ret/ptc2 depends on tyrosine 539, a docking site for phospholipase Cgamma. Mol Cell Biol 1996;16(5):2151–63.

[76] Jung HS, Kim DW, Jo YS, et al. Regulation of protein kinase B tyrosine phosphorylation by thyroid-specific oncogenic RET/PTC kinases. Mol Endocrinol 2005;19(11):2748–59.

[77] De Falco V, Castellone MD, De Vita G, et al. RET/papillary thyroid carcinoma oncogenic signaling through the Rap1 small GTPase. Cancer Res 2007;67(1):381–90.

[78] Uchida M, Enomoto A, Fukuda T, et al. Dok-4 regulates GDNF-dependent neurite outgrowth through downstream activation of Rap1 and mitogen-activated protein kinase. J Cell Sci 2006;119(Pt 15):3067–77.

[79] Segouffin-Cariou C, Billaud M. Transforming ability of MEN2A-RET requires activation of the phosphatidylinositol 3-kinase/AKT signaling pathway. J Biol Chem 2000;275(5): 3568–76.

[80] Melillo RM, Castellone MD, Guarino V, et al. The RET/PTC-RAS-BRAF linear signaling cascade mediates the motile and mitogenic phenotype of thyroid cancer cells. J Clin Invest 2005;115(4):1068–81.

[81] Castellone MD, Cirafici AM, De Vita G, et al. Ras-mediated apoptosis of PC CL 3 rat thyroid cells induced by RET/PTC oncogenes. Oncogene 2003;22(2):246–55.

[82] Jijiwa M, Fukuda T, Kawai K, et al. A targeting mutation of tyrosine 1062 in Ret causes a marked decrease of enteric neurons and renal hypoplasia. Mol Cell Biol 2004;24(18): 8026–36.

[83] Wong A, Bogni S, Kotka P, et al. Phosphotyrosine 1062 is critical for the in vivo activity of the Ret9 receptor tyrosine kinase isoform. Mol Cell Biol 2005;25(21):9661–73.

[84] Asai N, Fukuda T, Wu Z, et al. Targeted mutation of serine 697 in the Ret tyrosine kinase causes migration defect of enteric neural crest cells. Development 2006;133(22):4507–16.

[85] Brophy PD, Ostrom L, Lang KM, et al. Regulation of ureteric bud outgrowth by Pax2-dependent activation of the glial derived neurotrophic factor gene. Development 2001;128(23): 4747–56.

[86] Clarke JC, Patel SR, Raymond RM Jr, et al. Regulation of c-Ret in the developing kidney is responsive to Pax2 gene dosage. Hum Mol Genet 2006;15(23):3420–8.

[87] Kume T, Deng K, Hogan BL. Murine forkhead/winged helix genes Foxc1 (Mf1) and Foxc2 (Mfh1) are required for the early organogenesis of the kidney and urinary tract. Development 2000;127(7):1387–95.

[88] Grieshammer U, Le M, Plump AS, et al. SLIT2-mediated ROBO2 signaling restricts kidney induction to a single site. Dev Cell 2004;6(5):709–17.

[89] Miyazaki Y, Oshima K, Fogo A, et al. Bone morphogenetic protein 4 regulates the budding site and elongation of the mouse ureter. J Clin Invest 2000;105(7):863–73.

[90] Basson MA, Akbulut S, Watson-Johnson J, et al. Sprouty1 is a critical regulator of GDNF/RET-mediated kidney induction. Dev Cell 2005;8(2):229–39.

[91] Ishida M, Ichihara M, Mii S, et al. Sprouty2 regulates growth and differentiation of human neuroblastoma cells through RET tyrosine kinase. Cancer Sci 2007;98(6):815–21.

[92] Kim D, Dressler GR. PTEN modulates GDNF/RET mediated chemotaxis and branching morphogenesis in the developing kidney. Dev Biol 2007;307(2):290–9.

[93] Groussin L, Fagin JA. Significance of BRAF mutations in papillary thyroid carcinoma: prognostic and therapeutic implications. Nat Clin Pract Endocrinol Metab 2006;2(4):180–1.

[94] Shinohara M, Chung YJ, Saji M, et al. AKT in thyroid tumorigenesis and progression-Endocrinology 2007;148(3):942–7.

[95] Skinner MA, Moley JA, Dilley WG, et al. Prophylactic thyroidectomy in multiple endocrine neoplasia type 2A. N Engl J Med 2005;353(11):1105–13.

[96] Santoro M, Carlomagno F. Drug insight: small-molecule inhibitors of protein kinases in the treatment of thyroid cancer. Nat Clin Pract Endocrinol Metab 2006;2(1):42–52.

ELSEVIER
SAUNDERS

Endocrinol Metab Clin N Am
37 (2008) 375–387

ENDOCRINOLOGY
AND METABOLISM
CLINICS
OF NORTH AMERICA

Dysregulation of the Phosphatidylinositol 3-Kinase Pathway in Thyroid Neoplasia

John E. Paes, DO[a], Matthew D. Ringel, MD[a,b],*

[a]Division of Endocrinology, Diabetes, and Metabolism, The Ohio State University
Medical Center, The Ohio State University, 1581 Dodd Drive, 4th Floor,
McCampbell Hall, Columbus, OH 43210, USA
[b]Arthur G. James Comprehensive Cancer Center, The Ohio State University,
Columbus, OH 43210, USA

Activation of the phosphatidylinositol 3-kinase (PI3K) pathway is a common event in many cancers, including thyroid neoplasias. Class I PI3Ks are a family of proteins comprised of a regulatory and catalytic subunit (p85 and p110 subunits, respectively) that are activated by receptor tyrosine kinases and other signaling molecules, resulting in regulation of a wide variety of cellular functions [1]. Of the subfamilies of class I PI3Ks, PI3Kα is the best studied in thyroid cancer. Activation of PI3K results in the formation of phosphatidylinositol 3,4,5, triphosphate (PIP3), which subsequently recruits proteins with pleckstrin homology (PH) domains to the cytosolic membrane (Fig. 1). Several key PH domain-containing proteins transduce signaling through multiple downstream signaling cascades, including phosphoinositide-dependent kinase-1 (PDK1) and AKT [2,3]. PDK1 has been shown to phosphorylate a large number of kinases, including AKT, serum and glucocorticoid-induced kinase (SGK), protein kinase A, several protein kinase C isoforms, and others that are known to regulate cell growth, metabolism, and apoptosis. In addition to PH domains, several other phosphoinositide-binding domains have been described, supporting even broader consequences of PI3K signaling [2,3].

Dr. Ringel has received speaker honoraria from Genzyme Corporation and Abbott Laboratories.

This work was supported by NIH grant 5 R01 CA102572-02 to Dr. Ringel.

* Corresponding author. Division of Endocrinology, Diabetes, and Metabolism, The Ohio State University Medical Center, The Ohio State University, 1581 Dodd Drive, 4th Floor, McCampbell Hall, Columbus, OH 43210.

E-mail address: matthew.ringel@osumc.edu (M.D. Ringel).

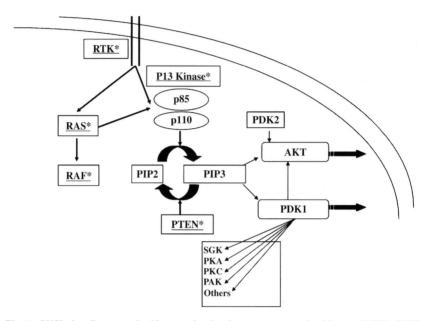

Fig. 1. PI3K signaling cascade. Upon activation by receptor tyrosine kinases (RTK), PI3K, which is comprised of a p85 regulatory and p110 catalytic domain, converts PIP2 to PIP3. PIP3 subsequently interacts with proteins containing PH domains, such as PDK1 and AKT, allowing for membrane recruitment (*dark arrows*). PDK1 phosphorylates AKT and other downstream targets including PKA, PKC isoforms, PAK, SGK, and other targets to regulate cell behavior. In the case of AKT, an additional phosphorylation by a PDK2 activity mediated by one of several kinases (see text) is required for full activation. PI3K signaling is inhibited by the lipid phosphatase activity of PTEN which converts PIP3 to PIP2. RTKs also activate the RAS/RAF/MEK signaling cascade, which has important biologic effects as well. RAS is also a site of cross-talk between these pathways through its ability to activate PI3K. Genetic alterations that result in constitutive signaling occur in thyroid cancer; the locations of these alterations in these pathways are underlined and notified with an asterisk.

The best studied downstream kinase in the PI3K pathway in thyroid cancer is AKT. After its recruitment to the membrane, AKT is phosphorylated at two critical sites for activation of the protein, threonine 308 by PDK1 and serine 473 by PDK2, an activity that has been ascribed to several kinases, including the rapamycin insensitive companion of target of rapamycin/target of rapamycin (rictor/TOR) complex [4], DNA-dependent kinase [5], PKCβII [6], intergin-linked kinase [7], and AKT [8] (ie, autophosphorylation). Phosphorylated AKT isoforms subsequently interact with effectors in the cytosol and nucleus to regulate cell proliferation, apoptosis, metabolism, and motility. A detailed discussion of the frequency and potential functional role of AKT activation in thyroid cancer and the potential importance of specific isoforms and subcellular localization in these effects has been recently published [9]. Although the importance of AKT as a key mediator of the downstream effects of PI3K has been demonstrated, other PI3K signaling pathways are also activated and regulate cell behavior [3].

One important negative regulator of this pathway is phosphatase and tensin homolog deleted on chromosome ten (PTEN). PTEN is a dual function lipid and protein phosphatase. Its lipid phosphatase function leads to the conversion of PIP3 to PIP2, thereby opposing the activity of PI3K, reducing membrane localization of PH domain-containing proteins such as PDK1 and AKT, and inhibiting subsequent signaling activity [3]. The importance of the function of the PH domain in regulating AKT activity was highlighted in a recent report by Carpten and colleagues [10] in which a glutamic acid to lysine substitution at amino acid 17 (E17K) in the PH domain of AKT1 was identified in 8% of breast, 6% of colorectal, and 2% of ovarian cancers that were analyzed. The AKT1 E17K mutant was shown to display altered subcellular localization to the plasma membrane, to exhibit enhanced levels of activity, and to transform fibroblasts and induce leukemia in a murine model.

In addition to upstream inhibition of the pathway by PTEN, downstream inhibition can occur through complex cross-signaling mechanisms, by the effects of protein phosphatases, or by disruption of protein stabilization. For example, AKT is stabilized by chaperone proteins, such as adaptor protein containing PH domain, phosphotyrosine-binding domain, leucine zipper region (APPL), Cdc37, and heat shock protein 90 (HSP90) [11,12]. Although not specific for AKT inhibition, compounds that disrupt Hsp90 binding to client proteins have been developed for potential therapeutic benefit and exhibit anti-proliferative effects in thyroid cells [13]. Inactivation of AKT activity also occurs via the activities of protein phosphatase 2A at Thr 308 and PHD leucine-rich repeat protein phosphatase (PHLPP) at Ser 473 [14–16]. A second isoform of PHLPP has recently been defined by Brognard and colleagues [17] that not only inactivates AKT but also inhibits cell cycle progression and promotes apoptosis through distinct AKT isoforms.

PTEN in thyroid cancer

PTEN in cowden syndrome

Perhaps the strongest evidence supporting a role for PI3K signaling in the development of thyroid neoplasia is Cowden syndrome (MIM#158350). Cowden syndrome is an autosomal dominant condition characterized by the development of benign hamartomas in multiple organ systems, such as the skin and gastrointestinal tract, as well as an increased risk of developing breast and thyroid cancer. Inactivating mutations of *PTEN* have been defined as the cause of Cowden syndrome [18] and can be identified in the majority of individuals meeting established diagnostic criteria [19]. Thyroid neoplasia can be identified in approximately two thirds of affected individuals. Thyroid cancer, most frequently follicular thyroid cancer (FTC), is identified in approximately 10% of individuals with Cowden syndrome; therefore, thyroid neoplasia is included as one of the major diagnostic criteria supporting a clinical diagnosis [19]. These genetic data provide strong evidence for a role of PI3K signaling in the development of FTC. Several groups have created murine models of generalized loss of *Pten* [20–22]. In these models, homozygous deletion of the *Pten* gene resulted in embryonic lethality, whereas *Pten* +/− mice developed neoplasias in multiple organ systems resembling Cowden syndrome, including thyroid tumors. In these tumors, loss of the remaining *Pten* allele was frequently identified, consistent with the role of *Pten* as a tumor suppressor gene that requires loss of expression of both alleles to result in tumor formation. Evidence of increased activation of PI3K signaling was also shown in the tumors, and the deficiency of *Akt1* reduced the formation of tumors in the *Pten* +/− mice in additional cross-breeding experiments [23]. These data confirm that loss of *Pten* expression can result in neoplastic transformation in vivo.

To analyze more specifically the ability of *Pten* loss to cause thyroid neoplasia, Yeager and colleagues [24] developed a mouse strain (Pten$^{L/L}$; TPO-Cre) using Cre-mediated recombination to delete *Pten* specifically in the thyroid. In these interesting studies, mice with complete loss of *Pten* expression in the thyroid gland developed hyperplastic euthyroid goiters in association with increased PI3K signaling. Over time, a number of mice developed nodular hyperplasia and benign follicular tumors, although cancers were not identified. There were phenotypic differences between the female and male mice. The female mice were reported to have a higher proliferative index in the follicular cells at younger ages when compared with the males and were more likely to develop follicular adenomas at 8 to 10 months of age. The researchers subsequently identified an increase in expression and phosphorylation of estrogen receptor α, a downstream target of AKT, in the *Pten* null thyroid glands of the female mice. In addition to these experiments, the researchers compared the findings in the Pten$^{L/L}$; TPO-Cre mice with that in *Pten* +/− mice that developed hyperplastic nodules at a lower frequency. They identified loss of expression of the remaining wild-type allele in the nodular tissue, further supporting the ability of increased PI3K signaling to induce thyroid nodules. Taken together, these data suggest that genetic loss of *Pten* is sufficient to induce thyroid neoplasia in vivo.

PTEN in sporadic thyroid cancer

Several groups have assessed sporadic benign and malignant thyroid cancers for mutations, deletions, and changes in expression levels of *PTEN*. Nearly all of these studies demonstrate that mutations or deletions in *PTEN* are rare events in sporadic thyroid cancer, occurring at a low frequency in most of the studies, particularly in differentiated thyroid cancers (Table 1) [25–28]. In addition to gene mutations, loss of heterozygosity (LOH) at one of the *PTEN* alleles also occurs in thyroid cancer [26,29,30]. Nevertheless, it has not been reported to occur in tumors with a mutation in the other allele; therefore, this LOH would not be predicted

Table 1
Frequency of gene abnormalities in *PTEN* and *PI3KCA* predicted to activate PI3K in sporadic thyroid cancers

Gene abnormality	Follicular adenoma	FTC	PTC	ATC	References
PTEN mutation[a]	0/183 (0%)	10/147 (6.8%)	3/163 (1.8%)	8/59 (13.6%)	[25–28,32]
PTEN reduction[b]	1/36 (2.7%)	17/76 (22.4%)	5/14 (35.7%)	9/22 (40.9%)	[29,39]
PIK3CA mutation	0/180 (0%)	13/167 (7.8%)	5/296 (1.7%)	22/133 (16.5%)	[28,32,47,48]
PIK3CA amplification	23/177 (13%)	38/137 (27.7%)	33/286 (11.5%)	20/48 (42%)	[28,32,48]

[a] Does not include studies demonstrating loss of heterozygosity or hypermethylation. These are noted in the text.

[b] Includes only data relating to mRNA levels. Western blot and immunohistochemical studies not included. They are noted in the text. In some cases, downstream signaling activity has been assessed. These studies are described in the text.

to result in complete loss of *PTEN* gene expression, as seems to be required for tumor formation, unless other mechanisms were involved in the loss of allelic expression. Indeed, it has been reported that reduced expression of PTEN protein occurs in a fairly high percentage of anaplastic thyroid cancers (ATCs) and less frequently in FTC and papillary thyroid cancer (PTC) samples when analyzing tumors at the protein level by immunohistochemistry [30,31]. This observation has been correlated with LOH and with the identification of *PTEN* promoter hypermethylation. For example, Gimm and colleagues [30] reported the common reduction of PTEN protein expression as well as differences in PTEN subcellular localization in a comparison with normal tissue in sporadic thyroid cancers associated with *PTEN* LOH in one allele, suggesting that both epigenetic and post-translational regulation of PTEN might be involved in thyroid cancers.

Several recent studies in follicular thyroid neoplasias have demonstrated that *PTEN* mutations rarely occur in tumors with other PI3K-activating genetic changes, such as mutations or amplification of *PIK3CA* [28,32], providing important genetic evidence that supports the role of PI3K signaling in sporadic follicular tumor formation. Activation of RAS and loss of PPARγ function, which may be involved in the activity of PPARγ/PAX8, have been reported to activate PI3K signaling [33–35] and are associated with follicular thyroid tumor development and AKT activation in human tumors [36]. Although *PTEN* mutations appear to be relatively uncommon in sporadic FTC, LOH, promoter methylation, and loss of protein expression may be more commonly identified. These data in combination with the lack of genetic overlap between *PTEN* mutations and other FTC-related genetic alterations support a role for PI3K signaling in follicular tumorigenesis.

The frequency of *PTEN* mutations has also been reported in PTC and ATC. In general, the reported mutation rate of *PTEN* in PTC is lower than in FTC (see Table 1) [25–28,32,37], and although the frequency of PTC with reduced *PTEN* mRNA expression appears to be higher than the number with mutations, it seems unlikely that PTEN loss itself has a central role early in PTC tumorigenesis based on the well-defined role for BRAF and ERK signaling in these tumors. When taken together, mutations in *PTEN* or other genetic abnormalities predicted to increase AKT activity in PTC occur at a less frequent rate than in FTC in general (see Table 1), and they do not appear to be mutually exclusive of known PTC-inducing mutations such as activating mutations of *BRAF* [28]. This overlap is distinct from mutations that result in enhanced activation of the RAS/RAF/ERK pathway that appear to be mutually exclusive in PTC [38]. These data suggest that genetic changes leading to increased PI3K pathway signaling may represent a later-stage event in PTC. Consistent with this hypothesis are the observations that enhanced activation of AKT appears to occur most notably in the invasive fronts of PTC [36] and that a higher frequency of PI3K-related genetic changes occurs in ATC in comparison with well-differentiated PTC (see Table 1). In addition, based on signaling data from human tumors, the degree of PI3K signaling may differ depending on the initiating oncogene in PTC [36].

When compared with the findings in differentiated FTC and PTC, loss of PTEN expression and mutations of the *PTEN* gene are reported to occur at a higher frequency in ATC [25,28,29,39]. This finding may not be surprising because these tumors harbor many genetic changes, suggesting overall genomic instability. The functional role of the loss of PTEN function and subsequent increased PI3K signaling in the development of ATC is uncertain, although in vitro data support a role for this pathway in proliferation, survival, and motility in thyroid cancer cell lines, especially those with loss of *PTEN* [39]. It appears that the loss of PTEN expression and function may be important both in the development of FTC and more broadly in the progression and dedifferentiation of thyroid cancers.

PI3K in thyroid cancer

PIK3CA mutations and amplification in sporadic thyroid cancer

The *PIK3CA* gene encodes the catalytic subunit of class 1A PI3K (p110α). As described previously, PI3K is comprised of a regulatory subunit (p85) which forms a heterodimer with the catalytic subunit (p110), leading to generation of PIP3 and initiation of its signaling cascade. Samuels and colleagues [40] and other groups identified cancer-related mutations in *PIK3CA* that largely resided in hot spot regions of the gene that encode the helical and kinase domains of the protein [1]. These mutations have been shown to cause the expression of constitutively active PI3Kα proteins that are capable of inducing malignant transformation in vitro and in vivo [41–43]. In addition to activating mutations, *PIK3CA* gene amplification has also been implicated in cancer and has been associated with increased PI3K signaling [44–46]. Over the past several years, the frequency of *PIK3CA* mutations and gene amplification has been analyzed in sporadic thyroid carcinomas.

In FTC, the frequency of mutations in the hot spot domains of *PIK3CA* has ranged from 6% to 13% depending on the population [28,32,47,48]. By contrast, 24% to 28% of FTCs are described to have gene amplification of *PIK3CA* (defined as four or more copies) [28,32,48]. Intriguingly, in studies in which mutations and amplification of *PIK3CA* were studied in conjunction with *PTEN* and *RAS* mutations, the presence of these changes appeared to be mutually exclusive; however, PPARγ/PAX8 analysis was not included in these studies. Overall, these studies support a potential genetic role for genetic abnormalities involving *PIK3CA* in FTC.

In PTC, the frequency of mutations in *PIK3CA* appears to be lower than in FTC in several studies, with occurrence rates ranging from 0% to 3% (see Table 1). Similarly, although gene amplification of *PIK3CA* is more common than mutations in PTC, its frequency is lower than in FTC, with occurrence rates ranging from 5% to 14% [28,32,47,48]. In addition, although these changes were rare and relatively exclusive from *PTEN* or *RAS* gene mutations, they were not found to be independent of activating mutations of *BRAF*, the most common pathogenic mutation in PTC.

Of significant interest has been the recent finding that ATC frequently harbors mutations and gene amplification in *PIK3CA*. Garcia-Rostan and colleagues [47] identified *PIK3CA* hot spot gene mutations in 23% of 70 ATCs. Levels of phosphorylated AKT (pAKT) were scored as moderate or high in the majority of ATCs regardless of whether a *PIK3CA* mutation was present, suggesting multiple mechanisms for enhanced AKT signaling in these tumors. Tumors with moderate or high levels of pAKT statistically had higher levels of markers of proliferation. Immunoactive pAKT was detected in both the cytosol and nucleus in the majority of cases with higher levels of AKT overactivation. *PIK3CA* gene amplification and *PTEN* mutations and expression levels were not assessed in this study. A second study that included samples from 50 patients with ATC was recently published by Hou and colleagues [28]. In that study, *PIK3CA* mutations were identified in 12% of cases, gene amplification in 42% of cases, and *PTEN* mutations in 16% of cases. Different from the well-differentiated thyroid cancers, these findings were not mutually exclusive in this group of ATCs. When considered as a group, 58% of ATCs harbored one of these three genetic abnormalities predicted to increase PI3K signaling. In comparison, 31% of benign follicular adenomas, 55% of FTCs, and 24% of PTCs in this study had one of these abnormalities. It was concluded that the data supported a role for PI3K signaling in thyroid tumorigenesis, particularly in follicular neoplasia, and in thyroid cancer progression toward ATC. Table 1 includes a summary of the mutation and published expression level data for *PTEN* and *PIK3CA* in human thyroid neoplasias.

Other potential mechanisms for PI3K activation in thyroid cancer

Activation by thyroid oncogenes and tyrosine kinase receptors

A variety of other mechanisms might also be responsible for activation of PI3K signaling in thyroid cancer, including signaling through oncogenes such as RET/PTC or RAS, and signaling through other receptor tyrosine kinases known to be commonly overexpressed in thyroid cancers. An association between expression of both RET/PTC and constitutively active N-RAS and enhanced PI3K signaling has been reported in human thyroid cancers at the level of cell signaling [36] and gene expression [49]. Although the activation of downstream targets in the classical PI3K signaling cascade is known to be initiated by RET/PTC and other receptor tyrosine kinases, recent evidence suggests that RET/PTC3 may also be capable of activating PDK1 and AKT through tyrosine phosphorylation in a PI3K-independent manner [50,51]. In addition to RET/PTC, activated RAS is known to interact with and activate PI3K directly [33]. In human tumors, *RAS* gene mutations have been associated with follicular neoplasias [52] and with the follicular variant of papillary cancer [53]. *RAS* mutations have been shown to be associated with AKT activation [36] and to be largely mutually exclusive of *PIK3CA* and *PTEN* genetic abnormalities in well-differentiated thyroid cancers [28,32,47]. Although the focus of this manuscript is on PI3K signaling, it is important to recognize that the relative importance of PI3K signaling versus other pathways in the action of the RET/PTC and activated RAS in thyroid cancer is not fully elucidated. The importance of RAF/ERK signaling in RET/PTC downstream effects has been demonstrated [54], and although there are distinct genetic signatures for thyroid cancer harboring specific oncogenes, there is overlap between the expression profiles for tumors with BRAF V600E mutations and RET/PTC rearrangements [49]. It seems likely that both (and other) pathways are important in the oncogenic action of RET/PTC and activated RAS in thyroid cancer.

In addition to oncogenes, PI3K signaling may be activated by other events that occur in thyroid cancer, such as overexpression of a variety of receptor tyrosine kinases (eg, cMET), the FGF, IGF-1, and VEGF receptors, and others [55]. Many of these receptors are known to regulate angiogenesis or cell proliferation and invasion through activation of PI3K and other pathways, including the RAS/RAF cascade, suggesting their potential suitability as therapeutic targets.

Activation of the PI3K regulatory domain

In addition to mutations or gene amplifications of *PIK3CA*, PI3K signaling can be increased through cell signaling at the level of the regulatory domain of PI3K (p85). Potentially relevant for thyroid cancer are in vitro studies that have demonstrated the ability of thyroid hormone to activate

PI3K through interactions between thyroid hormone receptors and p85 in the cytosol in several cell types [56,57]. In addition, a particular thyroid hormone receptor β mutant (TRβ$^{PV/PV}$ thyroid cancer) that is capable of inducing invasive and eventually dedifferentiated in vivo in association with PI3K activation in the setting of high TSH levels [58,59] also appears to activate PI3K signaling via interactions with the p85 subunit [60]. It has recently been reported that treating these thyroid cancer–prone mice with the PI3K inhibitor LY294002 retards growth of the primary tumors and inhibits tumor invasion and metastases [61]. Although the clinical relevance of this thyroid hormone receptor β mutant is uncertain, the data provide evidence that disruption of PI3K signaling is capable of reducing thyroid cancer progression in an endogenous model system of thyroid cancer characterized by enhanced PI3K signaling. Further studies in additional model systems are needed to determine if this is a more generalized finding.

Activation of downstream signaling molecules in the PI3K pathway

The role of non-AKT downstream effectors of PI3K in thyroid cancer is only now being elucidated. Important roles for mTOR activation in thyroid neoplasia that may be independent of AKT are being studied [62]. Recent data also suggest an important role for p21-activated kinases, a family of proteins activated by PDK1, in thyroid cancer cell motility [63]. Activation of additional effectors of PDK1 such as protein kinase A has also been shown to be associated with the development of thyroid cancer [64]. Protein kinase C signaling, which also can be activated through the activity of PDK1 [65], has been shown to be up-regulated in some thyroid tumors as well [66,67]. It is likely that new information regarding the key upstream regulators and downstream targets of PI3K involved in thyroid tumorigenesis and progression will help define important potential therapeutic targets for thyroid cancer.

PI3K as a target for thyroid cancer therapy

PI3K itself has been suggested to be a target for novel cancer therapy, although it has not yet been studied in clinical trials in thyroid cancer [68]. The recent development of PI3K isoform-specific inhibitors, including PI3Kα inhibitors, has further raised the possibility of targeting this pathway for the treatment of patients with cancers harboring *PIK3CA* mutations or that display increased PI3K signaling through other mechanisms, including those detailed previously [1,69,70]. Because PI3K signaling has important metabolic and neurologic effects, side effects such as insulin resistance or other off-target effects will need to be closely monitored and might impact the dosing strategies or the ultimate utility of this approach [2,68]. It may be reasonable to consider inhibition of PI3K as part of a combinatorial therapeutic strategy. Indeed, Berns and colleagues [71] recently reported that the PI3K pathway was crucial in predicting resistance to trastuzumab in breast cancer. Whether PI3K inhibition has a similar role in the therapeutic resistance of poorly differentiated thyroid cancer remains to be determined. In addition to inhibiting PI3K directly, inhibitors of several downstream effectors, such as mammalian target of rapamycin (mTOR) [72], are also being developed and will be interesting to test in preclinical thyroid cancer systems.

Summary

Dysregulated PI3K signaling is a common event in thyroid cancer. Genetic evidence supporting the ability of constitutive PI3K signaling to cause follicular neoplasia derives from observations studying Cowden syndrome, a genetic syndrome caused by inactivation of *PTEN,* and includes the mutually exclusive nature of loss of *PTEN* expression and activating mutations and amplifications of the *PIK3CA* gene in sporadic FTC. Genetic alterations that result in activated PI3K signaling have also been identified in sporadic well-differentiated PTC and ATC, particularly in the latter, suggesting a role for PI3K signaling in dedifferentiated thyroid cancers. PI3K activation can also occur through the action of receptor tyrosine kinases and through cross-talk from signaling molecules known to be activated in thyroid cancer. Taken together, these data suggest that dysregulated PI3K signaling has an important role in thyroid neoplasia.

References

[1] Vogt PK, Kang S, Elsliger MA, et al. Cancer-specific mutations in phosphatidylinositol 3-kinase. Trends Biochem Sci 2007;32(7):342–9.
[2] Cully M, You H, Levine AJ, et al. Beyond PTEN mutations: the PI3K pathway as an integrator of multiple inputs during tumorigenesis. Nat Rev Cancer 2006;6(3):184–92.
[3] Blanco-Aparicio C, Renner O, Leal JF, et al. PTEN, more than the AKT pathway. Carcinogenesis 2007;28(7):1379–86.
[4] Sarbassov DD, Guertin DA, Ali SM, et al. Phosphorylation and regulation of Akt/PKB by the Rictor-mTOR complex. Science 2005;307(5712):1098–101.
[5] Feng J, Park J, Cron P, et al. Identification of a PKB/Akt hydrophobic motif ser-473 kinase as DNA-dependent protein kinase. J Biol Chem 2004;279(39):41189–96.
[6] Kawakami Y, Nishimoto H, Kitaura J, et al. Protein kinase C beta II regulates Akt phosphorylation on Ser-473 in a cell type- and stimulus-specific fashion. J Biol Chem 2004;279(46):47720–5.
[7] Lynch DK, Ellis CA, Edwards PA, et al. Integrin-linked kinase regulates phosphorylation of serine 473 of protein kinase B by an indirect mechanism. Oncogene 1999;18(56):8024–32.
[8] Toker A, Newton AC. Akt/protein kinase B is regulated by autophosphorylation at the hypothetical PDK-2 site. J Biol Chem 2000;275(12):8271–4.
[9] Shinohara M, Chung YJ, Saji M, et al. AKT in thyroid tumorigenesis and progression. Endocrinology 2007;148(3):942–7.
[10] Carpten JD, Faber AL, Horn C, et al. A transforming mutation in the pleckstrin homology domain of AKT1 in cancer. Nature 2007;448(7152):439–44.

[11] Basso AD, Solit DB, Chiosis G, et al. Akt forms an intracellular complex with Hsp90 and Cdc37 and is destabilized by inhibitors of Hsp90 function. J Biol Chem 2002;277(42): 39858–66.

[12] Mitsuuchi Y, Johnson SW, Sonoda G, et al. Identification of a chromosome 3p14.3-21.1 gene, APPL, encoding an adaptor molecule that interacts with the oncoprotein-serine/threonine kinase AKT2. Oncogene 1999;18(35):4891–8.

[13] Braga-Basaria M, Hardy E, Gottfried R, et al. 17-Allylamino-17-demethoxygeldanamycin activity against thyroid cancer cell lines correlates with heat shock protein 90 levels. J Clin Endocrinol Metab 2004;89(6):2982–8.

[14] Cantley LC, Neel BG. New insights into tumor suppression: PTEN suppresses tumor formation by restraining the phosphoinositide 3-kinase/AKT pathway. Proc Natl Acad Sci U S A 1999;96(8):4240–5.

[15] Gao T, Furnari F, Newton AC. PHLPP: a phosphatase that directly dephosphorylates Akt, promotes apoptosis, and suppresses tumor growth. Mol Cell 2005;18(1):13–24.

[16] Trotman LC, Alimonti A, Scaglioni PP, et al. Identification of a tumour suppressor network opposing nuclear Akt function. Nature 2006;441(7092):523–7.

[17] Brognard J, Sierecki E, Gao T, et al. PHLPP and a second isoform, PHLPP2, differentially attenuate the amplitude of Akt signaling by regulating distinct Akt isoforms. Mol Cell 2007; 25(6):917–31.

[18] Liaw D, Marsh DJ, Li J, et al. Germline mutations of the PTEN gene in Cowden disease, an inherited breast and thyroid cancer syndrome. Nat Genet 1997;16(1):64–7.

[19] Pilarski R, Eng C. Will the real Cowden syndrome please stand up (again)? Expanding mutational and clinical spectra of the PTEN hamartoma tumour syndrome. J Med Genet 2004;41(5):323–6.

[20] Di Cristofano A, Pesce B, Cordon-Cardo C, et al. Pten is essential for embryonic development and tumour suppression. Nat Genet 1998;19(4):348–55.

[21] Podsypanina K, Ellenson LH, Nemes A, et al. Mutation of Pten/Mmac1 in mice causes neoplasia in multiple organ systems. Proc Natl Acad Sci U S A 1999;96(4):1563–8.

[22] Stambolic V, Tsao MS, Macpherson D, et al. High incidence of breast and endometrial neoplasia resembling human Cowden syndrome in pten+/− mice. Cancer Res 2000; 60(13):3605–11.

[23] Chen ML, Xu PZ, Peng XD, et al. The deficiency of Akt1 is sufficient to suppress tumor development in Pten+/− mice. Genes Dev 2006;20(12):1569–74.

[24] Yeager N, Klein-Szanto A, Kimura S, et al. Pten loss in the mouse thyroid causes goiter and follicular adenomas: insights into thyroid function and Cowden disease pathogenesis. Cancer Res 2007;67(3):959–66.

[25] Dahia PLM, Marsh DJ, Zheng Z, et al. Somatic deletions and mutations in the Cowden disease gene, PTEN, in sporadic thyroid tumors. Cancer Res 1997;57:4710–3.

[26] Halachmi N, Halachmi S, Evron E, et al. Somatic mutations of the PTEN/MMAC1 tumor suppressor gene in sporadic follicular thyroid tumors. Genes Chromosomes Cancer 1998; 23(3):239–43.

[27] Hsieh MC, Lin SF, Shin SJ, et al. Mutation analysis of PTEN/MMAC 1 in sporadic thyroid tumors. Kaohsiung J Med Sci 2000;16(1):9–12.

[28] Hou P, Liu D, Shan Y, et al. Genetic alterations and their relationship in the phosphatidylinositol 3-kinase/akt pathway in thyroid cancer. Clin Cancer Res 2007;13(4):1161–70.

[29] Frisk T, Foukakis T, Dwight T, et al. Silencing of the PTEN tumor-suppressor gene in anaplastic thyroid cancer. Genes Chromosomes Cancer 2002;35(1):74–80.

[30] Gimm O, Perren A, Weng LP, et al. Differential nuclear and cytoplasmic expression of PTEN in normal thyroid tissue, and benign and malignant epithelial thyroid tumors. Am J Pathol 2000;156(5):1693–700.

[31] Alvarez-Nunez F, Bussaglia E, Mauricio D, et al. PTEN promoter methylation in sporadic thyroid carcinomas. Thyroid 2006;16(1):17–23.

[32] Wang Y, Hou P, Yu H, et al. High prevalence and mutual exclusivity of genetic alterations in the phosphatidylinositol-3-kinase/akt pathway in thyroid tumors. J Clin Endocrinol Metab 2007;92(6):2387–90.

[33] Rodriguez-Viciana P, Warne PH, Dhand R, et al. Phosphatidylinositol-3-OH kinase as a direct target of Ras. Nature 1994;370(6490):527–32.

[34] Farrow B, Evers BM. Activation of PPAR-gamma increases PTEN expression in pancreatic cancer cells. Biochem Biophys Res Commun 2003;301(1):50–3.

[35] Aiello A, Pandini G, Frasca F, et al. PPAR-γ agonists induce partial reversion of epithelial-mesenchymal transition in anaplastic thyroid cancer cells. Endocrinology 2006;147(9): 4463–75.

[36] Vasko V, Saji M, Hardy E, et al. Akt activation and localization correlate with tumor invasion and oncogene expression in thyroid cancer. J Med Genet 2004;41(3):161–70.

[37] Gimm O, Attie-Bitach T, Lees JA, et al. Expression of the PTEN tumour suppressor protein during human development. Hum Mol Genet 2000;9(11):1633–9.

[38] Fagin JA. How thyroid tumors start and why it matters: kinase mutants as targets for solid cancer pharmacotherapy. J Endocrinol 2004;183(2):249–56.

[39] Bruni P, Boccia A, Baldassarre G, et al. PTEN expression is reduced in a subset of sporadic thyroid carcinomas: evidence that PTEN growth suppressing activity in thyroid cancer cells mediated by p27kip1. Oncogene 2000;19(28):3146–55.

[40] Samuels Y, Wang Z, Bardelli A, et al. High frequency of mutations of the PIK3CA gene in human cancers. Science 2004;304(5670):554.

[41] Bader AG, Kang S, Vogt PK. Cancer-specific mutations in PIK3CA are oncogenic in vivo. Proc Natl Acad Sci U S A 2006;103(5):1475–9.

[42] Gymnopoulos M, Elsliger MA, Vogt PK. Rare cancer-specific mutations in PIK3CA show gain of function. Proc Natl Acad Sci U S A 2007;104(13):5569–74.

[43] Kang S, Bader AG, Vogt PK. Phosphatidylinositol 3-kinase mutations identified in human cancer are oncogenic. Proc Natl Acad Sci U S A 2005;102(3):802–7.

[44] Bertelsen BI, Steine SJ, Sandvei R, et al. Molecular analysis of the PI3K-AKT pathway in uterine cervical neoplasia: frequent PIK3CA amplification and AKT phosphorylation. Int J Cancer 2006;118(8):1877–83.

[45] Byun DS, Cho K, Ryu BK, et al. Frequent monoallelic deletion of PTEN and its reciprocal association with PIK3CA amplification in gastric carcinoma. Int J Cancer 2003;104(3): 318–27.

[46] Wu G, Xing M, Mambo E, et al. Somatic mutation and gain of copy number of PIK3CA in human breast cancer. Breast Cancer Res 2005;7(5):R609–16.

[47] Garcia-Rostan G, Costa AM, Pereira-Castro I, et al. Mutation of the PIK3CA gene in anaplastic thyroid cancer. Cancer Res 2005;65(22):10199–207.

[48] Wu G, Mambo E, Guo Z, et al. Uncommon mutation but common amplifications of the PIK3CA gene in thyroid tumors. J Clin Endocrinol Metab 2005;90(8):4688–93.

[49] Giordano TJ, Kuick R, Thomas DG, et al. Molecular classification of papillary thyroid carcinoma: distinct BRAF, RAS, and RET/PTC mutation-specific gene expression profiles discovered by DNA microarray analysis. Oncogene 2005;24(44):6646–56.

[50] Kim DW, Hwang JH, Suh JM, et al. RET/PTC (rearranged in transformation/papillary thyroid carcinomas) tyrosine kinase phosphorylates and activates phosphoinositide-dependent kinase 1 (PDK1): an alternative phosphatidylinositol 3-kinase–independent pathway to activate PDK1. Mol Endocrinol 2003;17(7):1382–94.

[51] Jung HS, Kim DW, Jo YS, et al. Regulation of PKB tyrosine phosphorylation by thyroid-specific oncogene Ret/PTC kinases. Mol Endocrinol 2005;19(11):2748–59.

[52] Vasko V, Ferrand M, Di Cristofaro J, et al. Specific pattern of RAS oncogene mutations in follicular thyroid tumors. J Clin Endocrinol Metab 2003;88(6):2745–52.

[53] Adeniran AJ, Zhu Z, Gandhi M, et al. Correlation between genetic alterations and microscopic features, clinical manifestations, and prognostic characteristics of thyroid papillary carcinomas. Am J Surg Pathol 2006;30(2):216–22.

[54] Mitsutake N, Miyagishi M, Mitsutake S, et al. BRAF mediates RET/PTC-induced MAPK activation in thyroid cells: functional support for requirement of the RET/PTC-RAS-BRAF pathway in papillary thyroid carcinogenesis. Endocrinology 2005;147(2):1014–9.

[55] Kondo T, Ezzat S, Asa SL. Pathogenetic mechanisms in thyroid follicular cell neoplasia. Nat Rev Cancer 2006;6(4):292–306.

[56] Cao X, Kambe F, Moeller LC, et al. Thyroid hormone induces rapid activation of Akt/PKB-mTOR-p70S6K cascade through phosphatidylinositol 3-kinase in human fibroblasts. Mol Endocrinol 2005;19:102–12.

[57] Kenessey A, Ojamaa K. Thyroid hormone stimulates protein synthesis in the cardiomyocyte by activating the Akt-mTOR and p70S6K pathways. J Biol Chem 2006;281(30):20666–72.

[58] Suzuki H, Willingham MC, Cheng SY. Mice with a mutation in the thyroid hormone receptor beta gene spontaneously develop thyroid carcinoma: a mouse model of thyroid carcinogenesis. Thyroid 2002;12(11):963–9.

[59] Kim CF, Vasko VV, Kato Y, et al. AKT activation promotes metastasis in a mouse model of follicular thyroid carcinoma. Endocrinology 2005;146(10):4456–63.

[60] Furuya F, Hanover JA, Cheng SY. Activation of phosphatidylinositol 3-kinase signaling by a mutant thyroid hormone beta receptor. Proc Natl Acad Sci U S A 2006;103(6):1780–5.

[61] Furuya F, Lu C, Willingham MC, et al. Inhibition of phosphatidylinositol 3' kinase delays tumor progression and blocks metastatic spread in a mouse model of thyroid cancer. Carcinogenesis 2007;28(12):2451–8.

[62] Brewer C, Yeager N, Di Cristofano A. Thyroid-stimulating hormone initiated proliferative signals converge in vivo on the mTOR kinase without activating AKT. Cancer Res 2007;67(17):8002–6.

[63] Porchia LM, Guerra M, Wang YC, et al. 2-Amino-N-{4-[5-(2-phenanthrenyl)-3-(trifluoro-methyl)-1H-pyrazol-1-yl]-phenyl} acetamide (OSU-03012), a celecoxib derivative, directly targets p21-activated kinase. Mol Pharmacol 2007;72(5):1124–31.

[64] Sandrini F, Matyakhina L, Sarlis NJ, et al. Regulatory subunit type I-alpha of protein kinase A (PRKAR1A): a tumor-suppressor gene for sporadic thyroid cancer. Genes Chromosomes Cancer 2002;35(2):182–92.

[65] Dutil EM, Toker A, Newton AC. Regulation of conventional protein kinase C isozymes by phosphoinositide-dependent kinase 1 (PDK-1). Curr Biol 1998;8(25):1366–75.

[66] Shimizu T, Usuda N, Sugenoya A, et al. Immunohistochemical evidence for the overexpression of protein kinase C in proliferative diseases of human thyroid. Cell Mol Biol 1991;37(8):813–21.

[67] Eszlinger M, Krohn K, Berger K, et al. Gene expression analysis reveals evidence for increased expression of cell cycle–associated genes and Gq-protein-protein kinase C signaling in cold thyroid nodules. J Clin Endocrinol Metab 2005;90(2):1163–70.

[68] Hennessy BT, Smith DL, Ram PT, et al. Exploiting the PI3K/AKT pathway for cancer drug discovery. Nat Rev Drug Discov 2005;4(12):988–1004.

[69] Hayakawa M, Kaizawa H, Moritomo H, et al. Synthesis and biological evaluation of 4-morpholino-2-phenylquinazolines and related derivatives as novel PI3 kinase p110-alpha inhibitors. Bioorg Med Chem 2006;14(20):6847–58.

[70] Marion F, Williams DE, Patrick BO, et al. Liphagal, a selective inhibitor of PI3 kinase alpha isolated from the sponge akacoralliphaga: structure elucidation and biomimetic synthesis. Org Lett 2006;8(2):321–4.

[71] Berns K, Horlings HM, Hennessy BT, et al. A functional genetic approach identifies the PI3K pathway as a major determinant of trastuzumab resistance in breast cancer. Cancer Cell 2007;12(4):395–402.

[72] Abraham RT, Gibbons JJ. The mammalian target of rapamycin signaling pathway: twists and turns in the road to cancer therapy. Clin Cancer Res 2007;13(11):3109–14.

ELSEVIER
SAUNDERS

Endocrinol Metab Clin N Am
37 (2008) 389–400

ENDOCRINOLOGY
AND METABOLISM
CLINICS
OF NORTH AMERICA

Epigenetic Dysregulation in Thyroid Neoplasia

Tetsuo Kondo, MD, PhD[a], Sylvia L. Asa, MD, PhD[b,c],
Shereen Ezzat, MD[b,d],*

[a]Department of Pathology, University of Yamanashi, Japan
[b]Ontario Cancer Institute, University Health Network, 610 University Avenue
#8-327, Toronto, ON, M5P 2S3, Canada
[c]Department of Pathology and Laboratory Medicine, University of Toronto,
Toronto, ON, Canada
[d]Department of Medicine, University of Toronto, Toronto, ON, Canada

Gain-of-function mutations in oncogenes, including *RET*, *RAS,* and *BRAF*, have greatly aided our understanding of the molecular mechanisms of thyroid carcinogenesis [1]. It is also clear that mutations or deletions cause inactivation of tumor suppressor genes such as p53/*TP53* in thyroid carcinomas [1]. However, recent advances have further disclosed the significance of epigenetic events in the development and progression of human tumorigenesis [2]. Indeed, various tumor-suppressor genes and thyroid hormone–related genes are epigenetically silenced in thyroid tumors [3]. The epigenetic pattern of gene silencing is also associated with certain histologic types of thyroid tumors. This article reviews the evidence for epigenetic gene dysregulation in follicular cell–derived thyroid carcinomas including papillary thyroid carcinoma (PTC), follicular thyroid carcinoma (FTC), and undifferentiated thyroid carcinoma (UTC). We also discuss future applications of epigenetics as ancillary diagnostic tools and in the design of targeted therapies for thyroid cancer.

Epigenetic gene regulation

Epigenetic modification is responsible for regulation of gene expression by mammalian cells without involving changes in the underlying genomic DNA sequence (Fig. 1). The mechanisms include methylation of cytosine

* Corresponding author. Ontario Cancer Institute, 610 University Avenue #8-327, Toronto, ON, M5P 2S3, Canada.
  E-mail address: shereen.ezzat@utoronto.ca (S. Ezzat).

0889-8529/08/$ - see front matter © 2008 Elsevier Inc. All rights reserved.
doi:10.1016/j.ecl.2007.12.002   *endo.theclinics.com*

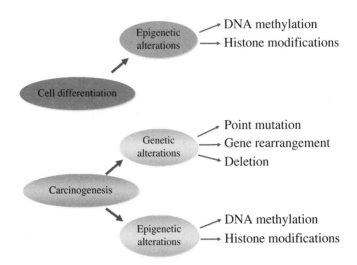

Fig. 1. Regulation of gene expression in cell differentiation and carcinogenesis. In normal mammalian cells, epigenetic changes play a role in the process of cellular differentiation, allowing cells to stably maintain different characteristics despite containing the same genomic material. In neoplastic cells, irreversible genetic changes including gain-of-function mutations and/or loss-of-function mutations are important in carcinogenesis and progression of transformed cells. Along with genetic events, reversible epigenetic changes of gene expression via DNA methylation and histone modification further govern the biological behavior of neoplastic cells.

residues of DNA and posttranslational modifications of the histone proteins associated with the DNA strand, resulting in selective gene activation and/or inactivation. DNA methylation occurs at CpG sites, cytosine-guanosine dinucleotide sequences, by covalent addition of a methyl group at the fifth position of the cytosine ring, resulting in methylcytosine. Clusters of CpGs, referred to as CpG islands, are typically located in and around the promoter region of genes. The methylation status of a promoter region can regulate downstream gene expression: hyper-methylated CpG islands repress gene expression by inhibiting transcription, while unmethylated CpG islands allow gene expression (Fig. 2). DNA methyltransferases (DNMTs) catalyze the transfer of a methyl group to DNA, resulting in CpG methylation. In contrast, DNMT inhibitors, such as 5′-aza-deoxycytidine (5′-Aza-dc), demethylate CpG islands.

Several methods are available for analyzing the methylation status of DNA in tissues and cell lines. Bisulphite-based cytosine methylation analysis using methylation-specific polymerase chain reaction (PCR) and/or DNA sequencing combined with restriction enzymes are popular techniques for methylation studies. In human cancers, certain tumor-suppressor genes are inactivated through promoter DNA methylation [4]. Genome-wide hypo-methylation has also been detected in cancer cells [5]. These findings suggest that aberrant patterns of DNA methylation play crucial roles in carcinogenesis and cancer progression.

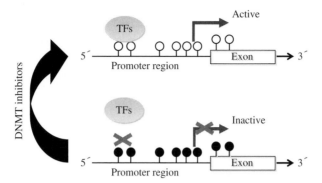

Fig. 2. DNA methylation inhibits gene transcription. DNA methylation is one of the most prevalent epigenetic modifications of DNA in mammalian genomes. The unmethylated status of CpG islands located in promoter regions corresponds with the ability of those genes to be transcribed in the presence of the necessary transcription-regulating factors. The transcriptional silencing of genes through hyper-methylation of CpG islands is a key contributor to tumor-suppressor inactivation. DNA methyltransferase (DNMT) inhibitors, such as 5′-aza-deoxycytidine, demethylate CpG islands. White circles, unmethylated CpG sites; black circles, hyper-methylated sites; TFs, transcriptional factors.

Although DNA methylation controls transcription, it alone is insufficient to silence gene expression. Chromatin modifications, such as histone acetylation and methylation, affect local chromatin structure that contributes to the determination of whether a gene is transcribed or repressed (Fig. 3). Nucleosomes, which are the fundamental repeating subunits of chromosomes in eukaryotes, consist of approximately 146 base pairs of DNA and four pairs of histones H2A, H2B, H3, and H4. Various histone modifications, including acetylation and methylation, work in concert with DNA methylation to regulate gene transcription. Generally, acetylation of lysine residues on histones H3 and H4 leads to the formation of an open chromatin structure that permits access to DNA of regulatory proteins such as transcriptional factors. Methylation of lysine 9 residues on H3 facilitates transcriptional repression, whereas methylation of lysine 4 on H3 is associated with transcriptionally active euchromatin.

The chromatin immunoprecipitation (ChIP) assay is commonly used to examine the status of histones [1,6]. Histone modification can also be suggested by the reexpression of silenced genes after treatment with histone deacetylase (HDAC) inhibitors. HDACs keep residues of histones deacetylated, and thus maintain transcriptional silencing. Conversely, HDAC inhibitors, such as trichostatin, inhibit histone deacetylation, leading to accumulation of acetylated histone proteins (see Fig. 3).

Epigenetic dysregulation of thyroid-specific genes

The main physiologic function of the thyroid gland is synthesis, storage, and secretion of thyroid hormones, triiodothyronine (T3) and L-thyroxine

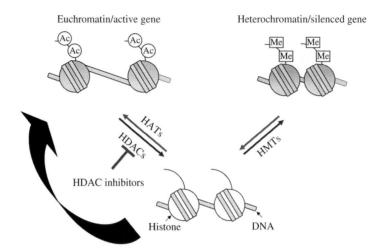

Fig. 3. Modifications of histone tails influence gene expression through chromatin remodeling. Histone deacetylases (HDACs) and histone acetyltransferases (HATs) exert opposing enzymatic activities that modulate the degree of acetylation of histones, thereby regulating the accessibility of chromatin and therefore gene expression and cellular differentiation. Administration of HDAC inhibitors, such as trichostatin, results in accumulation of acetylated histones and induces differentiation and/or apoptosis in transformed cells. Histone methyltransferases (HMT) are enzymes that catalyze the transfer of one to three methyl groups to lysine and arginine residues of histone proteins. Increased methylation of lysine residues of histone is a major factor in gene silencing. Ac, acetylation; Me, methylation.

(T4). The thyroid is composed of two distinct hormone-producing cell types that have been designated follicular cells and C cells. Follicular cells comprise follicles filled with colloid and are responsible for iodine uptake and thyroid hormone synthesis. C cells are scattered intrafollicular or parafollicular cells that are dedicated to the production of the calcium-regulating hormone calcitonin. The process of thyroid hormone synthesis requires a complex regulatory mechanism involving various thyroid-specific molecules such as the thyroid-stimulating hormone (TSH) receptor, thyroid peroxidase (TPO), thyroglobulin, the sodium/iodide symporter (NIS), and pendrin. In brief, iodine is actively trapped in follicular cells against an electro-chemical gradient across the plasma membrane, mediated by NIS protein in the basal membrane, and is transported into thyroid follicles presumably through pendrin in the apical membrane. During reaction with TPO, iodine is covalently bound to tyrosine residues within thyroglobulin, forming monoiodotyrosine (MIT) and diiodotyrosine (DIT). The follicular cells proteolytically cleave the iodinated tyrosines from thyroglobulin, forming T3 and T4, and releasing them into the blood. This process of synthesis and release of thyroid hormones is controlled by TSH receptor signaling, which is regulated by intricate feedback mechanisms via the hypothalamic-pituitary-thyroid axis.

Thyroid-specific genes involved in thyroid hormone synthesis are frequently dysregulated during thyroid cancer progression [7–10]. Down-regulation of these functional genes in thyroid carcinoma cells results in loss of the ability to concentrate iodine in follicles. Since radioactive iodine is an effective treatment for thyroid cancer only if carcinoma cells retain the ability to take up iodine [11], restoration of expression of thyroid-specific genes has a potential role in thyroid cancer therapeutics. Specifically, the promoter of the TSH receptor is hyper-methylated and silenced in thyroid carcinomas [12], the iodide transporters NIS and pendrin are methylated and down-regulated in thyroid tumors [12–14], and these may be targets for epigenetic targeting to promote the efficacy of radioactive iodine as a therapy.

The mechanisms underlying the epigenetic dysregulation of iodine metabolism in thyroid cancer are still unclear. Presumably, genetic events impact on loss of physical properties of neoplastic cells in parallel with tumor de-differentiation [15]. *BRAF* V600E mutation in PTC is associated with reduced expression of key genes involved in iodine metabolism [16]. This finding suggests that aberrant MAPK signaling alters the epigenetic environment in cancer cells. Indeed, suppression of the MAPK pathway by knockdown of mutant *BRAF* or administration of the MEK inhibitor, U0126, restores expression of iodide-metabolizing genes in a human thyroid carcinoma cell line expressing the V600E *BRAF* mutant, suggesting that the MAPK pathway will be a critical therapeutic target in restoring thyroid gene expression for effective radioiodine therapy [17].

Epigenetic dysregulation of tumor-suppressor genes

Inactivation of tumor suppressor genes is critical in tumorigenesis of thyroid follicular cells. Loss of function is mediated by irreversible processes such as gene deletion or mutation. Alternatively, tumor suppressor genes are inactivated via epigenetic processes. Cumulative epigenetic alterations may play a role in the sequential progression of indolent well-differentiated thyroid carcinomas to metastasizing carcinomas and through the spectrum of poorly differentiated to undifferentiated thyroid carcinoma.

Cell-cycle regulators that govern the growth activity of thyroid carcinomas are also controlled by epigenetics along with genetic changes such as point mutations and deletions. Cyclins heterodimerize with cyclin-dependent kinases (CDKs) and cooperate to control the G1 to S phase transition through inactivation of the tumor suppressor retinoblastoma (Rb) protein. The CDK inhibitors p16INK4A/*CDKN2A*, p21CIP1/*CDKN1B,* and p27KIP1/*CDKN1B* impair the activity of cyclin-CDK complexes, therefore the CDK inhibitors function as tumor suppressors. In thyroid cancers, CDK inhibitors, such as p27KIP1 and p16INK4A are commonly down-regulated [18]. Methylation of the CpG island of CDKN2A is detected in 30% of thyroid neoplasms [19].

Along with gain-of-function mutations in genes of MAPK pathway effectors, epigenetically silencing of tumor-suppressive Ras effector, RAS association domain family 1, splicing isoform A (*RASSF1A*) might be involved in thyroid carcinogenesis. RASSF1A protein lacks apparent enzymatic activity but contains a Ras association domain, and plays roles in regulation of cell cycle and apoptosis [20]. Aberrant methylation of the *RASSF1A* promoter region is one of the most frequent epigenetic inactivation events detected in human cancer and leads to silencing of *RASSF1A* [21]. In the thyroid, *RASSF1A* promoter methylation was present in more than 30% of benign and malignant thyroid tumors including PTC, FTC, and UTC [22,23]. The high frequency of *RASSF1A* hyper-methylation in both benign follicular adenomas (33% to 44%) and the increased occurrence of this phenomenon in FTC (70% to 100%) suggest that epigenetically silencing of *RASSF1A* is an early step in thyroid tumorigenesis [22–24]. A mutually exclusive relationship between *BRAF* mutation and *RASSF1A* methylation in PTC has been reported, but remains to be verified [22,23].

Also associated with MAPK pathway activation, fibroblast growth factors (FGFs) and FGF receptors (FGFRs) have been implicated in the progression of endocrine neoplasms including thyroid carcinoma [25,26]. FGFs, a family of 23 known heparin-binding proteins, signal through four high-affinity tyrosine kinase receptors, FGFR1 to FGFR4 [25]. Interestingly, tumor-suppressor properties of FGFR2 and its epigenetic down-regulation in thyroid cancers have been reported [26,27]. FGFR1, which is expressed mainly in neoplastic thyroid cells, propagates MAPK activation and promotes tumor progression [27]. In contrast, the FGFR2-IIIb isoform is expressed mainly in normal epithelial thyroid cells, but is significantly down-regulated in neoplastic cells. CpG methylation is associated with silencing of FGFR2 in thyroid cancer cells, and administration of the demethylating agent 5'-Aza-dc restores FGFR2 protein expression in those cells [6,27]. This reexpression of FGFR2-IIIb competes with FGFR1 for the adaptor immediate substrate FRS2 to impede signaling upstream of the RAS/BRAF/MAPK pathway, and also inhibits invasiveness of thyroid cancer cells [27].

Tumor cells are held together by direct cell-cell contact and by adhesion to the extracellular matrix. Loss of adhesion is considered to promote tumor invasiveness and increase the metastatic potential of thyroid carcinomas [28]. Cadherins belong to a family of single-transmembrane-calcium-dependent cell-cell adhesion molecules. There are three classical Cadherins: neuronal (N)-, placental (P)-, and epithelial (E)-cadherin. E-cadherin/*CDH1* is highly expressed in normal thyroid follicular cells. Expression of E-cadherin is maintained in some well-differentiated thyroid carcinomas, but is extremely low in undifferentiated thyroid carcinomas [29–31]. Silencing of E-cadherin is not likely to be attributable to intragenic mutation, since somatic mutations of *CDH1* are infrequent in thyroid carcinomas [32]. Instead, DNA methylation of the *CDH1* promoter is a more likely explanation for the down-regulation of this adhesion factor [33].

Epigenetic dysregulation of tumor-promoting genes

Tumor-promoting genes may also be deregulated in thyroid carcinoma cells through epigenetic mechanisms. One such example is reflected by the cancertestis/melanoma- associated antigens MAGE-A3/6. MAGE-A3/6 antigens are members of the MAGE-I family that includes the MAGE-A, -B, and -C subfamilies [34]. The MAGE-I family consists of a number of chromosome X-clustered genes, which are expressed mainly in testicular germ cells, placenta, and various malignant tumors. This feature provides the basis for the designation as "cancer/testis antigens" [34,35]. In the thyroid, MAGE-A3/6 is up-regulated in malignant tissues and carcinoma cell lines, and is silenced in normal thyroid tissues with CpG hyper-methylation of MAGE-A3/6 [1,36]. Although their function in thyroid cancer remains to be elucidated, tumor-promoting properties of MAGE-A3/6 have been reported. MAGE-A3/6-specific small interfering RNA suppresses growth of mast cells in vitro and in vivo in a murine model of mastcytosis [37]. MAGE-A3/6 targets wild-type p53 transactivation through HDAC recruitment, and suppresses apoptosis of human cancer cells [38,39]. Restrictive expression of MAGE-A3/6 suggests a putative therapeutic target for thyroid cancer. Interestingly, FGF7/FGFR2-IIIb signal activation results in histone H3 methylation and deacetylation of the same histone mark associated with the MAGE-A3/6 promoter to down-regulate gene expression in thyroid carcinoma [1].

Epigenetics as biomarker and therapeutic targets

The histologic diagnosis of PTC is based on nuclear features defined as "a distinctive set of nuclear characteristics" [40]. However, no one specific feature is absolutely diagnostic of PTC. In addition, considerable interobserver variation has been pointed out in the diagnosis of follicular lesions including follicular adenoma, FTC, and follicular variant of PTC [41,42]. Therefore, biomarkers are clearly needed as ancillary tools to aid in the histologic diagnosis of thyroid tumors. As described above, several molecules that are involved in the pathogenesis of thyroid cancers are epigenetically controlled. Moreover, the frequency of hyper-methylation of these genes is different among histologic subtypes of thyroid tumors. Differences in methylation patterns have emerged as potential biomarkers of thyroid tumors. For example, hyper-methylation of the TSH receptor gene may be a putative diagnostic marker of thyroid malignancy, as it is found in FTC, PTC, and UTC [12]. However, specific CpG methylation characteristic of each histologic subtype has not been found thus far. Similarly, the many targets that have been identified by microarray gene expression profiling [43,44] and immunohistochemical studies [45,46] as differentially expressed in normal and malignant thyroid tissues are likely to be dysregulated by epigenetic mechanisms. Further studies are required to clarify this issue.

Epigenetic regulation is a reversible event that promises to be more amenable to treatment by therapeutic agents. There are two opportunities for epigenetics as therapeutic targets in thyroid carcinoma. One is re-differentiation of cancer cells by restoring thyroid-specific genes for radioiodine therapy. The other is inhibiting tumor cell growth and/or invasiveness by reexpression of tumor-suppressive molecules. Several investigators demonstrated that DNMT inhibitors can be applied for reexpression of transcriptionally silenced genes and restoring thyroid function in carcinoma cells. NIS and TSH receptors are reexpressed by treatment of human thyroid carcinoma cell lines with demethylating agents [12,14,47]. As with DNA methylation, histone modification might be associated with down-regulation of thyroid-hormone-related genes. In the thyroid, HDAC inhibitors have been shown to restore the ability of radioiodide uptake and retention in poorly differentiated and undifferentiated carcinoma cells by reexpression of the NIS, TPO, and thyroglobulin genes [48–50]. These experimental studies provide future clinical applications of DNMT inhibitors and/or HDAC inhibitors in thyroid cancer patients who might otherwise not respond to radioiodide therapy.

Growth inhibition properties of HDAC inhibitors have been implicated. Several studies revealed HDAC inhibitors cause inhibition of cancer cell growth via cell cycle arrest and subsequent apoptosis with increase of CDK inhibitors in several human cancers [51–53]. In the thyroid, HDAC inhibitors suppress growth of human carcinoma cell lines including those with defects in the p53/*TP53* pathway, and induce caspase-mediated apoptosis with elevation of CDK inhibitors p21CIP1 and p27KIP1 [54–56]. Since p27KIP1 is a key modulator of metastatic potential of PTCs, HDAC inhibition for restoring p27KIP1 is a rational approach for thyroid carcinomas [18,57–59].

DNA methylation has a dominant effect on histone deacetylation. Analysis in vivo demonstrated that initial treatment with DNA methylation inhibitors, followed by HDAC inhibitors, can produce additive or synergistic effects for re-expression of transcriptionally silenced genes [60]. The combination usage of methylation inhibitors and HDAC inhibitors needs to be further investigated for effective application as an anti–thyroid cancer therapy.

Summary

Although aberrant MAPK signaling through genetic alterations is important in thyroid cell transformation, epigenetic events are emerging as significant contributors to carcinogenesis and tumor progression. This is particularly relevant in thyroid carcinomas that show a wide range of biological behaviors from indolence to highly aggressive, invasive, and metastatic cancers. Indeed, epigenetic silencing of growth inhibitory proteins can in some cases override the growth-promoting effects of activated oncogenes that represent early and frequent events in thyroid cancers [15]. However, the molecular mechanisms regulating epigenetic alterations are still unclear. The challenge will be to clarify the modifying factors that affect the epigenetic environment, and the relationships between genetic and epigenetic dysregulation.

Epigenetic dysregulation as a therapeutic target is becoming the new frontier for anti-cancer therapy in thyroid oncology. DNA methylation inhibitors and/or HDAC inhibitors induce reexpression of aberrantly silenced genes, resulting in growth arrest, apoptosis, and re-differentiation of thyroid carcinoma cells. Indeed, these agents have shown clinical activity in the treatment of certain human malignancies where tumor-suppressor genes are silenced through epigenetic mechanisms [61]. In the near future, the therapeutic application of these agents may provide new and effective options for patients with thyroid cancer.

References

[1] Kondo T, Zhu X, Asa SL, et al. The cancer/testis antigen melanoma-associated antigen-A3/A6 is a novel target of fibroblast growth factor receptor 2-IIIb through histone H3 modifications in thyroid cancer. Clin Cancer Res 2007;13:4713–20.

[2] Ozawa H, Iwatsuki K. Pharmacological properties of heterocyclic amidine derivatives. II. Pharmacological studies of phenylguanylpiperazine derivatives. Chem Pharm Bull (Tokyo) 1968;16:2482–7.

[3] Xing M. Gene methylation in thyroid tumorigenesis. Endocrinology 2007;148:948–53.

[4] Esteller M. Epigenetic gene silencing in cancer: the DNA hypermethylome. Hum Mol Genet 2007;16(Spec No 1):R50–9.

[5] Feinberg AP, Vogelstein B. Hypomethylation distinguishes genes of some human cancers from their normal counterparts. Nature 1983;301:89–92.

[6] Zhu X, Lee K, Asa SL, et al. Epigenetic silencing through DNA and histone methylation of fibroblast growth factor receptor 2 in neoplastic pituitary cells. Am J Pathol 2007;170:1618–28.

[7] Fabbro D, Di Loreto C, Beltrami CA, et al. Expression of thyroid-specific transcription factors TTF-1 and PAX-8 in human thyroid neoplasms. Cancer Res 1994;54:4744–9.

[8] Gerard AC, Daumerie C, Mestdagh C, et al. Correlation between the loss of thyroglobulin iodination and the expression of thyroid-specific proteins involved in iodine metabolism in thyroid carcinomas. J Clin Endocrinol Metab 2003;88:4977–83.

[9] Kondo T, Nakamura N, Suzuki K, et al. Expression of human pendrin in diseased thyroids. J Histochem Cytochem 2003;51:167–73.

[10] Mizukami Y, Hashimoto T, Nonomura A, et al. Immunohistochemical demonstration of thyrotropin (TSH)-receptor in normal and diseased human thyroid tissues using monoclonal antibody against recombinant human TSH-receptor protein. J Clin Endocrinol Metab 1994; 79:616–9.

[11] Maxon HR, Thomas SR, Hertzberg VS, et al. Relation between effective radiation dose and outcome of radioiodine therapy for thyroid cancer. N Engl J Med 1983;309:937–41.

[12] Xing M, Usadel H, Cohen Y, et al. Methylation of the thyroid-stimulating hormone receptor gene in epithelial thyroid tumors: a marker of malignancy and a cause of gene silencing. Cancer Res 2003;63:2316–21.

[13] Neumann S, Schuchardt K, Reske A, et al. Lack of correlation for sodium iodide symporter mRNA and protein expression and analysis of sodium iodide symporter promoter methylation in benign cold thyroid nodules. Thyroid 2004;14:99–111.

[14] Venkataraman GM, Yatin M, Marcinek R, et al. Restoration of iodide uptake in dedifferentiated thyroid carcinoma: relationship to human Na+/I-symporter gene methylation status. J Clin Endocrinol Metab 1999;84:2449–57.

[15] Kondo T, Ezzat S, Asa SL. Pathogenetic mechanisms in thyroid follicular-cell neoplasia. Nat Rev Cancer 2006;6:292–306.

[16] Durante C, Puxeddu E, Ferretti E, et al. BRAF mutations in papillary thyroid carcinomas inhibit genes involved in iodine metabolism. J Clin Endocrinol Metab 2007;92:2840–3.

[17] Liu D, Hu S, Hou P, et al. Suppression of BRAF/MEK/MAP kinase pathway restores expression of iodide-metabolizing genes in thyroid cells expressing the V600E BRAF mutant. Clin Cancer Res 2007;13:1341–9.

[18] Khoo ML, Beasley NJ, Ezzat S, et al. Overexpression of cyclin D1 and underexpression of p27 predict lymph node metastases in papillary thyroid carcinoma. J Clin Endocrinol Metab 2002;87:1814–8.

[19] Elisei R, Shiohara M, Koeffler HP, et al. Genetic and epigenetic alterations of the cyclin-dependent kinase inhibitors p15INK4b and p16INK4a in human thyroid carcinoma cell lines and primary thyroid carcinomas. Cancer 1998;83:2185–93.

[20] Donninger H, Vos MD, Clark GJ. The RASSF1A tumor suppressor. J Cell Sci 2007;120:3163–72.

[21] Dammann R, Schagdarsurengin U, Strunnikova M, et al. Epigenetic inactivation of the Ras-association domain family 1 (RASSF1A) gene and its function in human carcinogenesis. Histol Histopathol 2003;18:665–77.

[22] Nakamura N, Carney JA, Jin L, et al. RASSF1A and NORE1A methylation and BRAFV600E mutations in thyroid tumors. Lab Invest 2005;85:1065–75.

[23] Xing M, Cohen Y, Mambo E, et al. Early occurrence of RASSF1A hypermethylation and its mutual exclusion with BRAF mutation in thyroid tumorigenesis. Cancer Res 2004;64:1664–8.

[24] Schagdarsurengin U, Gimm O, Hoang-Vu C, et al. Frequent epigenetic silencing of the CpG island promoter of RASSF1A in thyroid carcinoma. Cancer Res 2002;62:3698–701.

[25] Ezzat S, Asa SL. FGF receptor signaling at the crossroads of endocrine homeostasis and tumorigenesis. Horm Metab Res 2005;37:355–60.

[26] St Bernard R, Zheng L, Liu W, et al. Fibroblast growth factor receptors as molecular targets in thyroid carcinoma. Endocrinology 2005;146:1145–53.

[27] Kondo T, Zheng L, Liu W, et al. Epigenetically controlled fibroblast growth factor receptor 2 signaling imposes on the RAS/BRAF/mitogen-activated protein kinase pathway to modulate thyroid cancer progression. Cancer Res 2007;67:5461–70.

[28] Liu W, Wei W, Winer D, et al. CEACAM1 impedes thyroid cancer growth but promotes invasiveness: a putative mechanism for early metastases. Oncogene 2007;26:2747–58.

[29] Brabant G, Hoang-Vu C, Cetin Y, et al. E-cadherin: a differentiation marker in thyroid malignancies. Cancer Res 1993;53:4987–93.

[30] Kato N, Tsuchiya T, Tamura G, et al. E-cadherin expression in follicular carcinoma of the thyroid. Pathol Int 2002;52:13–8.

[31] Scheumann GF, Hoang-Vu C, Cetin Y, et al. Clinical significance of E-cadherin as a prognostic marker in thyroid carcinomas. J Clin Endocrinol Metab 1995;80:2168–72.

[32] Soares P, Berx G, van Roy F, et al. E-cadherin gene alterations are rare events in thyroid tumors. Int J Cancer 1997;70:32–8.

[33] Rocha AS, Soares P, Seruca R, et al. Abnormalities of the E-cadherin/catenin adhesion complex in classical papillary thyroid carcinoma and in its diffuse sclerosing variant. J Pathol 2001;194:358–66.

[34] Xiao J, Chen HS. Biological functions of melanoma-associated antigens. World J Gastroenterol 2004;10:1849–53.

[35] van der BP, Traversari C, Chomez P, et al. A gene encoding an antigen recognized by cytolytic T lymphocytes on a human melanoma. Science 1991;254:1643–7.

[36] Milkovic M, Sarcevic B, Glavan E. Expression of MAGE tumor-associated antigen in thyroid carcinomas. Endocr Pathol 2006;17:45–52.

[37] Yang B, O'Herrin S, Wu J, et al. Select cancer testes antigens of the MAGE-A, -B, and -C families are expressed in mast cell lines and promote cell viability in vitro and in vivo. J Invest Dermatol 2007;127:267–75.

[38] Monte M, Simonatto M, Peche LY, et al. MAGE-A tumor antigens target p53 transactivation function through histone deacetylase recruitment and confer resistance to chemotherapeutic agents. Proc Natl Acad Sci U S A 2006;103:11160–5.

[39] Yang B, O'Herrin SM, Wu J, et al. MAGE-A, mMage-b, and MAGE-C proteins form complexes with KAP1 and suppress p53-dependent apoptosis in MAGE-positive cell lines. Cancer Res 2007;67:9954–62.

[40] DeLellis RA, Lloyd RV, Heitz PU, et al. Pathology and genetics of tumours of endocrine organs. WHO classification of tumours. Lyons (France): IARC Press; 2004.

[41] Hirokawa M, Carney JA, Goellner JR, et al. Observer variation of encapsulated follicular lesions of the thyroid gland. Am J Surg Pathol 2002;26:1508–14.

[42] Lloyd RV, Erickson LA, Casey MB, et al. Observer variation in the diagnosis of follicular variant of papillary thyroid carcinoma. Am J Surg Pathol 2004;28:1336–40.

[43] Huang Y, Prasad M, Lemon WJ, et al. Gene expression in papillary thyroid carcinoma reveals highly consistent profiles. Proc Natl Acad Sci U S A 2001;98:15044–9.

[44] Wasenius VM, Hemmer S, Kettunen E, et al. Hepatocyte growth factor receptor, matrix metalloproteinase-11, tissue inhibitor of metalloproteinase-1, and fibronectin are up-regulated in papillary thyroid carcinoma: a cDNA and tissue microarray study. Clin Cancer Res 2003;9:68–75.

[45] Cheung CC, Ezzat S, Freeman JL, et al. Immunohistochemical diagnosis of papillary thyroid carcinoma. Mod Pathol 2001;14:338–42.

[46] Prasad ML, Pellegata NS, Huang Y, et al. Galectin-3, fibronectin-1, CITED-1, HBME1 and cytokeratin-19 immunohistochemistry is useful for the differential diagnosis of thyroid tumors. Mod Pathol 2005;18:48–57.

[47] Tuncel M, Aydin D, Yaman E, et al. The comparative effects of gene modulators on thyroid-specific genes and radioiodine uptake. Cancer Biother Radiopharm 2007;22:281–8.

[48] Furuya F, Shimura H, Suzuki H, et al. Histone deacetylase inhibitors restore radioiodide uptake and retention in poorly differentiated and anaplastic thyroid cancer cells by expression of the sodium/iodide symporter thyroperoxidase and thyroglobulin. Endocrinology 2004;145:2865–75.

[49] Kitazono M, Robey R, Zhan Z, et al. Low concentrations of the histone deacetylase inhibitor, depsipeptide (FR901228), increase expression of the $Na(+)/I(-)$ symporter and iodine accumulation in poorly differentiated thyroid carcinoma cells. J Clin Endocrinol Metab 2001;86:3430–5.

[50] Zarnegar R, Brunaud L, Kanauchi H, et al. Increasing the effectiveness of radioactive iodine therapy in the treatment of thyroid cancer using Trichostatin A, a histone deacetylase inhibitor. Surgery 2002;132:984–90.

[51] Park WH, Jung CW, Park JO, et al. Trichostatin inhibits the growth of ACHN renal cell carcinoma cells via cell cycle arrest in association with p27, or apoptosis. Int J Oncol 2003;22:1129–34.

[52] Platta CS, Greenblatt DY, Kunnimalaiyaan M, et al. The HDAC inhibitor trichostatin A inhibits growth of small cell lung cancer cells. J Surg Res 2007;142:219–26.

[53] Wang ZM, Hu J, Zhou D, et al. Trichostatin A inhibits proliferation and induces expression of p21WAF and p27 in human brain tumor cell lines. Ai Zheng 2002;21:1100–5.

[54] Greenberg VL, Williams JM, Boghaert E, et al. Butyrate alters the expression and activity of cell cycle components in anaplastic thyroid carcinoma cells. Thyroid 2001;11:21–9.

[55] Greenberg VL, Williams JM, Cogswell JP, et al. Histone deacetylase inhibitors promote apoptosis and differential cell cycle arrest in anaplastic thyroid cancer cells. Thyroid 2001;11:315–25.

[56] Mitsiades CS, Poulaki V, McMullan C, et al. Novel histone deacetylase inhibitors in the treatment of thyroid cancer. Clin Cancer Res 2005;11:3958–65.

[57] Dackiw AP, Ezzat S, Huang P, et al. Vitamin D3 administration induces nuclear p27 accumulation, restores differentiation, and reduces tumor burden in a mouse model of metastatic follicular thyroid cancer. Endocrinology 2004;145:5840–6.

[58] Khoo ML, Freeman JL, Witterick IJ, et al. Underexpression of p27/Kip in thyroid papillary microcarcinomas with gross metastatic disease. Arch Otolaryngol Head Neck Surg 2002; 128:253–7.

[59] Liu W, Asa SL, Fantus IG, et al. Vitamin D arrests thyroid carcinoma cell growth and induces p27 dephosphorylation and accumulation through pten/akt-dependent and–independent pathways. Am J Pathol 2002;160:511–9.

[60] Wischnewski F, Pantel K, Schwarzenbach H. Promoter demethylation and histone acetylation mediate gene expression of MAGE-A1, -A2, -A3, and -A12 in human cancer cells. Mol Cancer Res 2006;4:339–49.

[61] Appleton K, Mackay HJ, Judson I, et al. Phase I and pharmacodynamic trial of the DNA methyltransferase inhibitor decitabine and carboplatin in solid tumors. J Clin Oncol 2007; 25:4603–9.

ELSEVIER
SAUNDERS

Endocrinol Metab Clin N Am
37 (2008) 401–417

ENDOCRINOLOGY
AND METABOLISM
CLINICS
OF NORTH AMERICA

Sonographic Imaging of Thyroid Nodules and Cervical Lymph Nodes

Stephanie A. Fish, MD[a], Jill E. Langer, MD[b],
Susan J. Mandel, MD, MPH[a],*

[a]Department of Medicine, University of Pennsylvania School of Medicine, 1 Maloney,
Endocrinology, HUP, 3400 Spruce Street, Philadelphia, PA 19104, USA
[b]Department of Radiology, University of Pennsylvania School of Medicine, Penn Tower,
Ground Floor, 300 South 33rd Street, Philadelphia, PA 19104, USA

The initial application of sonography for the evaluation of the neck, more than 30 years ago, was to differentiate cystic and solid thyroid nodules. With improvements in technology, ultrasound has been applied to characterize distinct features in the appearance of thyroid nodules. More recently, its function has been expanded to assess cervical lymph nodes for metastatic thyroid cancer. This review discusses the sonographic features of thyroid nodules associated with malignancy and the role of ultrasound in the management of patients with thyroid cancer.

Ultrasound imaging of thyroid nodules

When examined by ultrasound, rather than by palpation, thyroid nodules are commonly detected with a prevalence of 40% to 50% in the general population [1]. However, only 5% to 10% of thyroid nodules are malignant, even if found incidentally [2,3]. While fine-needle aspiration (FNA) is the cornerstone of the evaluation of thyroid nodules, ultrasound contributes significantly both to identify and to evaluate thyroid nodules. Multiple reports have examined the sonographic features of thyroid nodules as predictors of malignancy [2–12]. Table 1 lists the reported sensitivities and specificities of these features from 11 studies that analyzed over 100 nodules. Unfortunately, there is significant variability among these studies because of differing methodologies and because report of ultrasound features is highly operator

* Corresponding author. Division of Endocrinology, Diabetes, and Metabolism, 700 CRB, 415 Curie Blvd., Philadelphia, PA 19104.
  E-mail address: smandel@mail.med.upenn.edu (S.J. Mandel).

0889-8529/08/$ - see front matter © 2008 Elsevier Inc. All rights reserved.
doi:10.1016/j.ecl.2007.12.003

Table 1
Reported sensitivities and specificities of sonographic characteristics for detection of thyroid cancer

	Median sensitivity (range)	Median specificity (range)
Microcalcifications [3–5,7,10–12]	52% (26%–73%)	83% (69%–96%)
Absence of halo [4,8–10,12]	66% (46%–100%)	54% (30%–72%)
Irregular margins [2–6,9,12]	55% (17%–77%)	79% (63%–85%)
Hypoechoic [2–10,12]	81% (49%–90%)	53% (36%–66%)
Increased intranodular flow [2,5,7,10,12]	67% (57%–74%)	81% (49%–89%)

dependent [13]. However, there are certain ultrasound features that have been consistently associated with malignancy, including hypoechogenicity, increased vascularity, microcalcifications, irregular margins, and the absence of a halo.

The echogenicity of a thyroid nodule refers to its brightness relative to the normal thyroid parenchyma, which is homogeneously hyperechoic compared with the surrounding strap muscles of the neck (Figs. 1 and 2). Hypoechoic nodules are darker than the surrounding normal thyroid tissue and this finding is associated with malignancy (see Fig. 1A and Fig. 2A) [2–10,12]. This appearance is thought to result from the increased cellularity and cellular compaction seen in papillary thyroid cancer. In contrast, a follicular neoplasm, either a benign follicular adenoma or follicular carcinoma, is composed of small microfollicles with variable amounts of colloid. Therefore, the echogenicity of follicular carcinomas may depend on the colloid content that images as more hyperechoic (see Fig. 1B) [14]. Although echogenicity may appear to be a robust observation, the interobserver reproducibility is only moderate [13]. Nodule echogenicity is challenging to classify in two situations. First, the extranodular thyroid may be affected by

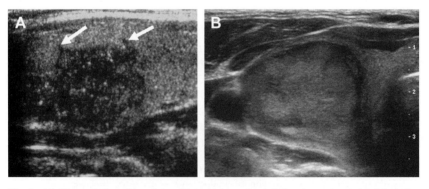

Fig. 1. (A) Hypoechoic solid nodule with irregular, microlobulated margins (microlobulation noted by arrows). Microcalcifications are present as the punctate white spots in the hypoechoic solid nodule. This was a papillary thyroid cancer. (B) Isoechoic solid nodule with a thick, irregular halo. No calcifications are present. This was a follicular cancer.

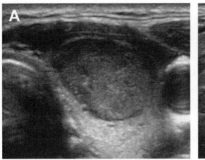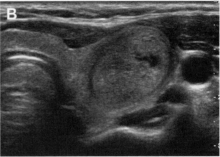

Fig. 2. (*A*) Hypoechoic solid nodule with a regular margin. A thin halo is noted posteriorly. This was a benign nodule. (*B*) Isoechoic nodule with a central cystic area. This nodule has a regular margin and is surrounded by a smooth, thin halo. This was a benign nodule.

Hashimoto's thyroiditis and therefore have a more heterogeneous appearance, making classification of the nodule's echogenicity more difficult. Second, one third of nodules are more than 25% cystic, and an additional quarter of nodules are up to 25% cystic [15]. Therefore, 55% of nodules have some cystic composition, which requires identification of the solid component to determine echogenicity.

The vascularity of a thyroid nodule is demonstrated with color flow Doppler (CFD) or power Doppler (PD) imaging. CFD is a measure of the directional component of the velocity of blood moving through the sample volume. The technical shortcomings of CFD include interference by noise and dependence on the angle of the probe. PD imaging is relatively independent of the angle of the probe and the sound beam and noise can be assigned to a homogeneous background rather than appearing as random color [7]. Since PD does not reflect directional flow, it is more sensitive for the detection of flow in small vessels. Nodule vascularity is categorized as absent, perinodular, or intranodular. Using PD, some authors have further subdivided intranodular flow into regular versus chaotic patterns [7]. Increased intranodular flow is associated with malignancy [2,4,5,7,10] and has good interobserver variability [13].

Calcifications are present in up to 30% of thyroid nodules. Microcalcifications image as echogenic foci smaller than 2 mm and are associated with malignancy (see Fig. 1A). The interobserver variability for the identification of microcalcifications is very good [13]. Microcalcifications are thought to represent aggregates of psammoma bodies, the laminated spherical concretions characteristic of many papillary cancers, and are rarely found in benign nodules or follicular neoplastic lesions [14,16]. Coarse or dense calcifications are larger than 2 mm and cause posterior acoustic shadowing. These dystrophic calcifications occur in both benign and malignant lesions in areas of fibrosis, tissue degeneration, and necrosis. Coarse calcifications may be associated with malignancy when they appear with microcalcifications or in the center of a hypoechoic nodule [12,17]. Peripheral calcifications surround a thyroid nodule and were once thought to indicate a benign process. However, this finding can be seen in malignant nodules [16], sometimes with interruption of the circumferential calcific rim that suggests malignant invasion of thyroid parenchyma.

The margins of a thyroid nodule can be regular and well defined (see Fig. 2) or irregular and microlobulated (see Fig. 1A). Interobserver variability for classification of nodule borders is the greatest of all sonographic features [13] and, thus, has limited utility. Irregular margins are seen with invasion of a malignant nodule into the surrounding thyroid parenchyma, eg, an unencapsulated papillary cancer. The irregular margin is less commonly observed with encapsulated follicular or Hürthle cell cancers [14].

A halo was first described as a thin hypoechoic rim that surrounds a nodule and is thought to represent compression of the extranodular blood vessels as a benign nodule slowly grows (see Fig. 2) [8–10,12]. An invasive malignancy, such as unencapsulated papillary cancer or medullary cancer, lacks a halo. However, follicular and Hürthle cell adenomas and cancers are generally surrounded by a fibrous avascular capsule. This capsule images sonographically as a thick, irregular hypoechoic rim, which is now recognized as a more worrisome, second type of halo (see Fig. 1B) [7]. In a recent study contrasting sonographic features of papillary versus follicular cancers, hypoechoic rims were demonstrated more frequently for follicular cancers (87%) rather than for papillary cancers (26%, $P < .05$) (see Fig. 1) [14].

There are several additional sonographic features of thyroid nodules that have been shown to be associated with malignancy in small studies, but these require further validation. First, two series have evaluated the shape of the nodule by looking at the ratio of the anteroposterior to transverse diameter (A/T). When the A/T ratio is greater than 1.0, indicating a spherical nodule, Cappelli and colleagues [5] found that this detected thyroid cancer with a sensitivity of 84% and a specificity of 82%. This is significantly higher than the sensitivity (33%) reported by the only other investigation of this feature [11]. Second, a recent study from Italy examined tissue stiffness as a risk factor for malignancy in a subset of nodules with indeterminate cytology using a technique called elastography. High elasticity scores, indicating stiffness, were found in 6 of 7 patients with malignant histology, and low scores in all 25 patients with benign lesions [18]. Finally, extrathyroidal invasion may be occasionally seen when the tumor growth extends through either the anterior or posterior thyroid capsule, which normally appears as a bright white outline surrounding the thyroid. In such instances, the margin of the tumor has an ill-defined edge that interrupts this capsule [19].

Because individual sonographic features have limited utility in predicting malignancy, some series have explored the association of combinations of features with cancer risk. In most series, as the specificity of a combination increases, the sensitivity decreases. For example, although fewer than 4% of benign nodules are hypoechoic with microcalcifications, only 26% to 31% of thyroid cancers will have this appearance [2,3,10]. Therefore, many

thyroid cancers would be missed if only the hypoechoic nodules with microcalcifications underwent FNA. The combination of sonographic features
that maximizes sensitivity and specificity is a solid, hypoechoic nodule, which
identifies approximately 70% of all cancers, but still describes the appearance
of 30% of benign nodules [3,6,9]. Additionally, as many as 66% of papillary
thyroid cancers have at least one sonographic feature not typically associated
with malignancy and 69% of benign nodules have one sonographic predictor
of malignancy [13,20].

Furthermore, as discussed previously, some of the variability associated
with the reported sensitivities of individual sonographic features for prediction of thyroid malignancy may depend on the histology of the thyroid
cancer. Papillary thyroid cancers are more likely to be solid, hypoechoic,
and lack a halo compared with follicular thyroid cancers. Follicular
cancers most commonly have a halo (90%), which is irregular (60%),
and are iso- to hyperechoic [14]. Therefore, it is critical to recognize that
ultrasound does not replace FNA cytology, rather the two modalities are
complementary.

Information obtained from sonography may be useful in two clinical situations. First, for nodules smaller than 1.5 cm where the cost-benefit analysis
of FNA is unclear, decision making for FNA based on suspicious sonographic features of hypoechogenicity, microcalcifications, irregular margins,
or increased vascularity is superior to using an arbitrary size cut-off of larger
than 1 cm [2,6]. In hypoechoic, solid small nodules, with or without microcalcifications, it is critical to examine the ipsilateral cervical lymph nodes
for metastases (see "Ultrasound imaging of normal and metastatic lymph
nodes"). If an abnormal lymph node is present, it is this lymph node that
should be targeted for FNA. From a series evaluating risks of recurrence
in patients with micropapillary thyroid cancer, patients with sonographically
or clinically detected abnormal lymph nodes have a higher chance of recurrence compared with those with confined intrathyroidal tumors [21]. Second,
if multiple thyroid nodules are present as potential candidates for FNA,
sonographic appearance can assist in nodule selection. For example, FNA
would be first performed for a 1.2-cm hypoechoic solid vascular nodule,
even in the presence of a large 4.1-cm complex nonvascular nodule.

Lymph nodes

In addition to providing excellent imaging for thyroid nodules, high-
frequency (10 to 14 MHz) ultrasound transducers allow for high-resolution
imaging of small anatomic structures such as cervical lymph nodes. Of the
approximately 800 lymph nodes in the human body, about 300 are located
in the neck, varying in size from 3 to 30 mm [22]. Most neck lymph nodes
are located superficially and are accessible to ultrasound imaging. Because
of the frequent metastatic involvement of these lymph nodes by differentiated
thyroid cancer (DTC), specifically papillary or Hürthle cell, their sonographic

examination is intrinsic to the care of these patients. For DTC patients, ultrasound provides an inexpensive and available means both to evaluate the lateral cervical lymph nodes before thyroidectomy and to monitor for recurrence in the central and lateral compartment lymph nodes and in the thyroid bed. In addition, ultrasound can also be a complementary modality in the surveillance of medullary thyroid cancer.

Classification of lymph nodes

Until the early 1990s, cervical lymph node classification was based on anatomic location, with the anterior nodal groups labeled as submental, submandibular, internal jugular, supraclavicular, posterior triangle, and parotid [23]. This classification was cumbersome and a better topographic classification was adapted to aide in mapping nodal surgical intervention. The most widely used classification is based on recommendations by the American Joint Committee on Cancer and the American Academy of Otolaryngology-Head and Neck Surgery and uses landmarks from cross-sectional anatomic imaging (Fig. 3) [22]. The lateral compartment neck nodes (levels II through IV) are found around the jugulocarotid vascular bundle and may be under the sternocleidomastoid muscle. Level II lymph nodes are located above the level of the hyoid bone to the base of the skull; level III nodes are between the levels of the hyoid bone and the cricoid cartilage; and level IV nodes are below the level of the cricoid cartilage extending to the clavicle. Level V includes the transverse cervical chain and posterior triangle lymph nodes. The central compartment or anterior neck lymph nodes, level VI, are located posterior and inferior to the thyroid gland, adjacent to the trachea and esophagus. This compartment, which is bordered laterally by the medial carotid sheaths, extends superiorly to the hyoid bone and inferiorly to the sternal notch. The level VII lymph nodes are the superior mediastinal lymph nodes, a portion of which may be imaged by ultrasound if the patient's neck is hyperextended. This bicompartmental approach to examination of the neck lymph nodes, lateral versus central, has clinical relevance in the evaluation and selection of the optimal surgical procedure as well as in the prognosis for thyroid cancer. This classification can be adapted to sonographic evaluation of lymph nodes. All of the necessary landmarks can be either imaged sonographically or palpated, with the exception of the hyoid bone whose location can be inferred.

Ultrasound protocol for lymph node evaluation

For imaging the cervical neck lymph nodes, a hyperextended neck position facilitates visualization of the low level IV and VI lymph nodes and a pillow may be placed under the patient's neck for support. The procedure for examining the lateral compartment regions of the neck is to orient the transducer in the transverse plane. The transducer is placed over the submandibular

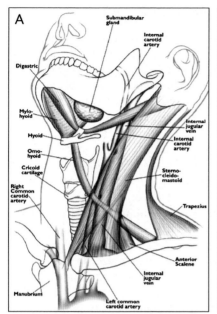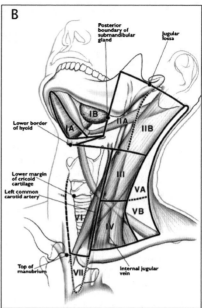

Fig. 3. (*A*) Note the anatomic landmarks that are used to divide the lateral and central lymph node compartments into Levels I to VI. (*B*) Lymph node mapping by levels, based on cross-sectional imaging. However, lymph node mapping can be approximated by sonographic imaging and knowledge of the necessary anatomic landmarks. (*From* Som PM, Curtin HD, Mancuso AA. An imaging-based classification for the cervical nodes designed as an adjunct to recent clinically based nodal classifications. Arch Otolaryngol Head Neck Surg 1999;125:388–96; with permission. Copyright © 1999, Massachusetts Medical Society. All rights reserved.)

gland and then moved inferiorly along the external carotid artery to the bifurcation of the common carotid artery. It is then centered over the jugulocarotid sheath and moved inferiorly until the carotid is visualized joining the subclavian artery on the right or disappears under the clavicle to enter the aortic arch on the left. The supraclavicular fossa and posterior triangle of the neck (level V) are then examined by moving the probe laterally along the supraclavicular region and then posteriorly and superiorly to the mastoid region along the course of the imputed track of the spinal accessory nerve, which approximates the posterior edge of the sternocleidomastoid muscle [23]. For imaging the central neck, the transducer is placed in transverse orientation above the tracheal cartilage at the approximate level of the hyoid bone and moved inferiorly along the anterior border of the trachea to the sternal notch. The more focused examination of the left and right paratracheal regions requires centering the probe between the trachea and respective carotid artery just inferior to the tracheal cartilage and scanning inferiorly to the sternal notch. Longitudinal imaging should be performed for any identified abnormal lymph node.

Ultrasound imaging of normal and metastatic lymph nodes

Normal lymph node morphology is characterized by a connective tissue capsule surrounding an outer cortex with the densely packed lymphocytes forming lymphoid follicles and an inner medulla containing the blood vessels, lymphatic sinuses, and connective tissue that provide guidance for the blood vessels to the more peripheral regions of the lymph node. The main artery to the lymph node enters at this central hilus and subsequently branches into smaller arterioles as it flows to the cortex (Fig. 4) [24]. A recent report of ultrasound examination of cervical lymph nodes in 1000 healthy volunteers documented the presence of one or more normal lymph nodes in almost 70% of subjects. The frequency of lymph node detection did not vary based on age, gender, or even recent infection [25].

Therefore, since detection of normal cervical lymph nodes is common and thyroid cancer often metastasizes to these same lymph nodes, it is essential to appreciate the different imaging characteristics of benign and malignant lymph nodes. The evaluated parameters should include size, shape, presence of an echogenic hilus and a hypoechoic cortex, vascularity, and other aspects of echogenicity, including cystic change and calcifications [23,24,26].

The size of normal lymph nodes may vary depending on neck region, with submandibular or level II lymph nodes tending to be larger, perhaps due to reactive hyperplasia from repeated oral cavity inflammation. Furthermore, thyroid cancer patients with radioiodine-induced sialadenitis may also develop large hyperplastic level II lymph nodes found in the submandibular and parotid regions. Large reactive lymph nodes in this area may exhibit a long axis measurement of up to 18 mm [27]. The short axis diameter varies less and the maximal short axis for a normal lymph node is reported to be 8 mm in level II and less than 5 mm in the other cervical regions [23,25].

The shape of a lymph node is assessed in numerical terms by the short-to-long axis ratio (S:L). A normal lymph node is oval, which translates into an S:L less than 0.5. Since neoplastic infiltration of a lymph node begins

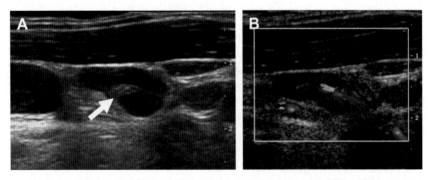

Fig. 4. (*A*) Normal lymph node. Note hypoechoic cortex and central hyperechoic fatty hilus (*arrow*). This lymph node has an oval shape. (*B*) Color flow Doppler imaging of this normal lymph node detects hilar vascularity.

in the cortex, malignant lymph nodes generally have a larger transverse diameter and a rounder shape, with an S:L of 0.5 or higher [23,24]. A round shape is suggestive of malignancy, but its specificity may depend on the region of the neck (Fig. 5). Submandibular and parotid lymph nodes may be round, as defined by the S:L. Furthermore, round reactive central neck lymph nodes just inferior to the thyroid are often imaged in patients with chronic autoimmune thyroiditis [27].

Sonographic imaging of a normal lymph node demonstrates an echogenic central hilus surrounded by a hypoechoic cortex (see Fig. 4). The echogenic hilus is more commonly present in larger (>5 mm transverse diameter) rather than smaller lymph nodes [23]. The echogenicity reflects two features: intranodal fatty tissue, which becomes more prominent with age, and the presence of intranodal arteries, veins, and lymphatic sinuses presenting acoustic interfaces that reflect sound waves. The likelihood of visualizing the fatty hilus increases with age reflecting the increased fatty deposition. Thyroid cancer metastases to lymph nodes begin with peripheral neoplastic infiltration and subsequent loss of the hypoechoic cortex that may be replaced by a hyperechoic appearance [26]. Early in the nodal invasion by thyroid cancer, the echogenic hilus may be preserved and the malignant cells are apparent as a small peripheral hyperechoic area in the otherwise normal hypoechoic cortex (Fig. 6). As the lymph node is progressively replaced by thyroid cancer, it assumes a more heterogeneous appearance and may demonstrate intranodal calcifications (both in papillary and medullary cancer) (Fig. 7) and cystic necrosis. Because metastatic lymph nodes in levels II to IV are situated adjacent to the carotid and jugular vessels, jugular compression (see Fig. 7) or displacement of the jugular vein from the carotid artery suggests malignancy [28].

Color or power Doppler examination of cervical lymph nodes allows for determination of vascularity patterns. To maximize sensitivity, Doppler settings should use both a low wall filter and a pulse repetition frequency of 850 Hz or lower to allow detection of low-flow vessels. Hilar vascularity

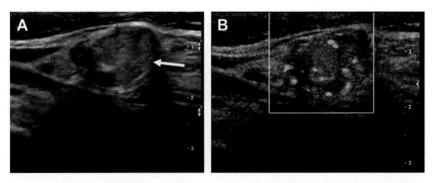

Fig. 5. (*A*) Rounded, hyperechoic metastatic thyroid cancer lymph node (*arrow*). (*B*) Increased vascularity of this lymph node by color flow Doppler.

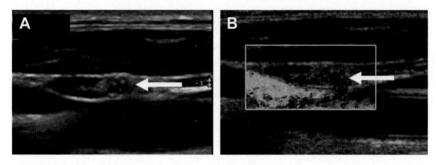

Fig. 6. (*A*) Lymph node that demonstrates involvement by metastatic thyroid cancer in the periphery (*arrow*). Note microcalcifications and hyperechogenicity of this area. However, the fatty hilus is still preserved in unaffected area. (*B*) Increased peripheral vascularity is demonstrated in the area corresponding to the metastatic involvement (*arrow*).

is detected in about 90% of normal lymph nodes with a transverse diameter larger than 5 mm (see Fig. 4B); smaller normal lymph nodes usually appear avascular [29,30]. Capillaries arising from these hilar vessels feed the nodal cortex [24]. Interestingly, the detection rate of hilar vascularity is higher in the elderly, which is thought to be caused by decreased vessel compressibility because of higher vessel stiffness in this group [23]. Furthermore, reactive lymph nodes may have prominent hilar vascularity because of both increased blood flow and vessel diameter [30]. In malignant lymph nodes, the vascular pattern is either peripheral (see Fig. 6B) or diffuse (hilar and peripheral) (see Fig. 5B), often with irregular distribution. The increase in peripheral nodal vascularity occurs because of initial deposition of the malignant cells in the marginal sinuses and the tumor-induced angiogenesis causes subsequent neovascularization. As tumor infiltration proceeds, increased vascularity is apparent throughout the lymph node [30].

Currently, the role of vascular resistance indices for determination of metastatic lymph node involvement is not well defined [26]. However, a recent

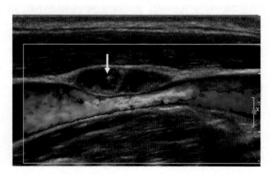

Fig. 7. Longitudinal view of a metastatic lymph node, with microcalcification (*arrow*). Note indentation of jugular vein with compression by the ultrasound transducer.

report demonstrated promising results from sonoelastography to differenti-ate malignant from benign lymph nodes based on their relatively higher tissue stiffness. This technique is relatively time intensive involving over 30 minutes of post–data acquisition analysis [31] and requires further validation; there-fore, its current applicability is limited.

No single sonographic feature is adequately sensitive for detection of lymph nodes with metastatic thyroid cancer. A recent study correlated the sonographic features acquired 4 days preoperatively directly with the histol-ogy of 56 cervical lymph nodes. Some of the most specific criteria were presence of cystic areas (100%), presence of hyperechoic punctations repre-senting either colloid or microcalcifications (100%), and peripheral vascular-ity (82%). Of these, the only one with sufficient sensitivity was peripheral vascularity (86%). All of the others had sensitivities less than 60% and would not be adequate to use as a single criterion for identification of malig-nant involvement [32]. As shown by earlier studies [27,33], the feature with the highest sensitivity was absence of a hilus (100%), but this had a low spec-ificity of only 29%.

Therefore, a reasonable approach to identify suspicious lymph nodes for further investigation would be to submit those without a fatty hilus to a care-ful Doppler examination for evaluation of vascularity. Peripheral or diffuse vascularization is worrisome. However, a rounded shape, an absent hilus, and heterogeneous echogenicity raise the suspicion of malignancy, especially when they coexist in the same lymph node. Last, lymph nodes with cystic change or microcalcifications should be considered as metastatic thyroid cancer. The location of the lymph nodes may also be useful for decision making. The incidence of malignant lymph nodes is much higher in levels III, IV, and VI than in level II [32,33].

Ultrasound-guided fine-needle aspiration

Ultrasound-guided FNA may be used to provide cytologic diagnosis and confirmation of metastatic disease. The reported sensitivities for FNA cytol-ogy range from 80% to 90% [27,34]; however, results may not be diagnostic in patients with cystic lymph nodes or if there is insufficient material in the needle hub. In these situations, the FNA material may be sent for thyroglob-ulin assay (FNA-Tg) by rinsing the needle in 1 mL of normal saline solution. The cut-off for a positive specimen is study specific [27,34,35]. However, each study confirms increased sensitivity (90% to 100%) for detection of thyroid cancer lymph node metastases if the FNA-Tg measurement is com-bined with cytology examination. Importantly, the presence of circulating anti-thyroglobulin antibodies does not invalidate FNA-Tg testing [28,34]. However, FNA-Tg may be undetectable if the malignancy does not itself produce thyroglobulin, such as poorly differentiated or anaplastic thyroid cancer [34]. FNA material may also be assayed for calcitonin if cytology is not revealing in patients with medullary thyroid cancer [36].

Clinical scenarios for ultrasound lymph node evaluation

Pre-thyroidectomy

At initial diagnosis of DTC, up to 30% of patients have clinically detected lymph node metastases [37,38]. However, centers performing routine ipsilateral and central neck dissections have documented lymph node metastases in up to 60% of patients [39–41]. Before thyroidectomy, the thyroid itself limits sonographic visualization of central neck lymph nodes, but level VI lymph nodes inferior to the lower lobes of the thyroid can be assessed. Ultrasound can evaluate the lateral neck compartments. Although the reported sensitivity for sonographic identification of metastatic lymph nodes in this setting may only be about 40% [42], ultrasound-detectable lymphadenopathy is clinically relevant. Sonographically identified lateral metastatic lymph nodes, but not those recognized microscopically only after pathologic examination of the resected specimen, are associated with worse relapse-free and overall survival [38,39]. Importantly, modified lateral neck dissection in these patients with clinical evidence of lateral lymph node metastases improves survival [38]. Hence, it is critical to know if metastatic lymph nodes are present before initial thyroidectomy.

Palpation alone of the lateral neck compartments is not adequate and does not substitute for sonographic evaluation. In a recent series, ultrasound evaluation identified nonpalpable lateral compartment lymph nodes in 14% of patients undergoing initial surgery [43]. Even when lymph nodes were palpable, sonographic assessment of the extent of lymph node involvement altered 40% of the operative procedures by changing the extent of resection [43,44]. Therefore, before thyroidectomy, sonographic evaluation of the lateral compartment and visible central compartment is recommended by the recently published guidelines of the American Thyroid Association and the American Association of Clinical Endocrinologists [45,46].

At the time of initial surgery, localization of metastatic lateral lymph nodes is usually ipsilateral to the primary tumor [40,41]. In fact, if a cancer is unilateral, it is unusual (18%) to have contralateral involvement of the lateral neck compartment [40]. The risk of contralateral lateral compartment lymph node involvement increases if the burden of ipsilateral lymph node involvement is high [40]. The location of the tumor within the thyroid may also influence lymph node spread. Lateral node involvement has been less frequently reported if the cancer is in the lower part of the thyroid lobe.

Surveillance for recurrent differentiated thyroid cancer

The primary goal of follow-up in DTC patients is the early discovery of persistent or recurrent disease. The overall risk of local recurrence of papillary thyroid cancer, either in cervical lymph nodes or in the thyroid bed, is up to 30% [37], but is as high as 25% even in low-risk (Stage I and II) patients [47]. Most recurrences appear in the first decade after initial therapy; however, a small number emerge decades after diagnosis.

In the past, a radioiodine whole-body scan was considered the main tool for disease detection during surveillance, but this has recently been discredited [48]. Three studies have confirmed that whole-body scans fail to identify the presence of metastatic cervical lymph nodes in almost 80% of cases when neck sonography accurately detects these abnormal lymph nodes (Fig. 8). And, for patients with undetectable serum thyroglobulin levels on levothyroxine suppression, the combination of a detectable stimulated serum thyroglobulin level with neck sonography identifies 95% of patients with metastatic lymph nodes and has a negative predictive value of 99% [49–51]. The recently published guidelines for DTC management by the American Thyroid Association support the use of only stimulated thyroglobulin and cervical ultrasound for surveillance of low-risk DTC patients rather than the use of radioiodine scanning [45].

The timing and interval for performance of neck ultrasound depends on the risk status of the patient. The American Thyroid Association DTC guidelines suggest that "cervical ultrasound to evaluate the thyroid bed and central and lateral cervical nodal compartments should be performed at 6 and 12 months and then annually for at least 3–5 years, depending on the patients' risk for recurrent disease and thyroglobulin status" [45]. Hence, if the serum thyroglobulin level remains detectable and other cross-sectional body imaging is negative, cervical ultrasound should continue to be done on regular intervals. However, if the stimulated serum thyroglobulin level is undetectable and a cervical ultrasound is negative, the utility of subsequent ultrasound imaging is low [52].

The distribution of persistent or recurrent lymph node metastases is most commonly the central compartment (35% to 50%), followed by the ipsilateral lateral neck (20% to 30%). Only rarely (8% to 15%) is the contralateral lateral neck compartment involved [41,44]. Within the levels of the lateral neck, a recent study reported that the pattern of metastatic lymph node involvement was approximately 50% for levels II and III, 40% for level IV, and only 20% for level V [53]. Again, palpation is insensitive for detection of recurrent or residual disease and sonographic identification of nonpalpable metastatic lymph nodes alters the extent of surgical resection in up to 70% of patients undergoing reoperation [43,44]. Cervical compartmental resection that is

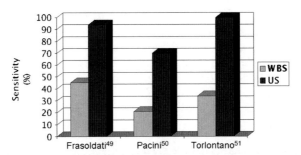

Fig. 8. The reported sensitivities of whole body scans (WBS) and ultrasound (US) for detection of metastatic lymph nodes from three different studies [49–51].

guided by sonographic findings is more likely to result in lower postoperative serum thyroglobulin levels and a subsequent negative neck ultrasound [54].

DTC neck recurrences represent a spectrum of clinical scenarios. The size of metastatic lymph nodes or local tumor recurrence varies from a few millimeters to several centimeters. At one end, there may be a 3-mm hypervascular lesion in the central neck at the site of a prior extensive debulking surgery for invasive local disease in the soft tissue. The utility of a reoperation to remove this small burden of disease is unknown and must be balanced against the morbidity of the reoperative procedure and the risk of continued sonographic surveillance. On the other end, sonography may detect multiple large metastatic lymph nodes in the lateral compartment for which a comprehensive modified lateral neck dissection is appropriate. In the near future, molecular marker analysis of the FNA material from metastatic lymph nodes may help to predict those with aggressive behavior. Future studies addressing the clinical relevance of different types of DTC neck recurrences are needed to refine therapeutic decision making.

Summary

Ultrasound is an important tool for the evaluation of the thyroid nodules and cervical lymph nodes. Certain sonographic features of thyroid nodules can be helpful in identifying those nodules most at risk for malignancy including hypoechogenicity, increased vascularity, microcalcifications, irregular margins, and the absence of a halo. These features alone do not have the sensitivity or specificity to diagnose thyroid cancer and FNA remains the procedure of choice to diagnose thyroid cancer. However, the sonographic appearance of a nodule can be helpful in determining which nodules should undergo FNA, especially when the nodule is small or there are multiple nodules present.

Ultrasound is also useful in identifying cervical lymph nodes. Normal lymph nodes have a typical appearance with an echogenic central hilus surrounded by a hypoechoic cortex. When lymph nodes are involved with metastatic thyroid cancer, the normal architecture is destroyed, leaving a heterogeneous appearance with possible calcifications, cystic spaces, or peripheral vascularity. Ultrasound is the best method to identify metastatic lymph nodes either at initial presentation of differentiated thyroid cancer or during surveillance for residual disease. When a suspicious lymph node is identified, fine-needle aspiration for both cytology and thyroglobulin measurement can be used to identify malignant lymph nodes and plan appropriate interventions.

Acknowledgments

We are grateful to Mr. Sherard Graham for his expert assistance in manuscript preparation.

References

[1] Mazzaferri EL. Management of a solitary thyroid nodule. N Engl J Med 1993;328(8):553–9.

[2] Papini E, Guglielmi R, Bianchini A, et al. Risk of malignancy in nonpalpable thyroid nodules: predictive value of ultrasound and color-Doppler features. J Clin Endocrinol Metab 2002;87(5):1941–6.

[3] Nam-Goong IS, Kim HY, Gong G, et al. Ultrasonography-guided fine-needle aspiration of thyroid incidentaloma: correlation with pathological findings. Clin Endocrinol (Oxf) 2004; 60(1):21–8.

[4] Kovacevic O, Skurla MS. Sonographic diagnosis of thyroid nodules: correlation with the results of sonographically guided fine-needle aspiration biopsy. J Clin Ultrasound 2007; 35(2):63–7.

[5] Cappelli C, Pirola I, Cumetti D, et al. Is the anteroposterior and transverse diameter ratio of nonpalpable thyroid nodules a sonographic criteria for recommending fine-needle aspiration cytology? Clin Endocrinol (Oxf) 2005;63(6):689–93.

[6] Leenhardt L, Hejblum G, Franc B, et al. Indications and limits of ultrasound-guided cytology in the management of nonpalpable thyroid nodules. J Clin Endocrinol Metab 1999; 84(1):24–8.

[7] Cerbone G, Spiezia S, Colao A, et al. Power Doppler improves the diagnostic accuracy of color Doppler ultrasonography in cold thyroid nodules: follow-up results. Horm Res 1999;52(1):19–24.

[8] Brkljacic B, Cuk V, Tomic-Brzac H, et al. Ultrasonic evaluation of benign and malignant nodules in echographically multinodular thyroids. J Clin Ultrasound 1994;22(2):71–6.

[9] Takashima S, Fukuda H, Nomura N, et al. Thyroid nodules: re-evaluation with ultrasound. J Clin Ultrasound 1995;23(3):179–84.

[10] Rago T, Vitti P, Chiovato L, et al. Role of conventional ultrasonography and color flow-Doppler sonography in predicting malignancy in 'cold' thyroid nodules. Eur J Endocrinol 1998;138(1):41–6.

[11] Kim EK, Park CS, Chung WY, et al. New sonographic criteria for recommending fine-needle aspiration biopsy of nonpalpable solid nodules of the thyroid. AJR Am J Roentgenol 2002;178(3):687–91.

[12] Frates MC, Benson CB, Doubilet PM, et al. Prevalence and distribution of carcinoma in patients with solitary and multiple thyroid nodules on sonography. J Clin Endocrinol Metab 2006;91(9):3411–7.

[13] Wienke JR, Chong WK, Fielding JR, et al. Sonographic features of benign thyroid nodules: interobserver reliability and overlap with malignancy. J Ultrasound Med 2003;22(10): 1027–31.

[14] Jeh SK, Jung SL, Kim BS, et al. Evaluating the degree of conformity of papillary carcinoma and follicular carcinoma to the reported ultrasonographic findings of malignant thyroid tumor. Korean J Radiol 2007;8(3):192–7.

[15] Alexander EK, Hurwitz S, Heering JP, et al. Natural history of benign solid and cystic thyroid nodules. Ann Intern Med 2003;138(4):315–8.

[16] Taki S, Terahata S, Yamashita R, et al. Thyroid calcifications: sonographic patterns and incidence of cancer. Clin Imaging 2004;28(5):368–71.

[17] Reading CC, Charboneau JW, Hay ID, et al. Sonography of thyroid nodules: a "classic pattern" diagnostic approach. Ultrasound Q 2005;21(3):157–65.

[18] Rago T, Santini F, Scutari M, et al. Elastography: new developments in ultrasound for predicting malignancy in thyroid nodules. J Clin Endocrinol Metab 2007;92(8):2917–22.

[19] Ito Y, Kobayashi K, Tomoda C, et al. Ill-defined edge on ultrasonographic examination can be a marker of aggressive characteristic of papillary thyroid microcarcinoma. World J Surg 2005;29(8):1007–11 [discussion: 1011–2].

[20] Chan BK, Desser TS, McDougall IR, et al. Common and uncommon sonographic features of papillary thyroid carcinoma. J Ultrasound Med 2003;22(10):1083–90.

[21] Ito Y, Tomoda C, Uruno T, et al. Preoperative ultrasonographic examination for lymph node metastasis: usefulness when designing lymph node dissection for papillary microcarcinoma of the thyroid. World J Surg 2004;28(5):498–501.

[22] Som PM, Curtin HD, Mancuso AA. Imaging-based nodal classification for evaluation of neck metastatic adenopathy. AJR Am J Roentgenol 2000;174(3):837–44.

[23] Ying M, Ahuja A. Sonography of neck lymph nodes. Part I: normal lymph nodes. Clin Radiol 2003;58:351–8.

[24] Solbiati L, Osti V, Cova L, et al. Ultrasound of thyroid, parathyroid glands and lymph nodes. Eur Radiol 2001;11:2411–24.

[25] Bruneton JN, Balu-Maestro C, Marcy PY, et al. Very high frequency (13 MHz) ultrasonographic examination of the normal neck: detection of normal lymph nodes and thyroid nodules. J Ultrasound Med 1994;13(2):87–90.

[26] Ahuja A, Ying M. Sonography of neck lymph nodes. Part II: abnormal lymph nodes. Clin Radiol 2003;58:359–66.

[27] Frasoldati A, Valcavi R. Challenges in neck ultrasonography: lymphadenopathy and parathyroid glands. Endocr Pract 2004;10:261–8.

[28] Baskin HJ. Detection of recurrent papillary thyroid carcinoma by thyroglobulin assessment in needle washout after fine-needle aspiration of suspicious lymph nodes. Thyroid 2004;14:959–63.

[29] Wu CH, Chang YL, Hsu WC, et al. Usefulness of Doppler spectral analysis and power Doppler sonography in the differentiation of cervical lymphadenopathies. AJR Am J Roentgenol 1998;171(2):503–9.

[30] Ahuja A, Ying M, King A, et al. Lymph nodes hilus. Gray scale and power Doppler sonography of cervical nodes. J Ultrasound Med 2001;20:987–92.

[31] Lyshchik A, Higashi T, Asato R, et al. Cervical lymph node metastases: diagnosis at sonoelastography—initial experience. Radiology 2007;243:256–67.

[32] LeBoulleux S, Girard E, Rose M, et al. Ultrasound criteria for malignancy for cervical lymph nodes in patients followed up for differentiated thyroid cancer. J Clin Endocrinol Metab 2007;92:3590–4.

[33] Kuna SK, Bracic I, Tesic V, et al. Ultrasonographic differentiation of benign from malignant neck lymphadenopathy in thyroid cancer. J Ultrasound Med 2006;25(12):1531–7, quiz 1538–40.

[34] Boi F, Baghino G, Atzeni F, et al. The diagnostic value for differentiated thyroid carcinoma metastases of thyroglobulin (Tg) measurement in washout fluid from fine-needle aspiration biopsy of neck lymph nodes is maintained in the presence of circulating anti-Tg antibodies. J Clin Endocrinol Metab 2006;91:1364–9.

[35] Cignarelli M, Abrosi A, Marino A, et al. Diagnostic utility of thyroglobulin detection in fine-needle aspiration of cervical cystic metastatic lymph nodes from papillary thyroid cancer with negative cytology. Thyroid 2003;13:1163–7.

[36] Kudo T, Miyauchi A, Ito Y, et al. Diagnosis of medullary thyroid carcinoma by calcitonin measurement in fine-needle aspiration biopsy specimens. Thyroid 2007;17(7):635–8.

[37] Schlumberger M. Papillary and follicular thyroid carcinoma. N Engl J Med 1998;338:297–306.

[38] Noguchi S, Maurakami N, Yamashita H, et al. Papillary thyroid carcinoma: modified radical neck dissection improves prognosis. Arch Surg 1998;133:276–80.

[39] Ito Y, Tomoda C, Uruno T, et al. Ultrasonographically and anatomopathologically detectable node metastases in the lateral compartment as indicators of wrose relapse-free survival in patients with papillary thyroid carcinoma. World J Surg 2005;29:917–20.

[40] Mirallie E, Vissert J, Sagan C, et al. Localization of cervical node metastasis of papillary thyroid carcinoma. World J Surg 1999;23:970–4.

[41] Machens A, Hinze R, Thomusch O, et al. Pattern of nodal metastasis for primary and reoperative thyroid cancer. World J Surg 2002;26:22–6.

[42] Ito Y, Uruno T, Nakano K, et al. An observation trial without surgical treatment in patients with papillary microcarcinoma of the thyroid. Thyroid 2003;13:381–7.

[43] Stulak JM, Grant CS, Farley DR, et al. Value of pre-operative ultasonography in the surgical management of initial and reoperative papillary thyroid cancer. Arch Surg 2006; 141:489–96.

[44] Kouvaraki MA, Shapiro SE, Fornage BD, et al. Role of preoperative ultrasonography in the surgical management of patients with thyroid cancer. Surgery 2003;134:946–55.

[45] Cooper DS, Doherty GM, Haugen BR, et al. Management guidelines for patients with thyroid nodules and differentiated thyroid cancer. Thyroid 2006;16(2):109–42.

[46] American Association of Clinical Endocrinologists and Associazone Medici Endocrinologi medical guidelines for clinical practice for the diagnosis and management of thyroid nodules. Endocr Pract 2006;12:63–99.

[47] Mazzaferri EL, Kloos RT. Current approaches to primary therapy for papillary and follicular thyroid cancer. J Clin Endocrinol Metab 2001;86:1447–63.

[48] Mazzaferri EL, Kloos RT. Is diagnostic iodine-131 scanning with recombinant human TSH useful in the follow-up of differentiated thyroid cancer after thyroid ablation. J Clin Endocrinol Metab 2002;87:1490–8.

[49] Frasoldati A, Pesenti M, Gallo M, et al. Diagnosis of neck recurrences in patients with differentiated thyroid carcinoma. Cancer 2003;97(1):90–6.

[50] Pacini F, Molinaro E, Castagna MG, et al. Recombinant human thyrotropin-stimulated serum thyroglobulin combined with neck ultrasonography has the highest sensitivity in monitoring differentiated thyroid carcinoma. J Clin Endocrinol Metab 2003;88(8):3668–73.

[51] Torlontano M, Attard M, Crocetti U, et al. Follow-up of low risk patients with papillary thyroid cancer: role of neck ultrasonography in detecting lymph node metastases. J Clin Endocrinol Metab 2004;89(7):3402–7.

[52] Kloos RT, Mazzaferri EL. Thyroid carcinoma. In: Cooper DS, editor. Medical management of thyroid disease. New York: Marcel Dekker, Inc.; 2001. p. 227–312.

[53] Kupferman ME, Patterson M, Mandel SJ, et al. Patterns of lateral neck metastasis in papillary thyroid carcinoma. Arch Otolaryngol Head Neck Surg 2004;130:857–60.

[54] BinYousef HM, Alzahrani AS, Al-Sobhi SS, et al. Preoperative neck ultrasonographic mapping for persistent/recurrent papillary thyroid cancer. World J Surg 2004;28:1110–4.

ELSEVIER
SAUNDERS

Endocrinol Metab Clin N Am
37 (2008) 419–435

ENDOCRINOLOGY
AND METABOLISM
CLINICS
OF NORTH AMERICA

Follow up Approaches in Thyroid Cancer: A Risk Adapted Paradigm

R. Michael Tuttle, MD[a,b,*], Rebecca Leboeuf, MD[a,b]

[a]Joan and Sanford I. Weill Medical College of Cornell University, Department of Medicine,
1300 York Avenue, New York, NY 10021, USA
[b]Memorial Sloan-Kettering Cancer Center, Zuckerman Research Building,
1275 York Avenue, New York, NY 10021, USA

Data from the Surveillance, Epidemiology, and End Results Program predicts that one out of every 136 people born in the United States today will be diagnosed with thyroid cancer at some point during their lifetime [1]. An estimated 33,550 cases of thyroid cancer will be diagnosed in 2007 (8,070 men and 25,480 women). While 30-year disease specific survival rates can exceed 95% [2,3], the 5-year survival rate in older patients presenting with distant metastatic disease can be as low as 56% [4]. Because most patients with thyroid cancer respond very well to treatment, it is not surprising that an estimated 366,466 thyroid cancer survivors are living in the United States as of January 2004 [5].

The primary goal of follow-up in these thyroid cancer survivors is to identify and appropriately treat the nearly 30% of patients who may experience a clinically significant recurrence (which may occur as long as 20 to 30 years after initial therapy), based on the assumption that early detection and treatment of recurrent disease lowers morbidity and prolongs life [3]. As the paradigm for disease detection in low-risk patients moves away from routine diagnostic whole-body radioactive iodine (RAI) scanning and toward a greater reliance on neck ultrasonography and serum thyroglobulin (Tg) determinations as primary tools for disease detection, it is critical to understand both the strengths and limitations of this new follow-up paradigm.

Recently, several international authorities on thyroid cancer have published guidelines outlining generally similar approaches to the treatment and follow-up of thyroid cancer patients [6–11]. In each of these guidelines,

* Corresponding author. Memorial Sloan Kettering Cancer Center, Zuckerman Research Building, Room 834, 1275 York Avenue, New York, NY 10021.
E-mail address: tuttlem@mskcc.org (R.M. Tuttle).

estimates of risk for recurrence and risk of disease-specific death are used to guide both initial treatment and follow-up recommendations.

By combining an understanding of the biology of the disease (response to initial therapy, likelihood of recurrence, common sites of recurrence, time to recurrence) with an improved understanding of the clinical utility of the specific test (sensitivity, specificity, and negative predictive value), we as health care providers can tailor the extent and intensity of our follow-up recommendations to the specific risk of disease-specific death and clinically evident recurrence in an individual patient. Therefore, the goal of this article is to describe a risk-adapted framework that will guide the practicing clinician in the selection and timing of appropriate follow-up tests for individual patients. The article will focus on the follow-up of patients with follicular-derived thyroid cancers (papillary and follicular thyroid cancers), leaving other rarer forms of thyroid cancer (medullary, anaplastic, lymphoma) for other investigators and articles.

Risk stratification

To begin to determine which tests would be appropriate for detection of disease-specific death or recurrent disease, it is critical to be able to appropriately risk stratify patients shortly after initial diagnosis, based on the likelihood of death or recurrence of thyroid cancer. Thereafter, just as importantly, one has to define likely sites of recurrence, as well as the likelihood that the recurrence will be RAI avid (or fluorodeoxyglucose [FDG] avid) and produce sufficient quantities of Tg to allow detection of recurrent disease. Fortunately, several different risk stratification systems have been published, each being very efficient at defining patients at high or low risk for disease-specific mortality (reviewed in Tuttle and colleagues [12]). Unfortunately, even in the best of these systems, there continues to be a small risk of death from disease in patients classified as low risk, warranting long-term follow-up. Several tumor-related and patient-related factors are commonly found in multivariate analysis to be predictors of disease-specific death in thyroid cancer: age at diagnosis, size of the primary tumor, histology of the tumor, locally invasive thyroid cancer (completeness of resection), and presence of distant metastases [12]. Lymph node involvement has been reported in some studies to increase disease recurrence without having an impact on disease-specific survival [13], while other studies demonstrate an increase in disease specific mortality in patients with lymph node involvement [3].

Each of these staging systems provides good risk stratification based on data available shortly after initial therapy. The authors refer to this as "initial risk stratification" and it certainly is a good starting point for initial decision making. However, in the follow-up, a patient's additional data is accumulated that may either increase or decrease this initial risk estimate. The authors refer to the integration of the predictive values of these additional data into the initial risk estimates as "ongoing risk stratification." Over the years, the ongoing risk stratification provides important additional information that may significantly alter the initial assessment of the risk of recurrence, risk of death, and likely sites of recurrences.

Initial risk stratification

Initial estimates of the risk of death from thyroid cancer

The American Joint Committee on Cancer (AJCC) staging system, while commonly used throughout oncology, is designed to risk stratify for death, but not necessarily for recurrence [14]. So while AJCC staging is useful in identifying patients likely to die of thyroid cancer, it is not particularly helpful in predicting recurrence. Therefore, the addition of a postoperative clinicopathologic staging system should be used in conjunction with the AJCC staging system to improve prediction of risk for recurrence and thereby inform the authors' follow-up testing paradigm [7]. While a wide variety of staging systems are useful, the MACIS (Metastasis, Age, Completeness of resection, Invasion, Size of primary tumor) scoring system has proven to be predictive of disease-specific death and is readily applied based on the usual clinical information available to the clinician, and therefore is most likely to be informative to clinicians caring for patients with thyroid cancer [15].

In the authors' experience, even without a mathematical scoring system, several readily available clinical factors quickly stratify patients into one of four groups, based on the likelihood of dying from thyroid cancer (very low, low, intermediate, high) (Table 1). This table is based upon the variables repeatedly shown to be significant in multivariate analysis predicting death from thyroid cancer. The intermediate risk group comprises patients in whom the patient factors and tumor factors present a combination of high-risk and low-risk features. While it is clear that these intermediate risk patients are neither truly high risk nor low risk, the precise risk of death is hard to quantify for an individual patient. Therefore, the authors classify them as an intermediate group that deserves concern greater than the low-risk group, but certainly does not have the death rate associated with patients with all of the high-risk features. So while no risk stratification system can identify a cohort of patients with a 0% risk of death from disease, it can separate patients into high, intermediate, low, and very low risk of death from disease, and therefore should have a major impact on both the extent and intensity of the authors' proposed follow-up and therapies.

Initial estimates of the risk of clinically evident recurrence

Unlike most other solid tumors, the risk of recurrence and the risk of death from thyroid cancer are not always concordant [3]. For example, young children with thyroid cancer have a very high recurrence rate (often exceeding 30%–40%) but 30-year disease specific death rates that are less

Table 1
Risk of death from thyroid cancer

	Very low risk	Low risk	Intermediate risk	High risk
Age at diagnosis	<45 years	<45 years	Young patients (<45 yrs) • Classic PTC >4 cm • Or vascular invasion • Or microscopic extrathyroidal extension • Or worrisome histology of any size[a]	>45 years
			Older patients (>45 yrs) • Classic PTC <4 cm • Or worrisome histology <1 cm–2 cm confined to the thyroid[a]	
Primary tumor size	<1 cm	1 cm–4 cm		>4-cm classic PTC
Histology	Classic PTC, confined to the thyroid gland[b]	Classic PTC, confined to the thyroid gland[b]	Histology in conjunction with age as above	Worrisome histology >1 cm–2 cm[a]
Completeness of resection	Complete resection	Complete resection	Complete resection	Incomplete tumor resection
Lymph node involvement	None apparent	Present or absent[c]	Present or absent[c]	Present or absent[c]
Distant metastasis	None apparent	None apparent	None apparent	Present

Only those patients meeting all criteria within the respect column would be classified as very low risk, low risk, or low risk. Older patients with either incomplete tumor resection or presence of distant metastasis are considered high risk, irrespective of tumor size and specific histology. Patients with a combination of risk factors (age, histology, and tumor size) crossing over between columns are classified as intermediate risk patients.

[a] Worrisome histologies includes histologic subtypes of PTC, such as tall cell variant, columnar variant, insular variant, and poorly differentiated thyroid cancers.

[b] Confined to the thyroid gland with no evidence of vascular invasion or extrathyroidal extension.

[c] Cervical lymph node metastases in older patients, but probably not in younger patients, may confer an increased risk of death from disease.

than 1% to 2%. However, older patients (more than 60 years old at diagnosis) have a high recurrence rate that is associated with an increase in disease-specific death. These differences likely reflect both the different biologies of papillary thyroid cancer (PTC) in young patients (classic PTC, RAI avid) compared with older patients (often more poorly differentiated tumors, RAI refractory), but also a difference in response to therapy (older patients more unlikely to be made disease free with additional surgery or RAI, compared with younger patients). While the overall goal of follow-up in thyroid cancer survivors is prevention of disease-specific death, it is critical that clinically significant recurrence be identified and appropriately treated. It is hoped that early detection and therapy of disease recurrence will prevent disease-specific death.

While the risk factors that predict recurrence are often the same as those that predict an increased risk of death from thyroid cancer, factors—such as presence of metastatic disease at diagnosis or incomplete surgical resection—are more difficult to apply to "disease recurrence" strategies, as these patients usually have persistent disease (despite initial therapy) and are dealt with as patients at very high risk of persistent disease, progressive disease, or new metastatic lesions. Therefore, these patients are excluded from the following follow-up paradigm because the intensity and tools for follow-up need to be formulated on an individual patient basis in patients with incomplete surgical resection or distant metastatic disease present at diagnosis.

The risk factors for development of recurrent disease in those patients who have had complete resection of the initial tumor and no evidence of distant metastases at initial evaluation are presented in Table 2. Age at diagnosis continues to be an important predictive factor, with the highest risk of recurrence in the very young and the elderly. Similarly, size of the primary tumor is also linked to risk of recurrence in most studies, as are the histology of the primary tumor and the presence of gross extrathyroidal extension at the time of initial surgery. Most, but not all, studies demonstrate that the presence of identifiable cervical lymph node metastases at diagnosis carries a higher risk of subsequent identification of recurrent disease.

Over the last several years, pathology reports are providing more detailed information regarding the subtypes of thyroid cancer, the presence of microscopic multifocal disease, and the presence of microscopic extrathyroidal extension. While these features likely are indicative of a more aggressive thyroid cancer, it remains unclear whether the presence or absence of these risk factors should convey a significant risk of recurrence independent of size of the primary tumor, the age of the patient, and the completeness of resection. To be conservative, the authors have used these factors to classify as moderate risk, but additional studies are needed to make sure that the authors are not unnecessarily up-staging these patients, particularly when the primary tumor is quite small.

Table 2
Risk stratification for the likelihood of clinically evident recurrence from thyroid cancer following complete resection of primary tumor in patients with no evidence of distant metastases at
initial evaluation

	Low risk	Intermediate risk	High risk
Age at diagnosis	Any age	20–60 years	<20 or >60 years
Primary tumor size	<1 cm[a]	1 cm–4 cm	>4 cm
Histology	Classic PTC, confined to the thyroid gland	Classic PTC, minor extrathyroidal extension, or vascular invasion	Other than classic PTC, gross extra-thyroidal extension or vascular invasion
Lymph node involvement	None apparent	Present or absent	Present

Patients with incomplete tumor resection or distant metastasis at diagnosis are very likely to
have persistent disease even after aggressive initial therapy, and therefore are dealt with differently than the more usual patient without evidence of distant metastasis, in which all gross evidence of disease has been resected and are therefore not included in this risk stratification scheme.

[a] Classic PTC less than 1 cm with microscopic extrathyroidal extension, vascular invasion,
or lymph node metastases would be considered intermediate risk.

Ongoing risk stratification

Ongoing estimates of the impact of therapy (treatment variable)

Though each of the published staging systems provides very good risk
stratification based on information obtainable within the first few weeks
(or months) after initial therapy, none of the staging systems include variables that reflect the effectiveness of initial therapy, the negative predictive
values of follow-up evaluations, or the impact of the length of time a patient
has been free of disease after initial therapy. In clinical practice, the authors
incorporate all of these additional factors into an ongoing reassessment of
risk for both recurrence and death from thyroid cancer as time passes. In
a simplistic fashion, an individual patient response to therapy can be classified as excellent, acceptable, or incomplete (Table 3).

Ideally, after initial therapy patients are rendered free of disease and, therefore, all follow-up studies will demonstrate no evidence of disease, in which
case the patient would be classified as having an excellent response to initial
therapy and be very unlikely to die from thyroid cancer or even develop clinically significant recurrence. However, an incomplete response to initial therapy that is manifest by early development of clinically significant recurrent
disease or markedly elevated (or rising) serum Tg after initial therapy would
place the patient at significant risk for continued disease progression.

In actual clinical practice, the authors' follow-up studies often are not absolutely definitive as to the presence or absence of low level disease. For example, very low level Tg (on suppression or stimulation) could represent
either residual normal thyroid tissue or low level thyroid cancer. Millimeter-sized abnormal lymph nodes in the neck found during the follow-up

Table 3
Response to therapy variables

	Excellent response[a]	Acceptable response	Incomplete response
Suppressed Tg[b]	Undetectable	Detectable but <1 ng/mL	>1 ng/mL
Stimulated Tg[b]	Undetectable	<10 ng/mL	>10 ng/mL
Trend in suppressed Tg[c]	Remains undetectable	Declining	Stable or rising
Anti-Tg antibodies	Absent	Absent or declining	Persistent or rising
Neck ultrasonography	No evidence of disease	Non-specific changes in thyroid bed; Probable inflammatory lymph nodes; Stable millimeter sized cervical lymph node even if abnormal by ultrasound criteria	Evidence of structurally significant recurrent or persistent disease in the thyroid bed (>1 cm); Cervical lymph nodes (>1 cm), or distant metastases, particularly if structurally progressive or FDG avid
Diagnostic RAI whole body scan[d]	No evidence for RAI-avid disease	No evidence for RAI-avid disease; Very faint uptake in thyroid bed only	Persistent or recurrent RAI-avid disease present
Cross sectional imaging (MRI, CT)[d]	No evidence of disease	Nonspecific changes	Structural disease present
FDG positron emission tomography (PET) scanning[d]	No evidence of disease	Nonspecific changes consistent with normal variants or inflammatory changes	FDG-avid disease present

[a] Patients deemed to have an excellent or acceptable response to therapy generally warrant observation without additional specific therapy, while patients with an incomplete response are likely to require additional evaluation and treatment.

[b] Stimulated and suppressed Tg value cut offs optimized for patients treated with total thyroidectomy and RAI remnant ablation.

[c] While most sensitive and specific in patients with total thyroidectomy and RAI remnant ablation, a rising Tg over time should also prompt further evaluation in patients treated with less than total thyroidectomy, or with total thyroidectomy without RAI remnant ablation. This highlights the crucial importance of measuring serum Tg in the same laboratory, to ensure comparability among the samples over time.

[d] While these studies are not routinely recommended for all patients without additional high-risk features or clinical suspicion of persistent or recurrent disease, results from these studies can be used as additional response to therapy measures, if done.

of many thyroid cancer patients could represent persistent low level disease or simply benign inflammatory lymph nodes. Similarly, FDG-PET scanning often cannot differentiate small inflammatory lymph nodes from small volume thyroid cancer. Even though the clinician cannot be 100% certain these patients have had an excellent response to therapy, at the worst they have low-level persistent disease that may or may not ever become clinically evident. Therefore, in the absence of other clinical indications, these indeterminate results can be considered an acceptable outcome that warrants continued follow-up, reserving additional treatments for evidence of disease progression. Most patients in this acceptable category will be there by virtue of suppressed Tg values detectable but less than 1 ng/mL or stimulated Tg values less than 10 ng/mL, usually with a neck ultrasonography that is either negative or nonspecific. In this setting, serum Tg values will often decline over time with levothyroxine suppression and observation alone [16], further supporting a cautious observation approach rather than an aggressive therapy.

Even though the acceptable response category probably includes many patients who will never develop clinically significant disease recurrence, common sense demands a closer follow-up of these patients, with low level Tg values or nonspecific imaging studies to identify the small number of patients in this category that will develop rising serum Tg values or increasing size of small metastatic lymph nodes that may require additional therapy.

When estimating the response to therapy, it is critical that sufficient time be allowed to pass to see both the effectiveness of initial therapy and to identify early clinical recurrences that may become manifest in the first 2 to 3 years after initial therapy. For example, serum Tg levels often fall for several years after RAI ablation in the absence of identifiable structural disease, which would result in down-staging of the patient from an "acceptable" response to an "excellent" response over the years. Conversely, small lymph nodes in the neck that are destined to develop into clinically significant recurrences may not be recognized for several years after initial therapy. Development of new abnormal cervical lymph nodes would result in up-staging the patient to an incomplete response and call for more careful observation and possibly additional therapy. Therefore, it is important to consider both the disease-free survival interval and the initial risk stratification when considering when response to therapy classification is most likely to yield reliable long-term prognostic information.

Influence of disease-free survival on risk of recurrence

Even though clinically evident disease recurrence can develop as many as 30 to 40 years after initial therapy, large retrospective studies consistently demonstrate that the majority of recurrences were detected in the first 10 to 15 years of follow-up [2,3]. Although not yet proven, it is likely that the increased sensitivity of the follow-up testing paradigm that the authors are currently using will identify most recurrences (or persistent disease) sooner than the techniques used in these older studies, resulting in higher rates of recurrence or persistent disease in the first 5 years after therapy, with low rates thereafter. Because thyroid cancer is a slow, progressive disease that plays out over 30 to 40 years, all patients require lifelong follow-up to identify those few patients who develop clinically significant recurrences years after their initial therapy. However, it seems likely that serum Tg on suppression will be an adequate screen for detection of late recurrences in patients who have had appropriate initial therapy with risk specific follow-up in the first few years after diagnosis.

Until long-term studies are completed, demonstrating the negative predictive values of undetectable Tg values and neck ultrasonography based on risk stratification and response to therapy at specific time points after initial therapy, the authors will be conservative in the approach to integrating disease-free survival into the ongoing re-risk stratification paradigm. It seems reasonable to use a 2 to 10 year disease-free survival period (depending on initial risk stratification) to identity those patients who are at lowest risk for development of clinically significant thyroid cancer recurrence. When considered as a continuous variable, the longer the disease-free survival period (with appropriate follow-up studies), the lower the risk of clinically significant recurrence.

It is important to emphasize that disease-free survival is defined not only by time since initial therapy, but also the use of appropriate follow-up testing (usually suppressed Tg with or without neck ultrasound). The authors are often referred patients 25 to 30 years after initial therapy for "recurrent disease" who have large volume metastatic disease with serum Tg values on suppression that exceed 1,000 ng/mL. In some retrospective studies, these patients would be considered to have recurrent disease 25 to 30 years after initial therapy, when in reality they likely have had persistent disease for several years. Therefore, the authors are only confident that patients have had prolonged disease-free survival and are at low risk of recurrence if there are adequate follow-up studies on the patient in addition to prolonged survival after initial therapy.

Influence of follow-up testing on risk of recurrence or death

In the follow-up of thyroid cancer patients, the focus is often on tests that have very high sensitivity for disease detection. And while this is certainly important, it is also important to understand the positive-preditive value and negative-predictive value of the various tests that are used to identify recurrent disease. A test result with a high negative-predictive value will lower the assessment of the risk for recurrence in an individual patient, while a test result with a high positive-predictive value would demand continued close follow-up and further evaluation.

One of the difficulties in assessing the predictive value of specific tests is that the test will perform differently based on the pretest probability of disease in an individual patient. For example, a normal neck ultrasound in a high-risk patient with a suppressed serum Tg of 800 ng/mL would not significantly lower the estimate of risk for recurrence. However, a normal neck ultrasound in a low-risk patient with an undetectable Tg on suppression has a negative-predictive value that exceeds 95%, and is therefore very reassuring [17]. Each of the published guidelines is similar in regard to the follow-up studies to be done in the first few years after initial therapy [6–10]. These generally include serum Tg on suppression every 6 months and neck ultrasound at 6 months to 12 months, and then yearly for 3 to 5 years based on the risk of the patient. Stimulated Tg values and diagnostic whole body scanning are used more selectively in patients at a high rather than a low risk of recurrence treated with total thyroidectomy and RAI ablation. Additional cross-sectional imaging and FDG-PET scanning are reserved for higher risk patients or clinical indications of non-RAI persistent disease. The similarities and differences in the published guidelines have been previously reviewed [12].

Therefore, while precise predictive values of individual tests in specific patients are hard to define, negative test results are generally reassuring and should lower the risk for development of recurrent disease. Because each of these tests are also used as a response-to-therapy variable in Table 3, they play a critical role in the assessment of how effective the initial therapy was, and therefore should reflect the risk of disease recurrence and death.

The primary follow up test predicting disease specific death from thyroid cancer is FDG-PET scanning [18]. Because FDG-PET scanning identifies metabolically active, non-RAI avid thyroid cancers, it is not surprising that patients with markedly positive FDG-PET scans have a poor prognosis, both in terms of progression of disease but also in terms of disease specific mortality. FDG-avid lesions seldom respond to RAI therapy [19], and as such FDG-PET scanning can be used as an adverse response to therapy variable.

Influence of initial therapeutic choices on estimating the impact of therapy

Obviously, the Tg values presented as excellent, acceptable, and incomplete are most sensitive and specific when patients have undergone total thyroidectomy and radioactive iodine ablation. However, by definition, less than total thyroidectomy is only recommended for low-risk patients [20], and as such intensive follow-up and highly sensitive and specific disease detection techniques are not required. In patients treated with less than total thyroidectomy, serial determinations of Tg—without thyroid stimulating hormone (TSH) stimulation—and serial neck ultrasound evaluating both the contralateral residual thyroid tissue and cervical lymph nodes would routinely be recommended. Excellent response to therapy would be a stable Tg over time (with similar TSH levels) and no evidence of structural disease in the contralateral lobe or neck lymph nodes. An example of an acceptable response could be a millimeter-sized colloid nodule in the contralateral lobe, or nonspecific lymph nodes on neck ultrasound. Obviously, the threshold for a complete thyroidectomy is low and would include development of significant abnormalities in the contralateral thyroid lobe, a rising serum Tg, or evidence of metastatic disease on neck ultrasound or other cross-sectional imaging.

Serum Tg values are also more difficult to interpret in patients treated with total thyroidectomy without radioactive iodine remnant ablation. Even though many of these patients will have Tg levels less than 1 ng/mL on suppression, values as high as 5 ng/mL to 10 ng/mL are likely to represent residual normal thyroid tissue and not necessarily persistent disease. Postoperative Tg values will vary with the completeness of the total thyroidectomy and the level of TSH suppression. Precise cut-off values that differentiate residual normal thyroid tissue from metastatic thyroid cancer are not well defined. In the authors' center, where the surgeons routinely leave less than 1% to 2% residual normal thyroid, a suppressed serum Tg 1 month after surgery that exceeds 10 ng/mL to 20 ng/mL raises concern for persistent thyroid cancer and would warrant additional imaging and RAI remnant ablation. Whether or not the patient underwent RAI ablation, a rising serum Tg on suppression over time with similar levels of TSH suppression would be suspicious for recurrent disease and defined as an incomplete response to therapy.

Secondary risk stratification

While continuous, ongoing risk stratification occurs at each follow-up visit, it seems reasonable to define a point in time where secondary risk stratification can be seen as a gateway to less intensive long-term follow-up consisting of yearly physical examination and suppressed Tg values. While the exact time point for secondary risk stratification remains to be defined, from a clinical perspective it seems reasonable to re-evaluate the risk of the patient based primarily on response to treatment approximately 2 years after initial therapy.

By 2 years after initial therapy, several additional pieces of data that were not available at the time of initial risk assessment are now available for incorporation into an updated risk classification scheme that incorporates several responses to therapy variables (eg, one or two neck ultrasounds, several suppressed Tg values, sometimes stimulated Tg values, and diagnostic whole-body follow-up scans). Additionally, serum Tg values often continue to decline for at least 12 to 18 months after RAI ablation, so a 2 year time point would allow a reasonable period of time to assess whether the Tg is rising or falling in a given patient. While a time point this early in the course of the disease may not accurately define which patients are "cured" of disease, it can certainly guide the recommendations regarding the types and intensity of follow-up studies that are likely to be cost effective.

It must be emphasized that the secondary risk stratification at 2 years after initial therapy is designed simply to guide the follow-up paradigm and not to accurately predict which patients are "cured" of disease. While all thyroid cancer patients are at risk of recurrence, the follow-up paradigm the authors recommend should be based both on the likelihood of recurrence and the likelihood that a minimal disease detection paradigm (suppressed Tg and physical examination) will identify recurrent disease at a time that the disease is still treatable with minimal morbidity and mortality.

From a practical standpoint, additional risk stratification time points could be considered at year 5 for moderate-risk patients, and at year 10 for high-risk patients before being entirely comfortable that a minimal follow-up paradigm of suppressed Tg and physical examination without additional studies is adequate for disease detection in these patients with more than low risk for recurrence. However, it is very likely that patients initially staged as moderate- and high-risk patients that have an excellent response to therapy as determined at the 2-year secondary risk stratification endpoint can be down staged to a lower risk category. Additional long-term studies incorporating both initial stage of disease and status of response to therapy variables at 2 years after diagnosis are needed before the authors can be comfortable down-staging these higher risk patients as early as 2 years after initial therapy.

Clearly, specific follow up recommendations will vary for individual patients, based on initial risk stratification, disease-free survival time, and response to therapy variables, but this method does provide an approach to secondary risk stratification several years after initial therapy and should guide the long-term follow-up approach.

A risk-adapted paradigm

From a clinical perspective, the intensity and methods of follow-up surveillance should be based on the individual patient's risk of recurrence or death from thyroid cancer. This follow-up paradigm is at first based on initial estimates of risk based on data available shortly after diagnosis and initial treatment. The paradigm is then modified as new data becomes available over time, continually adjusting the risk estimates based on the new information obtained: a risk-adapated follow-up paradigm. Based on the length of disease-free survival and the estimate of response to therapy, the intensity and methods of follow-up are adjusted to match the new risk estimates.

Initial risk assessment for death from disease and disease recurrence is done using one of the widely available prognostic staging systems. Patients with gross disease remaining despite aggressive initial therapy, or with distant metastases at diagnosis, may require additional therapy with RAI or external beam radiation therapy and more intensive follow-up with RAI imaging, FDG-PET imaging, and cross-sectional imaging. Because of the wide variety of presentations of these patients, it is difficult to develop a meaningful generalizable follow-up paradigm in this context. In general, cross-sectional imaging at 6-month intervals is appropriate with additional FDG-PET scanning and RAI scanning, as indicated by the specific clinical conditions.

However, a risk-adapted follow-up scheme is much more applicable to patients who had all evidence of gross disease resected and who have no evidence of distant metastases at diagnosis. In general, the authors expect the treatments to result in a very low disease-specific mortality and a low, but significant, risk of recurrent thyroid cancer. As described above, the follow-up scheme is begun by classifying patients based on the best estimate of risk of recurrence into low, moderate, or high risk (Table 4). In many aspects, the first 2 years of follow-up for all three risk groups is similar, with suppressed Tg values done every 6 months and neck ultrasonography on a yearly basis. Additional cross-sectional imaging, FDG-PET scanning, and routine diagnostic whole body scanning are reserved for high-risk patients. The occasional intermediate risk patient with low level Tg values and indeterminate ultrasonography may also undergo diagnostic whole body scanning looking for RAI-avid disease that may be amenable to a second dose of RAI.

Over this 2-year period, risk stratification is an ongoing process, incorporating additional data into the initial risk assessment and either lowering or raising the estimate of the risk of recurrence based on these follow-up tests. All patients then undergo a formal secondary risk assessment at 2 years after initial therapy. At that point, all data gathered over the last 2 years are reviewed and evaluated to determine the response to initial therapy. Patients with an excellent response to therapy should have a very low risk of recurrence and immediately enter into a long-term, minimal follow-up program of yearly physical examinations and suppressed serum Tg values. Additional neck ultrasonography, stimulated Tg, or other testing modalities are only used if there is some clinical suspicion of recurrent disease or the patient was at very high risk of recurrence in the initial staging evaluation.

At the time of secondary risk stratification, patients often have very low level Tg values, very small abnormal cervical lymph nodes, or nonspecific changes on cross-sectional imaging studies. While these findings would not be considered an excellent response to therapy, they can be considered an acceptable response to therapy that probably is best served with cautious observation. Additional neck ultrasonography is probably warranted in this group of patients on a yearly basis for up to 5 years. At that point, if there has been no structural disease progression and the Tg remains at a stable low level, it seems reasonable to transition to the long-term, minimal follow-up program of yearly physical examination, suppressed serum Tg, and occasional neck ultrasound every few years.

Patients with an incomplete response to therapy manifested by rising serum Tg values, structurally progressive disease, or persistent FDG-PET positive disease are at the highest risk for development of clinically evident recurrent disease and require continued intensive follow-up with neck ultrasonography, cross-sectional imaging, RAI imaging, and FDG-PET imaging.

Table 4

Risk-adapted follow-up paradigm for detecting recurrent disease in patients with complete tumor resection and no evidence of distant metastases at initial risk stratification

	Initial estimate of risk of recurrence First 2 years of follow-up		
	Low risk	Intermediate risk	High risk
Suppressed Tg[a]	Q 6 months	Q 6 months	Q 6 months
Stimulated Tg[a]	Not required	1–2 years	1–2 years
Neck ultrasonography[b]	Q year × 2	Q year × 2	Q year × 2
Diagnostic RAI whole body scan[b]	Not required	1–2 years	1–2 years
Cross sectional imaging (MRI, CT)[b]	Not required	Not required	If Tg elevated or high clinical suspicion
FDG-PET scanning[b]	Not required	Not required	If Tg elevated, RAI scan negative
	Secondary risk stratification Response to therapy assessment		
	Excellent	Acceptable	Incomplete
Ongoing follow-up	Yearly physical examination, yearly suppressed Tg[b]	Yearly physical examination, yearly suppressed Tg, stimulated Tg to document undetectable Tg on suppression, continued observation/assessment of indeterminate structural abnormalities for at least another 2–3 years[a]	Consider additional cross-sectional imaging, possibly FDG-PET scan and the need for additional therapy.

[a] Patients with stable low level Tg values and stable small structurally abnormal lymph nodes that have been stable for 5 years (and therefore still in the acceptable response category) can transition to yearly follow-up, suppressed Tg values, and occasional neck ultrasonography to document continued structurally stability.

[b] Intermediate or high-risk patients, even in the setting of an excellent treatment response at year 2, may still be periodically require neck ultrasonography, depending on the specifics of each individual case. Additionally, patients in whom the initial therapy was less than total thyroidectomy and RAI ablation may benefit from occasional neck ultrasounds over the next 5 to 10 years, because Tg on suppression is less sensitive for detection of recurrent disease in this setting.

The majority of patients with an incomplete response to therapy will require additional therapy, with appropriate use of surgical resection, RAI therapy, external beam irradiation, and systemic therapies.

While this risk-adapted approach will have better sensitivity and specificity in patients treated with total thyroidectomy and RAI ablation, it can also be readily applied to patients treated with either less than total thyroidectomy or total thyroidectomy without RAI ablation. At most centers, these will be patients initially classified as low or intermediate risk for recurrent disease. The authors follow these patients in a similar fashion to those patients treated with total thyroidectomy and RAI ablation, with a serum Tg on suppression every 6 months and with a neck ultrasound yearly for 2 years. By definition, these are rather low-risk patients, so whole body RAI scanning is not required, and without RAI ablation stimulated Tg values have little meaning and are therefore not done.

Even patients treated with less than total thyroidectomy and RAI ablation should undergo secondary risk stratification at 2 years. The definition of excellent and acceptable response to therapy must be modified because an undetectable Tg, while present in many of them, would not be a requirement for excellent response to therapy. Thus, the authors consider a stable Tg over time, in conjunction with an ultrasound that shows no evidence of recurrent disease, as an excellent response to therapy. Very few patients fall into an "acceptable response to therapy" category because concern by the patients (and clinicians) about even subtle changes in the contralateral lobe or cervical lymph node ultrasonography during the follow-up of these patients often leads to additional therapy. While the authors are comfortable following most of these low- and intermediate-risk patients without additional surgery or RAI, we recognize that many patients and clinicians are not, and would recommend additional diagnostic tests or treatment.

The other difference in the long-term follow-up recommendations in patients treated with less than total thyroidectomy and RAI ablation is that neck ultrasonography is recommended as part of their ongoing follow up for the next 5 to 10 years, usually done every 2 to 3 years, depending on the individual risks factors of each patient. The rationale for this additional testing is that Tg on suppression without total thyroidectomy and RAI ablation is less sensitive for detection of small volume recurrent disease in the contralateral lobe or in cervical lymph nodes in these patients. These recommendations reflect a decreased reliance in the sensitivity and specificity of serum Tg and an increase in the importance of neck ultrasonography in the follow-up of low- to intermediate-risk patients treated with less than total thyroidectomy and RAI ablation.

Summary

After initial therapy to remove all evidence of gross disease, the primary goal of follow-up of thyroid cancer patients is to detect and treat recurrent disease to minimize morbidity and mortality. The authors' recommendations regarding a follow-up paradigm should be informed by initial risk stratification, ongoing risk stratification, response to therapy variables, and disease-free survival interval. In this article, the authors provide a framework that begins to integrate each of these factors into the complex decision-making process that is clinical medicine. With appropriate selection of tests, based on a risk-adapted approach, physicians should be able to identify patients with clinically significant disease recurrence in a timely fashion, without subjecting every thyroid cancer survivor to needless, expensive, time-consuming, and worrisome tests that are unlikely to uncover clinically significant disease.

References

[1] Ries LA, Harkins D, Krapcho M, et al. SEER cancer statistics review, 1975–2003, based on November 2005 SEER data submission. Available at: http://seer.cancer.gov/csr/1975_2003/. Accessed November 1, 2006.

[2] Hay ID, Thompson GB, Grant CS, et al. Papillary thyroid carcinoma managed at the Mayo clinic during six decades (1940–1999): temporal trends in initial therapy and long-term outcome in 2444 consecutively treated patients. World J Surg 2002;26(8):879–85.

[3] Mazzaferri EL, Kloos RT. Clinical review 128: current approaches to primary therapy for papillary and follicular thyroid cancer. J Clin Endocrinol Metab 2001;86(4):1447–63.

[4] Hundahl SA, Cady B, Cunningham MP, et al. Initial results from a prospective cohort study of 5583 cases of thyroid carcinoma treated in the United States during 1996. U.S. and German thyroid cancer study group. An American college of surgeons commission on cancer patient care evaluation study. Cancer 2000;89(1):202–17.

[5] Ries LAG, Melbert D, Krapcho M, et al. SEER cancer statistics review, 1975–2004, national cancer institute. Based on November 2006 SEER data submission, posted to the SEER web site, 2007. Available at: http://seer.cancer.gov/csr/1975_2004/. Accessed November 23, 2007.

[6] Bta. British thyroid association and royal college of physicians: guidelines for the management of thyroid cancer in adults. Available at: www.british-thyroid-association.org. Accessed November 1, 2006.

[7] Cooper DS, Doherty GM, Haugen BR, et al. Management guidelines for patients with thyroid nodules and differentiated thyroid cancer. Thyroid 2006;16(2):109–42.

[8] Pacini F, Schlumberger M, Dralle H, et al. European consensus for the management of patients with differentiated thyroid carcinoma of the follicular epithelium. Eur J Endocrinol 2006;154(6):787–803.

[9] Sherman SI. National comprehensive cancer network, clinical practice guidelines in oncology, thyroid cancer V.2.2007. Available at: http://www.nccn.org/professionals/physician_gls/PDF/thyroid.pdf. Accessed November 23, 2007.

[10] Thyroid Carcinoma Task Force. AACE/AAES medical/surgical guidelines for clinical practice: management of thyroid carcinoma. American association of clinical endocrinologists. American college of endocrinology. Endocr Pract 2001;7(3):202–20.

[11] Watkinson JC. The British thyroid association guidelines for the management of thyroid cancer in adults. Nucl Med Commun 2004;25(9):897–900.

[12] Tuttle RM, Leboeuf R, Martorella AJ. Papillary thyroid cancer: monitoring and therapy. Endocrinol Metab Clin North Am 2007;36(3):753–78.

[13] Grebe SK, Hay ID. Thyroid cancer nodal metastases: biologic significance and therapeutic considerations. Surg Oncol Clin N Am 1996;5(1):43–63.

[14] American Joint Committee on Cancer Staging Manual. 6th edition. New York: Springer-Verlag; 2002.

[15] Dean DS, Hay ID. Prognostic indicators in differentiated thyroid carcinoma. Cancer Control 2000;7(3):229–39.
[16] Pacini F, Agate L, Elisei R, et al. Outcome of differentiated thyroid cancer with detectable serum Tg and negative diagnostic (131)I whole body scan: comparison of patients treated with high (131)I activities versus untreated patients. J Clin Endocrinol Metab 2001;86(9): 4092–7.
[17] Pacini F, Molinaro E, Castagna MG, et al. Recombinant human thyrotropin-stimulated serum thyroglobulin combined with neck ultrasonography has the highest sensitivity in monitoring differentiated thyroid carcinoma. J Clin Endocrinol Metab 2003;88(8):3668–73.
[18] Robbins RJ, Wan Q, Grewal RK, et al. Real-time prognosis for metastatic thyroid carcinoma based on 2-[18F]fluoro-2-deoxy-D-glucose-positron emission tomography scanning. J Clin Endocrinol Metab 2006;91(2):498–505.
[19] Wang W, Larson SM, Tuttle RM, et al. Resistance of [18f]-fluorodeoxyglucose-avid metastatic thyroid cancer lesions to treatment with high-dose radioactive iodine. Thyroid 2001; 11(12):1169–75.
[20] Shaha AR, Shah JP, Loree TR. Low-risk differentiated thyroid cancer: the need for selective treatment. Ann Surg Oncol 1997;4(4):328–33.

ELSEVIER
SAUNDERS

Endocrinol Metab Clin N Am
37 (2008) 437–455

ENDOCRINOLOGY
AND METABOLISM
CLINICS
OF NORTH AMERICA

Surgical Approaches to Thyroid Tumors

Jessica E. Gosnell, MD, Orlo H. Clark, MD*

*University of California, San Francisco, Mt. Zion Medical Center, 1600 Divisadero Street,
Box 1674, San Francisco, CA 94143-1674, USA*

The surgical approach to thyroid tumors has changed considerably since Samuel Gross' alarming but colorful description of thyroidectomy as "horrid butchery" in 1866, in which "every stroke of [the] knife will be followed by a torrent of blood..." [1]. Thanks to the contributions of Kocker, Billroth, Halstead, Mayo, Dunhill, and Crile, the last one hundred years have heralded improved anesthesia, antisepsis, and surgical technique, and with these advances have come dramatically improved outcomes. The last several decades have brought refinements in surgical technique, an improved understanding of anatomy and embryology, and advances in the molecular biology of thyroid tumors. Indeed, thyroid surgery today is associated with minimal morbidity and mortality. Today's patients often undergo minimally invasive or minimal incision surgery by an experienced thyroid surgeon, go home the same or the next day, and suffer few long-term complications. When appropriately treated, most patients who have thyroid disease do well and continue to enjoy long disease-free productive lives. For the minority of patients who have aggressive cancers, familial tumor syndromes, or recurrent disease, continued improvements in technique, multimodal treatment protocols, and clinical trials using novel diagnostic tools and designer drug therapies should improve outcomes and save lives.

This article includes discussions of the surgical approach to benign and malignant disease and the role of prophylactic thyroidectomy and nodal dissection for medullary thyroid cancer. The controversy regarding the extent of dissection for differentiated thyroid cancer and the role of lymph node dissection are reviewed also. A description of the authors' surgical technique for thyroidectomy is detailed. Finally, several emerging technologies are introduced.

---

* Corresponding author.
E-mail address: clarko@surgery.ucsf.edu (O.H. Clark).

0889-8529/08/$ - see front matter © 2008 Elsevier Inc. All rights reserved.
doi:10.1016/j.ecl.2008.02.002

Benign disease

Total thyroidectomy is gaining popularity in the treatment of benign conditions of the thyroid, because it decreases the risk of recurrent disease [2,3]. The most common indications for thyroidectomy for benign disease are euthyroid multinodular goiter with local compression or retrosternal extension, toxic goiter, and solitary thyroid nodule with (1) indeterminate/ follicular or Hurthle cell pattern by fine needle aspiration (FNA) cytology; (2) prior ionizing radiation to the head and neck; (3) family history of thyroid cancer; (4) worrisome ultrasound features, such as irregularity, micro-calcifications, and hypervascularity; and (5) ultrasound findings of cervical lymphadenopathy. Surgical options for these conditions include thyroid lobectomy, subtotal thyroidectomy, near-total thyroidectomy, total thyroidectomy, and unilateral lobectomy with contralateral subtotal lobectomy (Hartley-Dunhill procedure); each are associated with distinct advantages and limitations. Operations in which some, but not all, thyroid tissue is resected have been associated with lower reported rates of recurrent laryngeal nerve injury and hypoparathyroidism, and therefore, have been attractive options for benign disease. Unfortunately, patients can develop recurrent disease after these unilateral resections. They also may require completion thyroidectomy for cancer identified on permanent histologic analysis. In both situations, reoperations often involve scaring and loss of normal tissue planes and are associated with higher rates of postoperative complications. Total thyroidectomy has several distinct advantages. When performed correctly, it generally precludes disease recurrence in the thyroid. It also serves to remove occult cancers and cancers that may develop in the contralateral lobe. Total thyroidectomy also can simplify thyroid hormone replacement. Many endocrine centers are reporting low or comparable complication rates after total thyroidectomy for benign thyroid disease compared with thyroid lobectomy [4,5].

In summary, total thyroidectomy may be an attractive surgical approach in selected patients who have benign or malignant thyroid disease when it can be done with a low complication rate. Unilateral thyroid operations are appropriate for low-risk patients who have unilateral disease. Subtotal, near-total or Hartley-Dunhill procedures may avoid complications in certain intraoperative situations if nerve injury or hypoparathyroidism seems imminent. However, total thyroidectomy should be considered for patients who have benign disease and who are at high-risk for recurrence or findings of cancer. Detailed discussions with patients are an essential part of preoperative planning.

Differentiated thyroid cancer

The "best" surgical approach for differentiated thyroid cancer continues to be controversial, mainly with regard to the extent of thyroidectomy and management of regional lymph nodes. This debate has been ongoing for decades and is unlikely to be definitively resolved without large prospective studies and long-term follow-up. While the readers are likely familiar with this controversy, it is useful to briefly review the context of the controversy, discuss the arguments on either side, and describe the overall trends.

Differentiated thyroid cancer is quite common; there are approximately 33,000 new cases diagnosed in the United States each year, which result in 1,400 deaths a year [6,7]. Thyroid cancer is the most rapid increasing cancer in women and is now the 7th most common cancer in women. The vast majority of these cancers, 85%–95%, are differentiated thyroid cancers, either of follicular or papillary histology. Approximately 5% are parafollicular C-cell-derived medullary thyroid cancers [8,9].

Patients who have differentiated thyroid cancer generally do well. Mortality rates overall are 7%, with the majority of patients being either cured of the disease or living with recurrent disease for many years. However, recurrent disease occurs in up to 11% of patients, and up to half of these patients ultimately die of the disease. Recurrence in patients who have papillary thyroid cancer can occur up to four decades after initial surgical treatment, whereas recurrence of follicular thyroid cancer almost always occurs within 14 years of initial treatment.

A total of 17 risk stratifications systems have been developed around the world in an effort to better predict outcomes in patients who have differentiated thyroid cancer. Various systems, such as AMES, AGES, MACIS, DAMES, GAMES, and TNM, attempt to separate patients into low and high risk groups (Box 1), and include patient and tumor characteristics. Unfortunately, as the tumor characteristics are collected postoperatively, they do little to guide operative planning.

Box 1. Risk stratification systems for differentiated thyroid cancer

AGES
  Age, metastases, extent, size
AMES
  Age, metastases, extent, size
MACIS
  Metastases, age, completeness of resection
DAMES
  Diploid, age, metastases, extent, size
GAMES
  Grade, age, metastases, extent, size
TNM/IUAC
  Tumor size, nodal status, metastases

Extent of resection

Surgery is the primary treatment for differentiated thyroid cancer. Two general surgical approaches have been advocated among experts: unilateral thyroid lobectomy (including the isthmus) and total or near-total thyroidectomy. A consensus has been reached for certain subgroups of patients. For example, in high-risk patients, such as those who have bilateral tumors, distant metastases, extrathyroidal extension, and tumors with more aggressive histology (insular, tall cell), most doctors would favor total thyroidectomy. Similarly, in low-risk patients who have occult papillary thyroid cancer or minimally invasive follicular cancer or for non-compliant patients incapable of taking daily thyroid hormone replacement, lobectomy may be the favored procedure [10]. However, conflicting views persist for other low- to moderate-risk patients who have differentiated thyroid cancer.

Proponents of thyroid lobectomy/isthmusectomy cite several arguments. First, patients who have differentiated thyroid cancers generally do well [11]. Second, more extensive thyroidectomy has not resulted in a significant difference in either mortality or local recurrence in patients undergoing lobectomy versus total thyroidectomy in some reports [12]. Third, because unilateral thyroid operations expose only one recurrent laryngeal nerve (RLN) and only two of the four parathyroid glands to injury; advocates for this procedure suggest that complication rates are lower with lobectomy than with total thyroidectomy.

Proponents of total thyroidectomy include the following support for their technique. Total or near-total thyroidectomy facilitates the use of radioactive iodine postoperatively and allows for a lesser dose to detect and ablate residual thyroid tissue. Occult M1 (distant metastases) also can be identified. Thyroglobulin is a much more reliable tumor marker following more complete thyroid resections. Recurrent carcinoma is more common in patients treated with less than total or near-total thyroidectomy. Both DeGroot and Grant and their colleagues have documented fewer recurrences and deaths [13,14], even in low-risk patients. Up to 80% of patients who have differentiated thyroid cancer have multicentric tumors [15,16] with a rich bi-lobar lymphatic drainage pattern [17]. Total and near-total thyroidectomies resect any occult contralateral lesions and preclude development of new tumors within the thyroid. In doing so, total thyroidectomy also decreases the risk of the rare but devastating progression from differentiated thyroid cancer to anaplastic cancer. Whereas most patients who have differentiated thyroid cancer do well, up to 11% of patients recur, and half of these patients eventually die of their disease. It is has been difficult to identify these patients preoperatively, because they include patients in low-risk categories. In a recent retrospective study by Bilimoria and colleagues [18] of more than 50,000 patients, improved survival was documented with total thyroidectomy for patients who had papillary thyroid cancers larger than 1 cm. Finally, the contention that total or near-total thyroidectomy is associated with higher complication rates has not been supported by data from many experienced endocrine centers around the world. Numerous groups, including the authors' group, have reported comparable rates of RLN injury, hypoparathyroidism and postoperative bleeding for total thyroidectomy, near-total thyroidectomy, and thyroid lobectomy [19–22].

In summary, there are no class I data comparing extent of surgery for patients who have low-to moderate-risk differentiated thyroid cancer; however, several retrospective studies have suggested decreased recurrence and improved survival. In a recent international questionnaire, 90% of polled endocrine surgeons would perform a total thyroidectomy for differentiated thyroid cancers greater 1 cm, and 100% of surgeons would perform a total thyroidectomy for tumors greater than 2 cm [23]. The authors believe that the advantages to total or near-total thyroidectomy far outweigh the disadvantages. Total thyroidectomy, when performed by an experienced surgeon, offers the best treatment for differentiated tumors greater than 1 cm [18]. This is dependent, however, on the ability to perform these procedures with a complication rate of less than 2%. When a surgeon is concerned about the survival of the parathyroid glands or the RLN on the side of the initial lobectomy, he or she may do a subtotal or near-total thyroidectomy on the contralateral side to decrease the risk of complications.

Lymph node dissection

The surgical approach to regional lymph nodes in patients who have differentiated thyroid cancer is also controversial and plagued by a lack of prospective data. Important considerations include (1) lymphatic drainage patterns of the thyroid gland, (2) the incidence and prognostic significance of lymph node metastases in differentiated thyroid cancer, (3) the effect of lymph node metastases on survival and local recurrence, and (4) the complications of lymph node dissection.

The thyroid gland has a rich network of intrathyroidal lymphatic drainage with communication across the isthmus. Lymphatics from the thyroid accompany the vascular structures. Lymphatic flow, elegantly studied and published by Noguchi [17] in the 1970s, tends to be to the ipsilateral level VI nodes; this compartment is the most common site of metastatic papillary thyroid cancer in about 20% of patients who have nodal metastases.

Regional lymph node metastases in patients who have differentiated cancer can occur microscopically in up to 88% of patients who have papillary thyroid cancer and can occur in fewer than 10% of patients who have follicular thyroid cancer [24–27]. The prognostic significance of lymph node metastases in papillary thyroid cancer has been disputed. Several studies suggest that lymph node metastases are associated with an increased recurrence rate but have no adverse effect on cause-specific mortality [13,28]. Other studies show an increase in recurrence and mortality [29–31]. Authors in support of prophylactic lymph node dissection also describe reductions in thyroglobulin levels following prophylactic ipsilateral neck dissection, suggesting a higher cure rate [32].

Historically, lymph node dissections were morbid procedures with high rates of RLN injury, hypoparathyroidism, postoperative bleeding, and disability from loss of the internal jugular vein, spinal accessory nerve, and sternocleidomastoid muscle. With what were felt to be prohibitively high complication rates and unclear benefits, it is not surprising that prophylactic lateral lymph node dissection has not been adopted widely in North America and Europe. However, there has been a shift away from radical and modified neck dissections and a shift toward "functional" lymph node dissections that are more relevant for thyroid cancer (pre-tracheal, or level VI, and parajugular levels II, III, and IV).

So-called "berry picking" lymph node dissections, in which single or clustered palpable lymph nodes are resected, has been replaced by compartment-based lymph node dissections; large nodal metastases are almost always associated with smaller nodal metastases [27]. Compartment-based dissections are based upon the most commonly involved lymph node basins in thyroid cancer, rather than on those dissections originally described for epithelial-derived tumors of the aerodigestive tract. Ultrasound has emerged as an essential preoperative tool to identify clinically relevant cervical lymph node disease, because it often is used postoperatively to search for metastatic disease [33]. Less morbid than more radical operations, modified radical neck dissections and functional or selective lymph node dissections preserve important functional structures in the neck, such as the sternocleidomastoid muscle, the internal jugular vein, the spinal accessory nerve, and the cervical sensory nerves, and these dissections seem to reduce local recurrence and improve survival [34,35].

Follicular thyroid cancer

The surgical approach to follicular thyroid cancer has several distinctions. Pure follicular thyroid cancer is relatively rare, accounting for approximately 10% of patients who have thyroid cancer (see Box 1). In contrast to papillary thyroid cancers, follicular carcinomas tend to invade blood vessels and metastasize hematogenously. Lymph node metastases are uncommon (approximately 2%–13%) [36,37], while distant metastases are described in 5%–33% of cases at initial presentation [24]. Follicular thyroid cancer is characterized by generally benign cytologic features and often minimal invasion of the capsule or capsular blood vessels. FNA cytology cannot distinguish between benign or malignant follicular or Hurthle cell neoplasms. For this reason, patients who have follicular or Hurthle cell lesions often must undergo what is essentially a diagnostic operation, namely unilateral lobectomy and isthmusectomy. Frozen section evaluation rarely is diagnostic and, therefore, is not generally done. Findings of capsular or vascular invasion on permanent sections are indicative of carcinoma and prompt

consideration of completion thyroidectomy, followed by radioiodine ablation and thyroid suppression. Recent data suggest that minimal capsular
invasion and minimal vascular invasions may represent different disease;
the latter is of greater clinical significance [38]. Some authors advocate completion thyroidectomy in 7–10 days, while others wait 2–3 months. In either
case, lymph node dissection generally is not done because of the relatively
low incidence of lymph node metastases in follicular thyroid cancer, and
surgeons want to avoid complications such as recurrent laryngeal damage,
hypoparathyroidism, and bleeding in the reoperative field.

Medullary thyroid cancer

The surgical approach to medullary thyroid cancer (MTC) is guided by
its unique embryologic origins, its well-described genetic associations, its
relatively aggressive behavior, and the lack of effective adjuvant treatment.
Optimal outcomes for patients who have MTC depend on an attentive
preoperative work-up and meticulous thyroid and nodal operations by an
experienced surgical team.

MTC accounts for 5%–10% of all thyroid cancers, but it leads to a disproportionate number of thyroid cancer-related deaths (about 15%). While
most cases of MTC are sporadic, up to 25% of cases present as a component
of a hereditary disorder, such as multiple endocrine neoplasia (MEN) 2A,
MEN 2B or familial MTC. These disorders are associated with mutations
in the tyrosine-kinase rearranged during transcription (RET) proto-oncogene. All patients who have MTC need to undergo comprehensive RET
testing, because at least 10% of patients who have MTC have a de novo
germline mutation. Certain RET mutations also are associated with pheochromocytoma or primary hyperparathyroidism [39]. Clinically, MTC can
range from a very indolent sporadic disease to a very aggressive hereditary
form (such as those that occur with MEN-2B) with early local invasion and
rapid distant metastases.

In contrast to papillary and follicular thyroid cancers, which are derived
from follicular cells, MTC is derived from the parafollicular C-cell. Parafollicular C-cells are derived from the neural crest and produce and excrete
calcitonin. They do not secrete thyroglobulin. This embryologic distinction
has important diagnostic and therapeutic implications, because calcitonin
(rather than thyroglobulin) is the appropriate tumor marker in patients
who have MTC. Moreover, C-cells do not concentrate iodine, making postoperative radioactive iodine ablation an ineffective adjunctive therapy.
Thyroid suppression using thyroid hormones also appears to be ineffective,
because MTC cells do not have thyroid-stimulating hormone receptors.
Chemotherapy and radiation therapy have shown only limited success in
some small series [40–43].

As such, surgery remains the mainstay of therapy for MTC. The extent of
surgery is dictated by two important characteristics of MTC. First, familial

MTC tends to be bilateral, associated with C-cell hyperplasia, and multi-focal [44,45]. When Dralle and coworkers [46] reviewed the management of hereditary MTC in 1995, they reported biochemical normalization of serum calcitonin in 60% of patients who had undergone total thyroidectomy, whereas this occurred in only 10% of patients who underwent partial thyroidectomy. Other investigators have published similar findings. Second, postoperative radioactive ablation of remnants is ineffective in MTC. For these reasons, total thyroidectomy is indicated for all patients who have sporadic or hereditary MTC, irrespective of tumor size.

MTC is the first cancer for which prophylactic surgery was performed based on a genetic test. Patients who have hereditary forms of MTC can be identified early in the course of their disease or before MTC develops. Comprehensive mutational analysis of the RET proto-oncogene is recommended now for all patients who have MTC, even for apparently sporadic cases [39,47]. For at-risk kindred, genetic analysis has reassured mutation-negative family members. Because essentially all affected individuals will develop MTC, genetic analysis enables prophylactic thyroidectomy in mutation-positive patients at an earlier stage, which is associated with better outcomes [48]. Total thyroidectomy usually is performed in germline RET mutation carriers before the development of MTC or lymph node metastases.

The surgical approach to lymph nodes in patients who have MTC is considerably less controversial than that for the other differentiated thyroid cancers, largely because the number and size of lymph node metastases are of prognostic significance [49]. In addition, because these tumors do not concentrate iodine, nodal metastases cannot be ablated with radioiodine. Surgical clearance of involved nodes is the only effective treatment. Total thyroidectomy with meticulous bilateral removal of all central lymph nodes is essential for the best long-term results. An ipsilateral modified neck dissection (Levels II, III, and IV) is recommended for patients who have tumors over 1.5 cm, because nodal metastases are present in more than half of these patients [50–52]. Less aggressive approaches are associated with a higher recurrence rate [53]. For patients identified by RET testing, the approach to lymph node dissection is evolving as more is understood about genotype-phenotype correlations with individual codon mutations [54–57]. Historically, lymph node dissection (LND) was recommended for mutation-positive family members older than 5 years old, but it now should be based on which particular codon is involved, the serum calcitonin level, and the ultrasound findings [54,58]. Patients who have codon mutations known to be aggressive (such as codon 918 with MEN-2B) may merit an early aggressive lymph node dissection at diagnosis or at 1 year of age. In contrast, patients who have more indolent mutations likely can be treated with total thyroidectomy alone if the calcitonin level and neck ultrasound findings are normal. Studies by Skinner and colleagues and the Euromen Study Group suggest that total thyroidectomy should be done in familial MTC and MEN-2A before age 6 [55,59]. In a recent analysis of a large

MEN-2A family that had codon 804 mutations, central lymph node dissections were almost uniformly negative in young asymptomatic patients [56,57].

Anaplastic cancer

The surgical approach to anaplastic cancer has been in evolution as investigators have attempted to improve the dismal prognosis. Anaplastic cancer is a rare but lethal disease, accounting for less than 2% of all thyroid cancers, but accounting for a disproportionate 40% of thyroid cancer related deaths [9,60,61]. Survival often is measured in months rather than years, with a median survival rate of 4–6 months. The role of the surgeon has included providing adequate tissue for diagnosis only, providing a surgical airway for patients in extremis, or being the primary treatment followed by adjuvant chemotherapy and external beam radiation therapy (XRT). Unfortunately, single modality treatments have not been effective. More recently, a multimodal approach with neoadjuvant chemotherapy/XRT followed by surgery has showed modest improvements in survival. Patients are treated first with radiosensitizing chemotherapy and then treated with XRT. Surgery is reserved for patients who show an initial response and those patients for whom it is feasible to resect all macroscopic disease [62]. In a series from the authors' institution that was published in 2005, this approach led to a significant reduction in the disease-specific mortality [61]. However, most patients do not undergo surgery, either because they did not meet the eligibility requirements listed above, or because they were too debilitated from the neoadjuvant treatment. For patients in this category who had progressive airway compromise, tracheal stents can provide palliation [63].

Surgical technique

While the improvements in surgery for thyroid disease in the last century were profound, more recent refinements in surgical technique, lighting, and magnification continue to improve patient outcomes. An improved understanding of anatomy, an increased recognition of embryologic vestiges (such as the tubercle of Zuckerkandl), and thyrothymic rests have resulted in more complete resections, decreased recurrence rates, and decreased complications. There is an increased awareness of the external branch of the superior laryngeal nerve, the so-called "high note nerve," and the "neglected nerve" [64,65], which may result in decreased voice range and increased voice fatigue if injured during thyroidectomy. Newer innovations, such as nerve monitoring, laparoscopy, intraoperative ultrasound, and ultrasound localization of lymph node recurrence, continue to move the field of endocrine surgery forward.

A general description of thyroidectomy is as follows. The procedure usually is performed under general anesthesia by using either a laryngeal mask and local anesthetic infiltration or by keeping the patient intubated and ventilated. It generally is performed as an overnight (23 hours) stay. The patient position is supine, with the neck held in extension by putting a pillow or bean bag under the shoulders. For adequate illumination of the narrow operative field, an operating headlight is helpful. A cervical block with 0.25% Marcaine can be used. The exact length of the incision depends on the size of the tumor, the girth of the patient's neck, and the amount of neck extension. Patients who have thin necks, smaller tumors and necks that extend will require a smaller incision. A curvilinear incision is made in a natural skin crease, approximately 1 cm caudal to the cricothyroid cartilage, and extended through the skin, subcutaneous tissue, and platysma.

Once the skin and platysma have been incised, a subplatysmal space is developed using electrocautery. Dissection in this plane can be done without blood loss, because it is an avascular plane of loose areolar tissue. The dissection is carried superiorly to the level of the thyroid cartilage and inferiorly to the sternal notch. Skin and platysma flaps are retracted using a spring retractor. Then the midline raphe of the strap muscles is incised from the thyroid cartilage to the sternal notch. The sternohyoid muscle is dissected from the underlying sternothyroid muscle until the ansa hypoglossal nerve is encountered laterally. Then the sternothyroid is dissected from the underlying thyroid gland, working laterally until the medial border of the carotid sheath is reached. After appropriate dissection, the strap muscles usually can be retracted adequately. If necessary, in patients who have large or invasive tumors, the strap muscles can be divided with cautery. This should be done high on the muscles, because the ansa hypoglossal nerve innervates them from below. The middle thyroid vein (or veins) is ligated and divided. The space medial to the common carotid artery is dissected then, sweeping the fibrofatty tissue away from the thyroid. We usually do this cephalad to the cricoid cartilage first, because the recurrent laryngeal nerve enters the larynx caudate to this area. This dissection is continued until the prevertebral fascia is reached. The space between the posterior aspect of the thyroid gland and the prevertebral fascia is developed further by gentle dissection. This step in the dissection exposes almost the entire anatomy of the recurrent laryngeal nerve and parathyroid glands.

Then the upper pole of the thyroid gland is mobilized. The upper pole dissection is facilitated by retracting the thyroid gland laterally and caudad, to enter the avascular plane between the thyroid gland and the cricothyroid muscle. In most cases, this allows the external branch of the recurrent laryngeal nerve to be identified and preserved (Fig. 1). Then upper pole vessels are ligated and divided individually.

Next, attention is directed to the midline. The tracheal surface is identified above and below the isthmus, and a blunt clamp can be passed along the anterior aspect of the trachea. A pyramidal lobe, which is present in as much as 80% of patients, should be identified and dissected to be

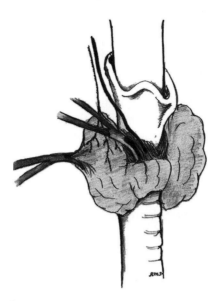

Fig. 1. Avascular plane between the thyroid gland and the cricothyroid muscle. (*Courtesy of* Robert M. Savio, MD, San Francisco, CA.)

included with the specimen. Failure to do so can result in recurrence or increase the dose of radioiodine postoperatively. An attempt also should be made to identify and resect the Delphian lymph node, which is found in the midline just cephalad to the cricoid cartilage. This midline dissection can be performed before the upper pole dissection as well. By providing identification of midline landmarks early in the case, this maneuver can be helpful in patients who have large tumors and distorted anatomy.

Then the inferior pole is mobilized. Inferior thyroid veins on the trachea in the midline can be ligated and divided. The thyrothymic ligament is detached from the thyroid, and a careful search for an inferior parathyroid gland can be undertaken.

At this stage, with all the prior mobilization, the thyroid nodule often can be delivered anteriorly and medially through the incision, allowing the critical lateral dissection to be undertaken close to the skin surface. As the lobe of the thyroid is retracted medially and the carotid sheath is retracted laterally, tension is placed on the inferior thyroid artery so the recurrent laryngeal nerve is encountered more easily where it crosses over or under the inferior thyroid artery at the midportion of the thyroid gland. The tubercle of Zuckerkandl is also an important landmark. Pay careful attention to any tubercle remnants, which, if left, can present as recurrence. In addition, the tubercle of Zuckerkandl can serve as an "arrow" to the RLN, which often runs just deep and medial to it [66]. The superior parathyroid often is situated at the end of the tubercle. Because the left and right recurrent nerves "recur" around different structures on the left and right, the anatomy of the recurrent laryngeal nerve is slightly different on the two sides of the neck. The right nerve tends to be more oblique in its trajectory, whereas the left nerve tends to be more medial, hugging the tracheoesophageal groove, before entering the cricothyroid muscle. In approximately 1% of the population, the right RLN is non-recurrent, thereby entering the cricothyroid muscle from a lateral or a superior direction. The recurrent nerves often can branch before they enter the cricothyroid muscle, and the medial branches usually contain the motor fibers. For this reason, identifying the nerve low in the neck and following it superiorly for any braches is often the safest approach. For patients who have bulky or invasive tumors or in those undergoing reoperative surgery, identifying the nerve medially and high in the neck as it enters the cricothyroid muscle is another useful maneuver. When the latter approach is used, one should not divide any tissue that could be the recurrent nerve.

The parathyroid glands should be dissected off the thyroid capsule on as broad a vascular pedicle possible to preserve their blood supply. The superior parathyroid glands most commonly are encountered close to the intersection of the inferior thyroid artery, the recurrent laryngeal nerve, and the tubercle of Zuckerkandl at the level of the cricoid cartilage. The inferior parathyroid glands are more variable in their location. They usually can be identified caudal to the inferior thyroid artery and anterior to the recurrent nerve; up to 15% of these glands are located in the thymus. Both parathyroid glands receive their blood supply from tertiary branches from the inferior and superior thyroid arteries; thus, it is important to ligate vessels directly on the thyroid capsule as opposed to main arterial trunks. Any parathyroid gland that cannot be preserved with its blood supply intact is removed and placed in iced physiologic saline for subsequent autotransplantation. A frozen section generally should be done to confirm parathyroid tissue. The parathyroid gland should be minced and autotransplanted in 1–3 pockets in the muscle. In most cases, this should be done in the sternocleidomastoid muscle on the same side and marked with a metal clip. When the thyroid cancer is extensive, highly invasive, or XRT is anticipated, the contralateral muscle is used. The forearm is used for parathyroid autotransplantation in patients at high risk for the development of hyperparathyroidism, such as MEN-1 or MEN-2A with high-risk codon mutations. Using this technique, it is easier to document which parathyroid gland is abnormal and to remove it.

With the nerves and the parathyroid glands in full view, the remaining dissection can be done relatively quickly. The ligament of Berry, a condensation of connective tissue that attaches the thyroid gland to the trachea, is divided then. Small arteries and veins are virtually always present. Because of the close proximity of the ligament of Berry to the recurrent laryngeal nerve, the nerve is most vulnerable to injury at this site during this dissection, and bleeding can be troublesome. No vessel should be clamped at this site until the recurrent laryngeal nerve is identified.

If a total thyroidectomy will be performed, the thyroid should be left intact, and an identical dissection is performed on the contralateral side. For patients in whom thyroid lobectomy alone is performed, the contralateral thyroid lobe should be palpated through the strap muscles or examined by ultrasound. The isthmus should be resected, with hemostatic control at the contralateral side. If carcinoma is present, this approach avoids recurrence and possible invasion of the trachea. In addition, it will help avoid unsightly midline masses in patients who may develop compensatory thyroid hypertrophy.

After thyroidectomy, the removed thyroid gland should be examined to ensure that no parathyroid glands have been excised inadvertently. If a parathyroid gland has been removed, it should be dissected off the thyroid gland, a small biopsy taken to confirm parathyroid tissue, and the gland should be autotransplanted as described above and marked with a clip. Once hemostasis is achieved, the skin incision is closed, using subcuticular sutures or butterfly clips.

Special topics

Postoperative care

Complications from thyroid surgery are rare but life-threatening. A threatened airway from hematoma or a bilateral RLN injury and hypoparathyroidism can be indolent, dramatic, or immediate in their presentation. A high index of suspicion, multidisciplinary training, and open lines of communication are essential. A preprinted order set, with hourly quantitative patient assessments (neck circumference, voice score), can provide early recognition of a hematoma. Serum calcium levels should be checked on the evening of surgery and on the first postoperative morning. Prophylactic calcium and vitamin D can be started in patients who are at high-risk for symptomatic hypocalcemia. Intact parathyroid hormone levels postoperatively have been suggested as good predictors of patients who will develop clinically significant hypoparathyroidism, but the authors doubt if it will prove to be cost effective.

Locally advanced thyroid cancer

Occasionally thyroid cancers may invade the trachea or esophagus [53,67]. Tracheal resection, rather than shaving the tumor from the trachea, may be indicated for patients who have intraluminal involvement of differentiated thyroid cancers, and tracheal resection has been associated with long-term survival [68–70]. Segmental tracheal resection for patients who do not have intraluminal involvement is controversial and should be individualized, depending on the patient's tumor biology, the presence of distant metastases, the patient's ability to be treated by nonoperative means, and individual patient priorities. Adjacent muscles, such as the strap muscles or latisimus dorsi, can be used to buttress repairs or plug small holes in the trachea [71]. The recurrent laryngeal nerves, when functioning, can be dissected free from the trachea or tumor and preserved. When any trachea is resected, the authors place a Penrose drain in case of air leakage, and antibiotics are recommended in this select group of patients.

Technology

The surgical approach to thyroid tumors has been energized by a number of emerging technologies over the last several years. While the analysis is ongoing, several newer techniques have stimulated spirited discussion at national and international meetings and have prompted important prospective studies. For example, nerve monitors have been introduced for identification and preservation of the recurrent laryngeal nerve. Intraoperative monitoring of the RLN was described fist in 1969 by Flisberg and Lindholm [72]. Since then, several forms of monitors have been proposed, including those that rely on palpation of the larynx while a nerve stimulator is used on the RLN to those that provide an audible signal when the RLN is approached. While some studies have suggested that the routine use of nerve monitors improves identification and decreases injury to the RLN [73,74], others have shown no prognostic benefit [75–78]. False positives and false negatives have been reported in approximately 5% of patients in whom nerve monitors were used, which, in the hands of most endocrine surgeons, is in excess of the rate of nerve injury to be prevented. Whereas no compelling data support its routine use yet, public awareness has grown, and an increasing number of Internet-savvy patients ask about nerve monitoring. The technique may prove useful for reoperative cases or in patients who have locally advanced disease. It also can be a useful teaching tool, by providing trainees visual and auditory confirmation of RLN anatomy and by providing "on-site" feedback to the surgeon about subtle surgical techniques (retraction, pressure) and their immediate impact on nerve function. The authors believe that nerve monitors are useful for confirming that a structure is the RLN, but they should not be relied upon for identification of the RLN. Routine identification of the recurrent laryngeal nerve, in contrast to avoidance, does appear to reduce RLN injury [79–82].

The role of ultrasound for the thyroid surgeon continues to evolve in each area of surgical decision-making. Preoperative ultrasound can provide helpful information for planning the extent of thyroid resection and lymph node resection. Lymph node dissection decreases recurrence and may improve survival. In addition, many recurrences are believed to represent persistent disease that was not appreciated or resected at the initial operation [83]. Since palpation is an imprecise tool for assessing lymph node involvement, preoperative ultrasound use is gaining acceptance. Intraoperative, pre-incision ultrasound is useful also; it can provide anatomic correlation for teaching, reconfirm thyroid pathology and recurrence, help to fashion the incision, and provide access for image-guided localization of recurrent disease (eg, wire and dye) [84]. A full discussion of postoperative ultrasound is not included here, but it is more sensitive than a whole body radioiodine scan for cervical recurrence in low-risk thyroid cancer patients [85].

Summary

Thyroidectomy has evolved from a dreaded "thankless" procedure with grim outcomes to a safe operation with excellent results, when performed by an experienced thyroid surgeon [86]. Much of the recent technical progress owes to an improved understanding of thyroid embryology and anatomy, which has fostered preservation of the recurrent laryngeal nerve, the external branch of the superior laryngeal nerve, and the parathyroid glands. Improved understanding of the natural history and biology of each distinct form of thyroid cancer and preoperative ultrasonography should allow the surgeon to tailor the operation appropriately, especially with regard to prophylactic or therapeutic lymph node dissection. More extensive initial surgery, such as total thyroidectomy, decreases tumor recurrence and appears to prolong life. Whether prophylactic ipsilateral central lymph node dissection, rather than just central lymph node exploration, is indicated is unknown and will require further investigation.

References

[1] Gross SD. A system of surgery, vol. 2. 4th edition. Philadelphia: HC Lea; 1886. p. 394.
[2] Reeve TS, Delbridge L, Cohen A, et al. Total thyroidectomy. The preferred option for multinodular goiter. Ann Surg 1987;206:782–6.
[3] Lal G, Ituarte P, Kebebew E, et al. Should total thyroidectomy become the preferred procedure for surgical management of Graves' disease? Thyroid 2005;15:569–74.
[4] Bellantone R, Lombardi CP, Bossola M, et al. Total thyroidectomy for management of benign thyroid disease: review of 526 cases. World J Surg 2002;26:1468–71.
[5] Zambudio AR, Rodriguez J, Riquelme J, et al. Prospective study of postoperative complications after total thyroidectomy for multinodular goiters by surgeons with experience in endocrine surgery. Ann Surg 2004;240:18–25.
[6] Greenlee RT, Murray T, Bolden S, et al. Cancer statistics, 2000. CA Cancer J Clin 2000;50: 7–33.
[7] Sherman SI, Angelos P, Ball DW, et al. Thyroid carcinoma. J Natl Compr Canc Netw 2007; 5:568–621.
[8] Hundahl SA, Fleming ID, Fremgen AM, et al. A National Cancer Data Base report on 53,856 cases of thyroid carcinoma treated in the U.S., 1985–1995 [see comments]. Cancer 1998;83:2638–48.
[9] Gilliland FD, Hunt WC, Morris DM, et al. Prognostic factors for thyroid carcinoma. A population-based study of 15,698 cases from the Surveillance, Epidemiology and End Results (SEER) program 1973–1991. Cancer 1997;79:564–73.
[10] Mazzaferri EL. Management of low-risk differentiated thyroid cancer. Endocr Pract 2007; 13:498–512.
[11] Hay ID. Management of patients with low-risk papillary thyroid carcinoma. Endocr Pract 2007;13:521–33.

[12] Schroder DM, Chambors A, France CJ. Operative strategy for thyroid cancer. Is total thyroidectomy worth the price? Cancer 1986;58:2320–8.

[13] DeGroot LJ, Kaplan EL, McCormick M, et al. Natural history, treatment, and course of papillary thyroid carcinoma. J Clin Endocrinol Metab 1990;71:414–24.

[14] Grant CS, Hay ID, Gough IR, et al. Local recurrence in papillary thyroid carcinoma: is extent of surgical resection important? Surgery 1988;104:954–62.

[15] Katoh R, Sasaki J, Kurihara H, et al. Multiple thyroid involvement (intraglandular metastasis) in papillary thyroid carcinoma. A clinicopathologic study of 105 consecutive patients. Cancer 1992;70:1585–90.

[16] Carcangiu ML, Zampi G, Pupi A, et al. Papillary carcinoma of the thyroid. A clinicopathologic study of 241 cases treated at the University of Florence, Italy. Cancer 1985;55: 805–28.

[17] Noguchi S, Noguchi A, Murakami N. Papillary carcinoma of the thyroid. I. Developing pattern of metastasis. Cancer 1970;26:1053–60.

[18] Bilimoria KY, Bentrem DJ, Ko CY, et al. Extent of surgery affects survival for papillary thyroid cancer. Ann Surg 2007;246:375–81 [discussion: 381–4].

[19] Clark OH. Total thyroidectomy: the treatment of choice for patients with differentiated thyroid cancer. Ann Surg 1982;196:361–70.

[20] de Roy van Zuidewijn DB, Songun I, Kievit J, et al. Complications of thyroid surgery. Ann Surg Oncol 1995;2:56–60.

[21] Reeve TS, Curtin A, Fingleton L, et al. Can total thyroidectomy be performed as safely by general surgeons in provincial centers as by surgeons in specialized endocrine surgical units? Making the case for surgical training. Arch Surg 1994;129:834–6.

[22] Perzik S. The place of total thyroidectomy in the management of 909 patients with thyroid disease. Am J Surg 1976;132:480–3.

[23] Shigematsu N, Takami H, Kubo A. Unique treatment policy for well-differentiated thyroid cancer in Japan: results of a questionnaire distributed to members of the Japanese Society of Thyroid Surgery and the International Association of Endocrine Surgeons. Endocr J 2006; 53:829–39.

[24] Emerick GT, Duh QY, Siperstein AE, et al. Diagnosis, treatment, and outcome of follicular thyroid carcinoma. Cancer 1993;72:3287–95.

[25] Noguchi M, Kumaki T, Taniya T, et al. Bilateral cervical lymph node metastases in well-differentiated thyroid cancer. Arch Surg 1990;125:804–6.

[26] Noguchi S, Murakami N. The value of lymph-node dissection in patients with differentiated thyroid cancer. Surg Clin North Am 1987;67:251–61.

[27] Noguchi S, Noguchi A, Murakami N. Papillary carcinoma of the thyroid. II. Value of prophylactic lymph node excision. Cancer 1970;26:1061–4.

[28] Grebe SK, Hay ID. Thyroid cancer nodal metastases: biologic significance and therapeutic considerations. Surg Oncol Clin N Am 1996;5:43–63.

[29] Noguchi S, Murakami N, Yamashita H, et al. Papillary thyroid carcinoma: modified radical neck dissection improves prognosis. Arch Surg 1998;133:276–80.

[30] Simon D, Goretzki PE, Witte J, et al. Incidence of regional recurrence guiding radicality in differentiated thyroid carcinoma. World J Surg 1996;20:860–6 [discussion: 866].

[31] Harwood J, Clark OH, Dunphy JE. Significance of lymph node metastasis in differentiated thyroid cancer. Am J Surg 1978;136:107–12.

[32] Sywak M, Cornford L, Roach P, et al. Routine ipsilateral level VI lymphadenectomy reduces postoperative thyroglobulin levels in papillary thyroid cancer. Surgery 2006;140:1000–5 [discussion: 1005–7].

[33] Rossi CR, Mocellin S, Scagnet B, et al. The role of preoperative ultrasound scan in detecting lymph node metastasis before sentinel node biopsy in melanoma patients. J Surg Oncol 2003; 83:80–4.

[34] Caron NR, Clark OH. Papillary thyroid cancer: surgical management of lymph node metastases. Curr Treat Options Oncol 2005;6:311–22.

[35] Cheah WK, Arici C, Ituarte PH, et al. Complications of neck dissection for thyroid cancer. World J Surg 2002;26:1013–6.

[36] Hirabayashi RN, Lindsays S. Carcinoma of the thyroid gland: a statistical study of 390 patients. J Clin Endocrinol Metab 1961;21:1596–610.

[37] Grebe SK, Hay ID. Follicular thyroid cancer. Endocrinol Metab Clin North Am 1995;24: 761–801.

[38] D'Avanzo A, Treseler P, Ituarte PH, et al. Follicular thyroid carcinoma: histology and prognosis. Cancer 2004;100:1123–9.

[39] Learoyd DL, Marsh DJ, Richardson AL, et al. Genetic testing for familial cancer. Consequences of RET proto-oncogene mutation analysis in multiple endocrine neoplasia, type 2. Arch Surg 1997;132:1022–5.

[40] Schlumberger M, Abdelmoumene N, Delisle MJ, et al. Treatment of advanced medullary thyroid cancer with an alternating combination of 5 FU-streptozocin and 5 FU-dacarbazine. The Groupe d'Etude des Tumeurs a Calcitonine (GETC). Br J Cancer 1995;71:363–5.

[41] Brierley J, Tsang R, Simpson WJ, et al. Medullary thyroid cancer: analyses of survival and prognostic factors and the role of radiation therapy in local control. Thyroid 1996;6:305–10.

[42] Scherubl H, Raue F, Ziegler R. Combination chemotherapy of advanced medullary and differentiated thyroid cancer. Phase II study. J Cancer Res Clin Oncol 1990;116:21–3.

[43] Orlandi F, Caraci P, Berruti A, et al. Chemotherapy with dacarbazine and 5-fluorouracil in advanced medullary thyroid cancer. Ann Oncol 1994;5:763–5.

[44] Russell CF, Van Heerden JA, Sizemore GW, et al. The surgical management of medullary thyroid carcinoma. Ann Surg 1983;197:42–8.

[45] van Heerden JA, Grant CS, Gharib H, et al. Long-term course of patients with persistent hypercalcitoninemia after apparent curative primary surgery for medullary thyroid carcinoma. Ann Surg 1990;212:395–400 [discussion: 400].

[46] Dralle H, Scheumann GF, Proye C, et al. The value of lymph node dissection in hereditary medullary thyroid carcinoma: a retrospective, European, multicentre study. J Intern Med 1995;238:357–61.

[47] Machens A, Ukkat J, Brauckhoff M, et al. Advances in the management of hereditary medullary thyroid cancer. J Intern Med 2005;257:50–9.

[48] Wells SA Jr, Chi DD, Toshima K, et al. Predictive DNA testing and prophylactic thyroidectomy in patients at risk for multiple endocrine neoplasia type 2A. Ann Surg 1994;220: 237–47 [discussion: 247–50].

[49] Saad MF, Ordonez NG, Rashid RK, et al. Medullary carcinoma of the thyroid. A study of the clinical features and prognostic factors in 161 patients. Medicine (Baltimore) 1984;63: 319–42.

[50] Moley JF, DeBenedetti MK. Patterns of nodal metastases in palpable medullary thyroid carcinoma: recommendations for extent of node dissection. Ann Surg 1999;229:880–7 [discussion: 887–8].

[51] Chong GC, Beahrs OH, Sizemore GW, et al. Medullary carcinoma of the thyroid gland. Cancer 1975;35:695–704.

[52] Russell WO, Ibanez ML, Clark RL, et al. Thyroid carcinoma. Classification, intraglandular dissemination, and clinicopathological study based upon whole organ sections of 80 glands. Cancer 1963;16:1425–60.

[53] Duh QY, Sancho JJ, Greenspan FS, et al. Medullary thyroid carcinoma. The need for early diagnosis and total thyroidectomy. Arch Surg 1989;124:1206–10.

[54] Machens A, Gimm O, Hinze R, et al. Genotype-phenotype correlations in hereditary medullary thyroid carcinoma: oncological features and biochemical properties. J Clin Endocrinol Metab 2001;86:1104–9.

[55] Machens A, Niccoli-Sire P, Hoegel J, et al. Early malignant progression of hereditary medullary thyroid cancer. N Engl J Med 2003;349:1517–25.

[56] Gosnell JE, Sywak MS, Sidhu SB, et al. New era: prophylactic surgery for patients with multiple endocrine neoplasia-2a. ANZ J Surg 2006;76:586–90.

[57] Learoyd DL, Gosnell J, Elston MS, et al. Experience of prophylactic thyroidectomy in multiple endocrine neoplasia type 2A kindreds with RET codon 804 mutations. Clin Endocrinol (Oxf) 2005;63:636–41.

[58] Machens A, Brauckhoff M, Holzhausen HJ, et al. Codon-specific development of pheochromocytoma in multiple endocrine neoplasia type 2. J Clin Endocrinol Metab 2005;90: 3999–4003.

[59] Skinner MA, Moley JA, Dilley WG, et al. Prophylactic thyroidectomy in multiple endocrine neoplasia type 2A. N Engl J Med 2005;353:1105–13.

[60] Kitamura Y, Shimizu K, Nagahama M, et al. Immediate causes of death in thyroid carcinoma: clinicopathological analysis of 161 fatal cases. J Clin Endocrinol Metab 1999; 84:4043–9.

[61] Kebebew E, Greenspan FS, Clark OH, et al. Anaplastic thyroid carcinoma. Treatment outcome and prognostic factors. Cancer 2005;103:1330–5.

[62] Green LD, Mack L, Pasieka JL. Anaplastic thyroid cancer and primary thyroid lymphoma: a review of these rare thyroid malignancies. J Surg Oncol 2006;94:725–36.

[63] Noppen M, Poppe K, D'Haese J, et al. Interventional bronchoscopy for treatment of tracheal obstruction secondary to benign or malignant thyroid disease. Chest 2004;125: 723–30.

[64] Delbridge L. The 'neglected' nerve in thyroid surgery: the case for routine identification of the external laryngeal nerve. ANZ J Surg 2001;71:212–4.

[65] Delbridge L, Samra J. Editorial: the 'neglected' nerve in thyroid surgery–the case for routine identification of the external laryngeal nerve. ANZ J Surg 2002;72:239.

[66] Pelizzo MR, Toniato A, Gemo G. Zuckerkandl's tuberculum: an arrow pointing to the recurrent laryngeal nerve (constant anatomical landmark). J Am Coll Surg 1998;187:333–6.

[67] Cody HS 3rd, Shah JP. Locally invasive, well-differentiated thyroid cancer. 22 years' experience at Memorial Sloan-Kettering Cancer Center. Am J Surg 1981;142:480–3.

[68] Yang CC, Lee CH, Wang LS, et al. Resectional treatment for thyroid cancer with tracheal invasion: a long-term follow-up study. Arch Surg 2000;135:704–7.

[69] Sywak M, Pasieka JL, McFadden S, et al. Functional results and quality of life after tracheal resection for locally invasive thyroid cancer. Am J Surg 2003;185:462–7.

[70] McCaffrey TV, Bergstralh EJ, Hay ID. Locally invasive papillary thyroid carcinoma: 1940–1990. Head Neck 1994;16:165–72.

[71] Shigemitsu K, Naomoto Y, Haisa M, et al. A case of thyroid cancer involving the trachea: treatment by partial tracheal resection and repair with a latissimus dorsi musculocutaneous flap. Japn J Clin Oncol 2000;30:235–8.

[72] Flisberg K, Lindholm T. Electrical stimulation of the human recurrent laryngeal nerve during thyroid operation. Acta Otolaryngol 1969;263:63–7.

[73] Randolph GW, Kobler JB, Wilkins J. Recurrent laryngeal nerve identification and assessment during thyroid surgery: laryngeal palpation. World J Surg 2004;28:755–60.

[74] Thomusch O, Sekulla C, Walls G, et al. Intraoperative neuromonitoring of surgery for benign goiter. Am J Surg 2002;183:673–8.

[75] Dralle H, Sekulla C, Haerting J, et al. Risk factors of paralysis and functional outcome after recurrent laryngeal nerve monitoring in thyroid surgery. Surgery 2004;136:1310–22.

[76] Chan WF, Lang BH, Lo CY. The role of intraoperative neuromonitoring of recurrent laryngeal nerve during thyroidectomy: a comparative study on 1000 nerves at risk. Surgery 2006;140:866–72 [discussion: 872–3].

[77] Loch-Wilkinson TJ, Stalberg PL, Sidhu SB, et al. Nerve stimulation in thyroid surgery: is it really useful? ANZ J Surg 2007;77:377–80.

[78] Dackiw AP, Rotstein LE, Clark OH. Computer-assisted evoked electromyography with stimulating surgical instruments for recurrent/external laryngeal nerve identification and preservation in thyroid and parathyroid operation. Surgery 2002;132:1100–6 [discussion: 1107–8].

[79] Chiang FY, Wang LF, Huang YF, et al. Recurrent laryngeal nerve palsy after thyroidectomy with routine identification of the recurrent laryngeal nerve. Surgery 2005;137:342–7.

[80] Karlan MS, Catz B, Dunkelman D, et al. A safe technique for thyroidectomy with complete nerve dissection and parathyroid preservation. Head Neck Surg 1984;6:1014–9.

[81] Mattig H, Bildat D, Metzger B. [Reducing the rate of recurrent nerve paralysis by routine exposure of the nerves in thyroid gland operations.] Zentralbl Chir 1998;123:17–20 [in German].

[82] Wagner HE, Seiler C. Recurrent laryngeal nerve palsy after thyroid gland surgery. Br J Surg 1994;81:226–8.

[83] Kouvaraki MA, Lee JE, Shapiro SE, et al. Preventable reoperations for persistent and recurrent papillary thyroid carcinoma. Surgery 2004;136:1183–91.

[84] Triponez F, Poder L, Zarnegar R, et al. Hook needle-guided excision of recurrent differentiated thyroid cancer in previously operated neck compartments: a safe technique for small, nonpalpable recurrent disease. J Clin Endocrinol Metab. 2006;91:4943–7.

[85] Torlontano M, Attard M, Crocetti U, et al. Follow-up of low risk patients with papillary thyroid cancer: role of neck ultrasonography in detecting lymph node metastases. J Clin Endocrinol Metab 2004;89:3402–7.

[86] Dieffenbach JHDie operative Chirugie: Die operation des Kropfes, vol. 2. Leipzig (Germany): FA Brokhaus; 1848. p. 340.

ELSEVIER
SAUNDERS

Endocrinol Metab Clin N Am
37 (2008) 457–480

ENDOCRINOLOGY
AND METABOLISM
CLINICS
OF NORTH AMERICA

An Updated Systematic Review and Commentary Examining the Effectiveness of Radioactive Iodine Remnant Ablation in Well-Differentiated Thyroid Cancer

Anna M. Sawka, MD, PhD, FRCPC[a,b,*],
James D. Brierley, MBBS, FRCP, FRCR, FRCP(C)[c,d],
Richard W. Tsang, MD, FRCP(C)[c,d],
Lehana Thabane, PhD[e,f],
Lorne Rotstein, MD, FRCSC[g,h], Amiram Gafni, PhD[e,i],
Sharon Straus, MD, MSc, FRCPC[j,k],
David P. Goldstein, MD, FRCSC[l]

[a]Division of Endocrinology and Department of Medicine, University Health
Network, Toronto, ON, Canada
[b]Division of Endocrinology and Department of Medicine, University of Toronto, Toronto, ON, Canada
[c]Department of Radiation Oncology, University Health Network Toronto, ON, Canada
[d]Department of Radiation Oncology, University of Toronto, Princess Margaret Hospital,
610 University Avenue, Toronto, ON M5G 2M9, Canada
[e]Department of Clinical Epidemiology and Biostatistics, McMaster University, Hamilton, ON, Canada
[f]Centre for Evaluation of Medicines, St. Joseph's Healthcare, 105 Main Street East, Level P1,
Hamilton, ON L8N 1G6, Canada
[g]Department of Surgery, University of Toronto, Toronto General Hospital, 200 Elizabeth Street,
Toronto, ON M5G 2C4, Canada
[h]Department of Surgery, University Health Network Toronto, ON, Canada
[i]Centre for Health Economics and Policy Analysis, McMaster University, 1200 Main Street West,
3H29, Hamilton, ON L8N 3Z5, Canada
[j]Department of Knowledge Translation, University of Toronto, 30 Bond Street, Toronto, ON M5B
1W8, Canada
[k]Division of Geriatrics and Department of Medicine, University of Calgary, Calgary, AB, Canada
[l]Department of Otolaryngology Head and Neck Surgery, University of Toronto, Princess Margaret
Hospital, 610 University Avenue, Toronto, ON M5G 2M9, Canada

Anna Sawka is a New Investigator supported by the Canadian Institutes of Health Research (CNI-80701).

* Corresponding author. Toronto General Hospital, 200 Elizabeth Street, 12-212 Eaton North, Toronto, ON M5G 2C4, Canada.

E-mail address: sawkaam@yahoo.com (A.M. Sawka).

Well-differentiated thyroid cancer (WDTC), including papillary and follicular carcinoma, is the most common endocrine malignancy [1]. The incidence of WDTC is rising [1–3], yet the majority of cases of WDTC are
diagnosed at an early stage [1–4]. Factors, such as advanced stage of disease
and older age, are associated with an increased risk of thyroid cancer-related
mortality [5]. After the first-line of treatment of thyroidectomy, additional
treatments for WDTC include thyroid hormone suppressive therapy and
often, following bilateral thyroidectomy, therapeutic radioactive iodine. Radioactive iodine (RAI) may be administered as a form of adjuvant therapy
(remnant ablation) or in the treatment of residual or recurrent thyroid cancer [6–10]. Radioactive iodine remnant ablation (RRA) refers to the destruc-
tion of residual normal thyroid tissue after complete gross surgical resection
of cancer. The goals of RRA are to destroy any residual microscopic thyroid
cancer (in an effort to decrease the risk of persistent or recurrent disease),
and to facilitate follow-up and early detection of persistent or recurrent disease by measurement of serum thyroglobulin (with or without thyrotropin
stimulation) or radioactive iodine scanning. There have been no long-term
randomized, controlled trials proving the treatment efficacy of adjuvant
RAI therapy on thyroid cancer-related outcomes; the best quality existing
evidence relating to this intervention is observational in nature and subject
to methodologic limitations [11]. Previously, the authors conducted a systematic review and meta-analysis examining long-term thyroid cancer-
related outcomes after RRA [11]. The work presented herein represents an
updated systematic review examining the effect of RRA on the risk of thyroid
cancer-related mortality and disease recurrence in early stage WDTC.

Selection of relevant studies for the systematic review

The inclusion and exclusion criteria for studies in the review have been
previously described [11]. Studies were eligible for inclusion if they were
randomized, controlled trials or cohort studies of adult patients that had:

Well differentiated thyroid cancer (defined as either papillary, follicular
or follicular variant of papillary);
Surgical treatment involving bilateral resection, such as total, near-total,
or subtotal thyroidectomy (ie, surgery that was more extensive than
ipsilateral lobectomy and isthmectomy);
Radioactive iodine ablation given within 1 year after the operation;
A median or mean follow-up period of at least 5 years; and
Reporting of the outcomes of any cancer-related deaths, cancer recurrence, local-regional recurrence in the thyroid bed or regional lymph
nodes, or distant metastases (all at 10 years for data unadjusted for
prognostic factors or interventions).

In summarizing the results of multivariable analyses adjusted for important prognostic factors, the authors included data on eligible subgroups of

interest whenever possible. However, if a minority of patients had disease that was more extensive or surgery that was less complete than that described above, such data was summarized if these variables were adjusted for in the relevant multivariable analysis. When studies of overlapping groups of patients were identified (ie, updates of previously published cohort studies), only the report with the largest number of eligible patients was included unless additional reports provided nonoverlapping information (such as reports of different outcomes). The authors included all studies in the original systematic review [11], unless a more recent update for the population of interest was available.

Search strategy for the updated systematic review

One investigator performed an updated search of seven different electronic databases for the time period spanning from the prior review (original search in late 2002) until August 2007. The databases searched included: Medline and other nonindexed citations, the Cochrane Database for Systematic Reviews, Database of Abstracts and Reviews, the Controlled Clinical Trials Database, American College of Physicians Journal Club, the Cochrane Clinical Trials Registry, and Embase. The search was restricted to English language publications involving adults and included the following terms: papillary thyroid carcinoma, follicular thyroid carcinoma, radioactive iodine, iodine radio-isotopes, and thyroid neoplasms.

All of the retrieved abstracts and citations were independently reviewed by two different investigators to assess relevance. Any abstract or citation deemed potentially relevant by either reviewer was obtained and assessed independently by two reviewers to determine eligibility for inclusion. Disagreements were resolved by consensus; both reviewers agreed completely on the studies deemed relevant for abstraction. The authors' approach to overlapping studies was to include the largest, most recent published studies for the study population of interest reporting the outcomes of interest, including data from the authors' original systematic review [11]. One reviewer assessed overlap of data among studies.

Data abstraction

One investigator abstracted the data. If detailed information on completeness of resection of gross disease in the primary surgery was not reported, data from "low-risk" postsurgical stage subgroups were abstracted (as defined by the individual author or reported standard staging systems). The definitions of "low risk" staging (if not provided by individual authors within the included articles) were defined as in the original review [11]. If "completely resected" or "low risk" were not specified by the original authors, summaries of multivariable analyses were still summarized, as long as stage of disease or completeness of resection was adjusted for within the statistical models. Data that had been obtained from primary investigators was included in the updated review if relevant. The quality assessment was restricted to the categorization of articles with respect to the reporting of analyses adjusted for important prognostic factors (such as the postsurgical pathologic stage of disease, surgical extent, or cointerventions).

Statistics

Data adjusted for prognostic factors or cointerventions were tabulated as reported in the primary studies without pooling because of important clinical and methodologic heterogeneity among studies. The criterion for statistical significance was set at alpha $= 0.05$, with the exception of heterogeneity assessments, for which alpha $= 0.10$. The authors pooled unadjusted data for the 10-year outcomes of thyroid cancer-specific mortality, any recurrence, local recurrence (in the neck or upper mediastinum), and distant metastases, respectively, using random effects models. A chi-squared analysis was performed to assess for heterogeneity of treatment effect for each pooled outcome. Another measure of statistical heterogeneity was the I^2 value, measuring the variability in treatment effect estimate because of heterogeneity rather than sampling error, such that a value exceeding 50% was considered significant. The risk difference (with 95% confidence intervals or CI) was used to estimate treatment outcomes. The reason for selecting a risk difference (as opposed to an odds ratio or relative risk) for measurement of pooled treatment effects was that this approach allowed the authors to include data from studies with zero event rates in the pooled analyses. Review Manager 4.2.10 software was used for all pooled analyses.

Results

In this updated systematic review, two reviewers independently reviewed 863 unique abstracts and citations and 74 potentially relevant full-text published articles. The authors included data from 28 studies, seven studies published since the time of the original review [12–18] (Fig. 1). The authors had planned to include data from all nonoverlapping studies from the original review [13,19–39]; however, updated data from the Princess Margaret Hospital (University Health Network, Toronto) [13] replaced data from a prior Princess Margaret Hospital publication [40], as well as an overlapping population from Mount Sinai Hospital (Toronto) [34] (some patients from Mount Sinai had been referred for external beam radiation therapy to Princess Margaret [J. Brierley, MD, personal communication, 2007]). Thus, the final updated review included data from 20 studies from the authors' original review [19–33,35–39], the original review [11], and seven newer studies [12–18].

There were no long-term randomized, controlled trials examining thyroid cancer-related outcomes after RRA identified; thus, this updated review is restricted to observational data. The updated prognostically unadjusted

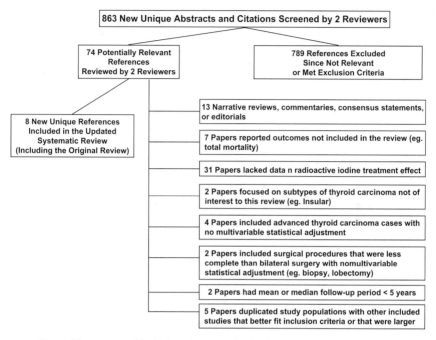

Fig. 1. The process of inclusion of new studies in the updated systematic review.

data from Princess Margaret Hospital included in this review was from WDTC patients whose disease was of pathologic stages 1 and 2 (American Joint Committee of Cancer, 5th edition) and who were treated with bilateral thyroidectomy and had grossly complete resection of disease (J. Brierley, MD, and R.W. Tsang, MD, unpublished data, 2007). It is important to mention that the updated analyses reported in a recent publication from the National Thyroid Cancer Treatment Cooperative Study Group [4] needed to be excluded from this update, as the mean duration of follow-up was only 3 years and below the authors' threshold of a minimum of 5 years [4]. The authors excluded raw unadjusted data from some recently up-dated studies for the following reasons: inclusion of patients who had less than bilateral surgery [13,41,42], inclusion of patients who had advanced disease [41,42], duplicate publication of a smaller subgroup of patients that was included in the original review [43], and timing of outcomes at a time point that was different than that of the authors' original interest (10 years) [44].

Summary of analyses statistically adjusted for prognostic factors or cointerventions

Because thyroid cancer-related outcomes are dependent upon important prognostic variables, the authors examined the results of studies in which the treatment effect of RRA was examined after statistical adjustment for such factors (or intended adjustment in the case of conditional analyses) (Tables 1–4). Some form of statistical adjustment of important prognostic factors was considered a methodologic quality indicator. The authors observed that in 12 prognostically adjusted studies examining the risk of thyroid cancer-related mortality after radioactive iodine treatment [12–17,19–24], a significant treatment benefit was observed in three studies, including the largest study (which was from Ohio State) [19], a registry-based study from Sweden [16], and a study from Turkey [17] (see Table 1). In the registry-based study from Sweden, there was a one to one matching of individuals who died from thyroid carcinoma with survivors (nested case-control design within a cohort), such that by design the thyroid cancer-related mortality rate was 50% [18]. Furthermore, in the study from Turkey [17], although a statistical adjustment was made for extent of disease, the thyroid cancer-related mortality rate after a mean follow-up of 7.2 years was the highest, at 24.2%. The high mortality rate in the study from Turkey may be explained by a high proportion of high-risk individuals included in the study (15.9% with distant metastases at initial presentation) [17]. In the remaining eight studies examining thyroid cancer-related mortality after radioactive iodine and adjusting for important prognostic factors, no significant treatment benefit was observed [12–15,20–24].

In six studies reporting adjusted analyses for the outcome of any thyroid cancer recurrence [19,24–28], a significant treatment benefit of postsurgical radioactive iodine was observed in three studies [11,19,24–28] (see Table 2). In the studies reporting an adjusted treatment benefit for the outcome of thyroid cancer recurrence, the event rate was generally over 20% [19,24,27]. Four studies examined the outcome of loco-regional recurrence, after adjustment for prognostic factors or cointerventions [8,13,20,21], and a significant treatment benefit was observed in three of these [13,20,21] (see Table 3). It is also important to note that the study in which no significant benefit was observed on the outcome of loco-regional recurrence, papillary microcarcinoma was the focus, such that the event rate was only 2% after a mean follow-up of 6.5 years [18].

There were three studies in which the effect of RRA on distant metastatic recurrence was evaluated after adjustment for prognostic factors or cointerventions [19–21]. The event rates for distant metastatic recurrence ranged from 1.6% in a study of exclusively papillary cancer patients (median follow-up 9.2 years) [20] up to 9% in a study of exclusively follicular carcinoma patients (mean follow-up 10.8 years) [21]. RRA was associated with a decreased risk of distant metastatic recurrence in two studies including papillary patients [19,20], but not in one study comprised of exclusively follicular carcinoma patients [21] (see Table 4).

Unadjusted pooled analyses

No newer nonoverlapping unadjusted thyroid cancer-related mortality data was found in the authors' updated review, so the original pooled analysis [11] was not redone. The authors originally reported [11] that there was significant statistical heterogeneity of treatment effect among 16 analyses examining the effect of RRA on 10-year thyroid cancer-related mortality in a total of 6,464 patients (chi-square 27.44, 15 degrees of freedom, $P = .025$) [19–21,24,26,29–33,35–39] (papillary and follicular data reported separately for [29,33]). Moreover, for the thyroid cancer-related mortality outcome, several studies reported thyroid cancer-related mortality rates as low as 0% in both treatment and control groups [26,31,39], highlighting the relatively low death rate because of thyroid carcinoma in early stage cases of papillary cancer [11]. Based on data from review of five studies of exclusively papillary patients [11], the authors estimate the ten-year incidence of thyroid cancer-related death to be 1.7% (45 out of 2,627) (original data from [20,29–31,33]).

In unadjusted analyses for the subgroup of patients composed entirely of papillary cancer survivors, the overall 10-year recurrence rates are estimated as follows: 9.3% (154 out of 1,652) any recurrence, 7.3% (50 out of 684) loco-regional recurrence, and 1.3% (9 out of 684) distant metastatic recurrence (numbers not additive as the same studies did not report all three outcomes) [11] (Figs. 2–4). In the updated unadjusted pooled analyses examining the outcome of any recurrence, there was statistically significant heterogeneity of RRA treatment effect among studies of WDTC patients for the outcome of any recurrence (chi-squared 122.71, 11 degrees of freedom, $P < .00001$, $I^2 = 91.0\%$) (data from 5,307 patients), precluding meaningful estimation of an overall treatment effect (see Fig. 2). Similarly, for the outcome of loco-regional recurrence, there was statistically significant heterogeneity of treatment effect of RRA among studies (chi-squared 20.36, 5 degrees of freedom, $P = .001$, $I^2 = 75.4\%$) (data from 1,244 patients summarized), also precluding meaningful estimation of treatment effect (see Fig. 3). RRA was associated with a statistically significant reduction in risk of distant metastatic recurrence with a risk difference of −2% (95% CI −4%, −1%) ($Z = 3.49$, $P = .0005$, pooled data from 2,263 patients) (see Fig. 2).

Commentary

Upon carefully examining the best existing long-term observational evidence, the authors could not confirm a significant, consistent, benefit of RRA in decreasing cause specific mortality or recurrence in early stage WDTC. RRA use was associated with a significantly decreased risk of distant metastases; however, this event was relatively rare in papillary cancer. The relatively low risk of thyroid cancer-related death in early stage thyroid carcinoma patients may limit the ability to prove a significant treatment benefit for this outcome. Previously, Hay [31,44] has reported a 20-year thyroid cancer-related mortality of 0.4% in papillary thyroid cancer patients with a MACIS score of less than 6 (Metastasis [distant], Age, Completeness

Table 1
Summary of adjusted analyses of thyroid cancer-related deaths

Study (type of analysis) [Ref]	Number of patients in model (% events)	Number of patients treated with radio-iodine ablation	Histology	Median follow-up period (years)	Prognostic variables adjusted for in model	Cointerventions adjusted for in model	Reported result for effectiveness of RAI treatment
Ohio State, United States Air Force 2001[a] (multivariable Cox regression) [19]	1,510[d] (unclear)	Unclear	Papillary, follicular	16.6 years	Time to treatment, age, follicular histology, lymph node metastases, tumor size, local tumor invasion, gender	Surgery more extensive than lobectomy	RAI remnant ablation: Hazard ratio 0.5 (0.4–0.7) $P < .0001$
Royal Liverpool University Hospital , UK 1994[a] (univariate, chi-square but planned multivariable model if significant) [22]	249 (15.3%)	81 (ablation), 75 (therapy of residual or recurrent disease)	Papillary, follicular	8.7 years	None	None	Not entered in multivariable model because not significant in univariate analysis (a priori design).
University of California at San Francisco 1997[b] (Cox proportional hazards model) [24]	187 (7% at 10 years)	305	Papillary, follicular, Hürthle cell	10.6 years	None	Extent of surgery, other modalities (external radiation, immunotherapy, chemotherapy)	No RAI: risk ratio 1.1 (0.5–2.3) $P = .76$

Study			Type	Follow-up	Variables adjusted for	Factor	Result
Hong Kong Queen Elizabeth (follicular) 2002[c] (multivariable Cox regression) [21]	135 (1.9% at 10 years)	123[d]	Follicular	10.8 years	Age, gender, tumor size, extrathyroidal extension, lymph node metastases, distant metastases at presentation, postsurgical loco-regional disease	Type of thyroid surgery	Not significant
Hong Kong Queen Elizabeth (papillary) 2002[c] (multivariable Cox regression) [20]	587 (1.3% at 10 years)	444	Papillary	9.2 years	Age, gender, tumor size, multicentric disease, extrathyroidal extension, lymph node metastases, distant metastases at presentation, and postsurgical loco-regional residual disease	Type of thyroid surgery	Not significant
Illinois Registry 1990 (Cox proportional hazards model) [23]	2,282 (not reported)	1,278	Papillary, follicular	6.5 years	Age, stage (American Joint Commission – tumor, node, metastasis or TNM staging), race, sex	Postoperative thyroid hormone	No RAI: Relative odds ratio of thyroid cancer-related survival 1.54 (1.01–2.35) $P = .05$

(continued on next page)

Table 1 (continued)

Study (type of analysis) [Ref]	Number of patients in model (% events)	Number of patients treated with radio-iodine ablation	Histology	Median follow-up period (years)	Prognostic variables adjusted for in model	Cointerventions adjusted for in model	Reported result for effectiveness of RAI treatment
Toronto Princess Margaret Hospital 2005 (Cox proportional hazards model) [13]	729 (12.7%; 7.1% papillary, 29.7% follicular)	528	Papillary, follicular (excluding Hürthle cell)	11.3 years	Age, tumor size, poor differentiation, postoperative residuum, distant metastatic disease at presentation	Total or near-total compared with subtotal thyroidectomy, external beam radiation therapy	RAI: hazard ratio 0.7 (0.4, 1.1) P = .14
Hong Kong Queen Mary 2007 [14]	760 (9.5% at 10 years, 8.7% papillary, 6.8% follicular)	472	Papillary (including tall cell), follicular	9.8 years	Papillary cancer model: age (≥50 years), tumor size (≥3.5 cm), cervical lymph node metastases, distant metastases, extrathyroidal extension, multifocality, capsular invasion, tall cell variant, completeness of resection. Follicular cancer model: age (≥50 years), distant metastases, completeness of resection	Papillary and follicular cancer models: external beam radiation therapy. Surgical extent was not significant in respective univariate models so not entered in multivariable analyses (a priori design)	Papillary and follicular analyses: not entered in multivariable model since not significant in univariate analysis (a priori design).

Study	N		Histology	Follow-up	Adjustment	Other factors	Result
Padova, Italy 2007[d], 2008 (Cox proportional hazards model) [15]	1,858 (unclear, estimate 5.4%)	1,568	Papillary	Mean 21.4 years	Gender, age at initial treatment (≥45 years), primary tumor size (>1.5 cm), disease stage according to the International Union Against Cancer TNM classification, metastatic disease being positive at I-131 scan	Surgical extent (total or subtotal thyroidectomy)	Not significant
Swedish Cancer Registry 2007 (conditional logistic regression) [16]	1,190 (595 cases who died of thyroid carcinoma and 595 matched controls who did not) (1:1 matching so event rate was 50% by design)	549 estimated	Differentiated thyroid carcinoma (excluding medullary and anaplastic)	Nested case-control study within a cohort. Mean 6.7 year follow-up for cases.	Matching for age, sex, and calendar period of diagnosis for each analysis. Respective multivariable analyses adjusted for: TNM stage, or completeness of resection.	Type of surgery, external beam radiation therapy, chemotherapy	Analysis adjusted for TNM stage of disease, RAI: odds ratio 1.5 (1.1, 1.9) Analysis adjusted for completeness of resection, type of surgery, external beam radiation therapy, and chemotherapy - RAI: odds ratio 1.4 (1.1, 1.8)

(continued on next page)

Table 1 (*continued*)

Study (type of analysis) [Ref]	Number of patients in model (% events)	Number of patients treated with radio-iodine ablation	Histology	Median follow-up period (years)	Prognostic variables adjusted for in model	Cointerventions adjusted for in model	Reported result for effectiveness of RAI treatment
Anakara, Turkey 2005 (Cox proportional hazards model) [17]	347 (24.2%)	267	Papillary, follicular	7.2 years	Age (≥45 years), primary tumor (continuous), angio-invasion, distant metastases at presentation	Type of thyroidectomy (total versus subtotal)	Adjuvant RAI: hazard ratio 0.5 (0.2, 0.8) $P = .0001$
Royal Marsden Hospital, UK 2003 (Cox proportional hazards model) [12]	111 (50.0% at 10 years); all patients aged ≥70 years at time of diagnosis	22 (20%) received 3 GBq for ablation 58 (22%) received 6.6–29.0 GBq for further treatment	Papillary, follicular, Hürthle cell	9 years	Age, gender, tumor stage, nodal status, distant metastatic status, histology (thyroid cancer subtype)	Surgical extent, external beam radiation therapy	Not entered in multivariable model because not significant in univariate analysis (a priori design).

Some data from the original systematic review included [11].
[a] Excluded patients with distant metastases at presentation from analysis.
[b] Includes only patients with primary tumors larger than 1 cm.
[c] Excluded patients with distant metastases, no gross nor microscopic residual disease after thyroid surgery.
[d] Information previously obtained from author.

of resection, Invasion [local], Size of primary tumor) who were treated with total or near-total thyroidectomy in absence of RRA. Based on the review of multiple studies [11], the authors estimate that in early stage papillary thyroid cancer, the thyroid cancer-related mortality rate is roughly 1.7% at 10 years. Thus, the majority of patients with early stage papillary thyroid carcinoma are unlikely to die from their disease. This finding should not be considered generalizable to higher risk patients, particularly those with gross residual tumor, complex features, or advanced postsurgical pathologic stage of disease, which were not specifically addressed in this review.

Given that thyroid cancer-related mortality is relatively uncommon in early stage disease, recurrence of disease is the primary concern. Conflicting findings on the benefit of RRA were found for the outcome of any thyroid cancer recurrence among prognostically adjusted and unadjusted analyses. However, RRA was associated with a decreased risk of distant metastatic recurrence in two adjusted analyses, as well as the pooled unadjusted analysis (pooled risk difference −2% for all WDTC subgroups combined). The extremely low event rate for distant metastatic recurrence, particularly in papillary cancer patients, is a limitation of these analyses. The pooled data on distant metastases directly conflict with the data for the outcome of any recurrence, highlighting the fact that different clinical centers chose to report different thyroid cancer outcomes (any recurrence or respective loco-regional and distant metastatic recurrences) and reflecting some uncertainty about the treatment benefit of RRA in decreasing recurrence of disease.

It is important to note that in exclusively early stage papillary thyroid cancer patients treated with bilateral thyroidectomy, the 10-year absolute risk of any recurrence was estimated to be about one in ten; the 10-year risk of loco-regional recurrence (7.3%) is about six times that of distant metastatic recurrence (1.3%) in this group. Hay has previously reported that that papillary cancer patients of a MACIS score less than 6 with positive lymph nodes resected at surgery have a risk of recurrence that is approximately double that of lymph node negative counterparts. Moreover, Hay did not observe a significantly decreased risk of 20-year recurrence in patients who had a MACIS score of less than 6 treated with RRA, regardless of lymph node status at presentation [31,44]. In a prospective study recently published by the National Thyroid Cancer Treatment Cooperative Group (TCTCG), in patients classified as having postsurgical Stage 1 disease (using the TCTCG classification system), a significant treatment benefit of RRA was not observed using propensity analysis for the outcomes of overall survival, disease-specific survival, and disease-free survival, respectively [4]. The relatively short mean follow-up period of 3 years [4] is an important limitation of the TCTCG study.

The authors did not address the issue of optimal activity dosing of radioactive iodine for remnant ablation in this review. Recently, Hackshaw and colleagues [45] performed a systematic review comparing the success of remnant ablation after various dose activities of radioactive iodine. In pooling

Table 2
Summary of individual multivariable analyses of any thyroid cancer-related tumor recurrence

Study (type of analysis) [Ref]	Number of patients in model (% events if given)	Patients treated with radio-iodine ablation	Histology	Median follow-up period (years)	Prognostic variables adjusted for in model	Cointerventions adjusted for in model	Reported result for effectiveness of radio-iodine ablation
Ohio State, United States Air Force 2001[a] (multivariable Cox regression) [19]	1,510[c] (23.5% for 1,528 patients, including patients with distant metastases)	Unclear	Papillary, follicular	16.6 years	Age, follicular histology, tumor size, local tumor invasion	Surgery more extensive than lobectomy, therapy with I131 for residual disease	RAI: hazard ratio 0.8 (0.7–0.97) $P = .016$ (in patients with completely resected disease)
Gunderson/ Lutheran Medical Center 1997 (multivariable logistic regression) [25]	177 (13% papillary, 8% follicular, 7% Hürthle cell)	"Frequently"	Papillary, follicular, Hürthle cell	7.2 years	Age, tumor size, presence of cervical lymph node metastases, local neck invasion, gender	Operation less extensive than near-total thyroidectomy	Not significant
Gustave-Roussy Institute (France) 1998[a,b] (multivariable logistic regression) [26]	273 (3.9%)	117	Papillary, follicular	7.3 years	Previous external radiation therapy, gender, mode diagnosis (incidental), neck lymph node metastases, histology, extrathyroidal and extranodal extent, multifocality, uni-or bilaterality, vascular invasion	Extent of surgery (total thyroidectomy compared with loboisthmectomy or isthmectomy), lymph node dissection	Not significant

University of California at San Francisco 1997[b] (Cox proportional hazards model) [24]	187 (20.5%)	305[c]	Papillary, follicular, Hürthle cell	10.6 years	None	Extent of surgery, ther modalities (external radiation, immunotherapy, chemotherapy)	No RAI: Risk Ratio (1.5–3.1) $P = .0001$
MD Anderson 1992 (multivariable Cox regression) [27]	1,599 (23%)	447	Papillary, follicular, Hürthle cell	11 years	Gender, pathology, extent of disease, age	Surgery, external radiotherapy	The most significant single factor was RAI treatment ($P <.001$).
Mexico 1996 (Cox proportional hazards model) [28]	229 (15% at 10 years)	149	Papillary, follicular	5 years	Sex, age, extent and size of tumor, nodal metastases, coexistence benign thyroid nodules or thyroiditis, presence Hürthle cells or tall cells, ploidy	Type of surgical resection, thyroid hormone suppression	Not significant

Some data from the original systematic review included [11].

[a] Excluded patients with distant metastases at presentation from analysis.

[b] Primary tumor ≤ 1 cm in diameter.

[c] Information previously obtained from authors.

Table 3
Summary of adjusted analyses of loco-regional recurrences

Study (type of analysis) [Ref]	Number of patients in model (% events if given)	Patients treated with radio-iodine ablation	Histology	Median follow-up period (years)	Prognostic variables adjusted for in model	Cointerventions adjusted for in model	Reported result for effectiveness of radio-iodine ablation
Hong Kong Queen Elizabeth (follicular) 2002[a] (multivariable Cox regression) [21]	135 (3.6% at 10 years)	123[b]	Follicular	10.8 years (provided for a larger group of 215 patients)	Age, gender, tumor size, extrathyroidal extension, lymph node metastases, distant metastases at presentation, postsurgical loco-regional disease	Type of thyroid surgery	RAI: Relative Risk 0.05 (0.005–0.51) P = .01
Hong Kong Queen Elizabeth (papillary) 2002[a] (multivariable Cox regression) [20]	587 (7.4% at 10 years)	444	Papillary	9.2 years	Age, gender, tumor size, multicentric disease, extrathyroidal extension, lymph node metastases, distant metastases at presentation, and postsurgical loco-regional residual disease	Type of thyroid surgery	RAI: relative risk 0.29 (0.17–0.51) P<.001
Toronto Princess Margaret Hospital 2005 (Cox proportional hazards model) [13]	729 (15.1%, 14.6% papillary, 16.8% follicular)	528	Papillary, follicular (excluding Hürthle cell)	11.3 years	Tumor size, age, metastastes in the neck	Total compared with subtotal thyroidectomy, external beam radiation therapy	RAI: hazard ratio 0.5 (0.3, 0.8) (P = .007)

| Padova, Italy 2007 (Cox proportional hazards model) [18] | 149 (2%) | 76 RAI remnant ablation, 19 radioactive iodine treatment of lymph node metastases at presentation | Papillary (microcarcinoma) | Mean 6.5 years | Gender, age at initial treatment (≥45 years), preoperative diagnosis of papillary cancer, presence of lymph node metastases at surgery or I-131 scan, coexistence of thyroid or parathyroid diseases, histopathologic findings (tumor size, multifocality, thyroid capsular invasion, presence of peritumoral sclerotic capsule) | Surgical extent (total versus partial thyroidectomy), lymphadenectomy, concurrent treatment with L-thyroxine or methimazole | Not significant |

Some data from the original systematic review included [11].

[a] Excluded patients with distant metastases, no gross nor microscopic residual disease after thyroid surgery.

[b] Information obtained from author.

Table 4
Summary of adjusted analyses of distant metastases

Study (type of analysis) [Ref]	Number of patients in model (% events if given)	Patients treated with radio-iodine ablation	Histology	Median follow-up period (years)	Prognostic variables adjusted for in model	Cointerventions adjusted for in model	Reported result for effectiveness of radio-iodine ablation
Ohio State, United States Air Force 2001[a] (multivariable Cox regression) [19]	1,510[c] (7.5% of 1,528 patients, including distant metastases at diagnosis)	Unclear	Papillary, follicular	16.6 years	Age, follicular histology, lymph node metastases, tumor size, local tumor invasion, gender	Surgery more extensive than lobectomy, therapy with I-131 (presumably for residual disease)	RAI: hazard ratio 0.6 (0.5–0.8) P = .002
Hong Kong Queen Elizabeth (follicular) 2002[b] (multivariable Cox regression) [21]	135 (9% at 10 years)	123[c]	Follicular	10.8 years	Age, gender, tumor size, extrathyroidal extension, lymph node metastases, distant metastases at presentation, postsurgical loco-regional disease	Type of thyroid surgery	Not significant
Hong Kong Queen Elizabeth (papillary) 2002[b] (multivariable Cox regression) [20]	587 (1.6% at 10 years)	444	Papillary	9.2 years	Age, gender, tumor size, multicentric disease, extrathyroidal extension, lymph node metastases, distant metastases at presentation, and postsurgical loco-regional residual disease	Type of thyroid surgery	RAI ablation: relative risk 0.2 (0.07–0.64) P = .006

Some data from the original systematic review included [11].

[a] Excluded patients with distant metastases at presentation from analysis.

[b] Excluded patients with distant metastases, no gross nor microscopic residual disease after thyroid surgery.

[c] Information obtained from author.

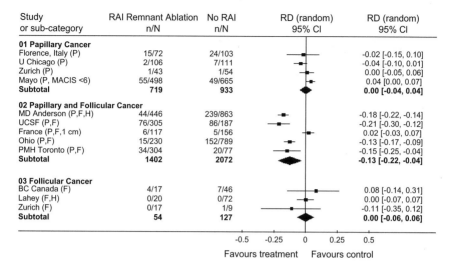

Study or sub-category	RAI Remnant Ablation n/N	No RAI n/N	RD (random) 95% CI	RD (random) 95% CI
01 Papillary Cancer				
Florence, Italy (P)	15/72	24/103		-0.02 [-0.15, 0.10]
U Chicago (P)	2/106	7/111		-0.04 [-0.10, 0.01]
Zurich (P)	1/43	1/54		0.00 [-0.05, 0.06]
Mayo (P, MACIS <6)	55/498	49/665		0.04 [0.00, 0.07]
Subtotal	**719**	**933**		**0.00 [-0.04, 0.04]**
02 Papillary and Follicular Cancer				
MD Anderson (P,F,H)	44/446	239/863		-0.18 [-0.22, -0.14]
UCSF (P,F)	76/305	86/187		-0.21 [-0.30, -0.12]
France (P,F,1 cm)	6/117	5/156		0.02 [-0.03, 0.07]
Ohio (P,F)	15/230	152/789		-0.13 [-0.17, -0.09]
PMH Toronto (P,F)	34/304	20/77		-0.15 [-0.25, -0.04]
Subtotal	**1402**	**2072**		**-0.13 [-0.22, -0.04]**
03 Follicular Cancer				
BC Canada (F)	4/17	7/46		0.08 [-0.14, 0.31]
Lahey (F,H)	0/20	0/72		0.00 [-0.07, 0.07]
Zurich (F)	0/17	1/9		-0.11 [-0.35, 0.12]
Subtotal	**54**	**127**		**0.00 [-0.06, 0.06]**

-0.5   -0.25   0   0.25   0.5

Favours treatment   Favours control

Fig. 2. Pooled analysis examining the risk difference for any thyroid cancer recurrence after radioactive iodine remnant ablation. *Abbreviations:* BC Canada, British Columbia, Canada; DF, degrees of freedom; F, follicular; P, papillary; PMH Toronto, Princess Margaret Hospital, University of Toronto; RAI, radioactive iodine; RD (random), risk difference calculated using a random effects model; U Chicago, University of Chicago. Some data from the original systematic review included [11].

data from observational studies, Hackshaw and colleagues observed that the success rate for ablation using activity of 100 mCi was significantly higher than for 30 mCi, but these findings were not confirmed in a pooled analysis of randomized, controlled trials [45]. Thus, Hackshaw and colleagues [45] concluded that "from the published data, it is not possible to reliably

Study or sub-category	RAI Remnant Ablation n/N	No RAI n/N	RD (random) 95% CI	RD (random) 95% CI
01 Papillary				
Zurich (P)	1/43	1/54		0.00 [-0.05, 0.06]
Hong Kong QE (P)	24/444	24/143		-0.11 [-0.18, -0.05]
Subtotal	**487**	**197**		**-0.05 [-0.20, 0.09]**
02 Papillary and Follicular				
PMH Toronto (P,F)	21/230	16/77		-0.12 [-0.21, -0.02]
Subtotal	**230**	**77**		**-0.12 [-0.21, -0.02]**
03 Follicular				
Lahey (F,H)	0/20	0/72		0.00 [-0.07, 0.07]
Zurich (F)	0/17	0/9		0.00 [-0.15, 0.15]
Hong Kong QE (F)	2/123	2/12		-0.15 [-0.36, 0.06]
Subtotal	**160**	**93**		**-0.03 [-0.13, 0.07]**

-0.5   -0.25   0   0.25   0.5

Favours treatment   Favours control

Fig. 3. Pooled analysis examining the risk difference for loco-regional thyroid cancer recurrence after radioactive iodine remnant ablation. Some data from the original systematic review included [11].

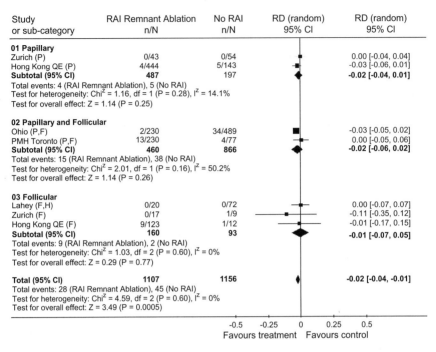

Study or sub-category	RAI Remnant Ablation n/N	No RAI n/N	RD (random) 95% CI	RD (random) 95% CI
01 Papillary				
Zurich (P)	0/43	0/54		0.00 [-0.04, 0.04]
Hong Kong QE (P)	4/444	5/143		-0.03 [-0.06, 0.01]
Subtotal (95% CI)	**487**	**197**		**-0.02 [-0.04, 0.01]**
Total events: 4 (RAI Remnant Ablation), 5 (No RAI)				
Test for heterogeneity: Chi² = 1.16, df = 1 (P = 0.28), I² = 14.1%				
Test for overall effect: Z = 1.14 (P = 0.25)				
02 Papillary and Follicular				
Ohio (P,F)	2/230	34/489		-0.03 [-0.05, 0.02]
PMH Toronto (P,F)	13/230	4/77		0.00 [-0.05, 0.06]
Subtotal (95% CI)	**460**	**866**		**-0.02 [-0.06, 0.02]**
Total events: 15 (RAI Remnant Ablation), 38 (No RAI)				
Test for heterogeneity: Chi² = 2.01, df = 1 (P = 0.16), I² = 50.2%				
Test for overall effect: Z = 1.14 (P = 0.26)				
03 Follicular				
Lahey (F,H)	0/20	0/72		0.00 [-0.07, 0.07]
Zurich (F)	0/17	1/9		-0.11 [-0.35, 0.12]
Hong Kong QE (F)	9/123	1/12		-0.01 [-0.17, 0.15]
Subtotal (95% CI)	**160**	**93**		**-0.01 [-0.07, 0.05]**
Total events: 9 (RAI Remnant Ablation), 2 (No RAI)				
Test for heterogeneity: Chi² = 1.03, df = 2 (P = 0.60), I² = 0%				
Test for overall effect: Z = 0.29 (P = 0.77)				
Total (95% CI)	**1107**	**1156**		**-0.02 [-0.04, -0.01]**
Total events: 28 (RAI Remnant Ablation), 45 (No RAI)				
Test for heterogeneity: Chi² = 4.59, df = 2 (P = 0.60), I² = 0%				
Test for overall effect: Z = 3.49 (P = 0.0005)				

-0.5   -0.25   0   0.25   0.5
Favours treatment   Favours control

Fig. 4. Pooled analysis examining the risk difference for distant metastatic thyroid cancer recurrence after radioactive iodine remnant ablation. Some data from the original systematic review included [11].

determine whether ablation success rates using 30 mCi are similar to 100 mCi" and suggested that "large randomized trials are needed to resolve the issue and guide clinical practice." In a subsequent single-center randomized controlled trial, including 72 patients with WDTC pretreated with recombinant human thyrotropin, Pilli and colleagues [46] observed that short-term remnant ablation rates were the same (88.9%) after administering 50 mCi, compared with 100 mCi of radioactive iodine.

In several recent clinical practice guidelines, including those from the American [6], European [8], and British [10] Thyroid Associations, selective use of RRA is suggested, such that the use of adjuvant radioactive iodine is particularly advocated for patients considered at high risk of thyroid cancer-related mortality (as classified by postsurgical pathologic status) or those in whom complex features may suggest an increased risk of recurrence. Thus, RRA should not be considered mandatory in patients with early stage thyroid carcinoma, particularly young individuals with relatively small primary tumors in the absence of complicating features. It should be noted that some physicians recommend RRA in early stage well-differentiated thyroid carcinoma in an effort to facilitate disease follow-up [47] and that some patients may have a preference for this approach.

The effect of RRA on long-term outcomes in early stage papillary thyroid carcinoma could be clarified in a randomized, controlled trial. However, a primary treatment outcome of thyroid cancer-related mortality is not feasible for use in a randomized, controlled trial, given the low rate of this event expected in early stage papillary thyroid cancer. In contrast, an outcome of any thyroid cancer recurrence or loco-regional recurrence may be reasonable for study. For example, in a 5-year randomized, controlled trial of RRA in early stage papillary thyroid cancer, in which the event rate is assumed to be 5% at 5 years and in which the hazard ratio is 0.60 after RRA, a total of 528 patients would be needed for study (time to event analysis, 4-year accrual and 5-year follow-up for all patients, power of 0.8, 2-sided alpha 0.05, one to one ratio of treatment and control patients) (Power and Precision Version 2, available at http://www.power-analysis.com).

About half of thyroid cancer specialists that the authors recently surveyed in Canada (226) and the United States (456) strongly supported the concept of a randomized, controlled trial of RRA in papillary thyroid cancer [47]. The authors are hopeful that such a trial may be designed and implemented such that one day this data could be included in an update of this systematic review. In the mean time, it is important for physicians treating early stage WDTC to evaluate the clinical, pathologic, biochemical, and radiologic data of each case carefully, advise patients about the uncertainty of the existing evidence supporting RRA, and disclose all acceptable treatment options (and their risks), including either declining or administering RRA. The implications of either declining or accepting RRA on long-term follow-up strategies need to be fully outlined to patients at the time of RRA decision making. In an age of freely available information, patients themselves may have strong opinions about accepting or declining RRA and it is important for physicians to be sensitive to such concerns. The current reality is that decision making about RRA in early stage thyroid carcinoma is a complex, evolving issue and long term higher quality evidence is needed to inform future clinical practice.

Acknowledgments

The authors would like to thank the following investigators for providing us with information related to their studies: Adil Al-Nahhas (Padova University, Italy), David Brams (Lahey Clinic, United States), Steve Hyer (Royal Marsden Hospital, United Kingdom), and Tony Panzarella (Princess Margaret Hospital, Canada).

References

[1] Canadian Cancer Society, National Cancer Institute of Canada, Statistics Canada, Public Health Agency of Canada. Canadian cancer statistics 2005. Available at: http://www. cancer.ca. Accessed August 2, 2005.

[2] Hayat MJ, Howlader N, Reichman E, et al. Cancer statistics, trends, and multiple primary cancers from the Surveillance, Epidemiology, and End Results (SEER) Program. Oncologist 2007;12:20–37.

[3] Davies L, Welch HG. Epidemiology of head and neck cancer in the United States. Otolaryngol Head Neck Surg 2006;135:451–7.

[4] Jonklaas J, Sarlis NJ, Litofsky D, et al. Outcomes of patients with differentiated thyroid carcinoma following initial therapy. Thyroid 2006;16:1229–42.

[5] Eustatia-Rutten CFA, Corssmit EPM, Biermasz NR, et al. Survival and death causes in differentiated thyroid carcinoma. J Clin Endocrinol Metab 2006;91:313–9.

[6] Cooper DS, Doherty GM, Haugen BR, et al. The American Thyroid Association Guidelines Task Force. Management guidelines for patients with thyroid nodules and differentiated thyroid cancer. Thyroid 2006;16:109–42.

[7] National Cancer Institute. Thyroid cancer (PDQ): treatment. 2006. Available at: http://www.cancer.gov/cancertopics/pdq/treatment/thyroid/healthprofessional/allpages. Accessed July 23, 2006.

[8] Pacini F, Schlumberger M, Dralle H, et al, The European Thyroid Cancer Task Force. European consensus for the management of patients with differentiated thyroid carcinoma of the follicular epithelium. Eur J Endocrinol 2006;154:787–803.

[9] American Association of Clinical Endocrinologists, American College of Endocrinology, American Association of Endocrine Surgeons. AACE/AAES medical/surgical guidelines for clinical practice: management of thyroid carcinoma. Endocr Pract 2001;7:202–20.

[10] British Thyroid Association, Royal College of Physicians. 2007 Guidelines for the management of thyroid cancer. 2nd edition. Available at: http://www.british-thyroid-association.org. Accessed October 20, 2007.

[11] Sawka AM, Thephamongkhol K, Brouwers M, et al. Clinical review 170: a systematic review and metaanalysis of the effectiveness of radioactive iodine remnant ablation for well-differentiated thyroid cancer. J Clin Endocrinol Metab 2004;89:3668–76.

[12] Vini L, Hyer SL, Marshall J, et al. Long-term results in elderly patients with differentiated thyroid carcinoma. Cancer 2003;97:2736–42.

[13] Brierley J, Tsang R, Panzarella T, et al. Prognostic factors and the effect of treatment with radioactive iodine and external beam radiation on patients with differentiated thyroid cancer seen at a single Canadian institution over 40 years. Clin Endocrinol (Oxf) 2005;63:418–27.

[14] Lang BH, Lo CY, Chan WF, et al. Prognostic factors in papillary and follicular thyroid carcinoma: their implications for cancer staging. Ann Surg Oncol 2007;14:730–8.

[15] Pelizzo MR, Boschin IM, Toniato A, et al. Papillary thyroid carcinoma: 35-year outcome and prognostic factors in 1858 patients. Clin Nucl Med 2007;32:440–4.

[16] Lundgren CI, Hall P, Dickman PW, et al. Influence of surgical and postoperative treatment on survival in differentiated thyroid cancer. Br J Surg 2007;94:571–7.

[17] Yildrim E. A model for predicting outcomes in patients with differentiated thyroid cancer and model performance in comparison with other classification systems. J Am Coll Surg 2005;200:378–92.

[18] Pelizzo MR, Boschin IM, Toniato A, et al. Natural history, diagnosis, treatment and outcome of papillary thyroid microcarcinoma (PTMC): a mono-institutional 12-year experience. Nucl Med Commun 2004;25:547–52.

[19] Mazzaferri EL, Kloos RT. Clinical Review 128: current approaches to primary therapy for papillary and follicular thyroid cancer. J Clin Endocrinol Metab 2001;86:1447–63.

[20] Chow SM, Law SC, Mendenhall WM, et al. Papillary thyroid carcinoma: prognostic factors and the role of radioiodine and external radiotherapy. Int J Radiat Oncol Biol Phys 2002;52(3):784–95.

[21] Chow SM, Law SC, Au SK, et al. Differentiated thyroid carcinoma: comparison between papillary and follicular carcinoma in a single institute. Head Neck 2002;24:670–7.

[22] Balan KK, Raouf AH, Critchley M. 1994 Outcome of 249 patients attending a nuclear medicine department with well differentiated thyroid cancer; a 23 year review. Br J Radiol 1994;67(795):283–91.

[23] Cunningham MP, Duda RB, Recant W, et al. Survival discriminants for differentiated thyroid cancer. Am J Surg 1990;160(4):344–7.

[24] Loh KC, Greenspan FS, Gee L, et al. Pathological tumor-node-metastasis (pTNM) staging for papillary and follicular thyroid carcinomas: a retrospective analysis of 700 patients. J Clin Endocrinol Metab 1997;82(11):3553–62.

[25] Martins RG, Caplan RH, Lambert PJ, et al. Management of thyroid cancer of follicular cell origin: Gundersen/Lutheran Medical Center, 1969–1995. J Am Coll Surg 1997;185(4): 388–97.

[26] Baudin E, Travagli JP, Ropers J, et al. Microcarcinoma of the thyroid gland the Gustave-Roussy Institute experience. Cancer 1998;83:553–9.

[27] Samaan NA, Schultz PN, Hickey RC, et al. The results of various modalities of treatment of well differentiated thyroid carcinoma: a retrospective review of 1599 patients. J Clin Endocrinol Metab 1992;75:714–20.

[28] Herrera MF, Lopez-Graniel CM, Saldana J, et al. Papillary thyroid carcinoma in Mexican patients: clinical aspects and prognostic factors. World J Surg 1996;20(1):94–9.

[29] Simpson WJ, Panzarella T, Carruthers JS, et al. Papillary and follicular thyroid cancer: impact of treatment in 1578 patients. Int J Radiat Oncol Biol Phys 1988;14(6):1063–75.

[30] Carcangiu ML, Zampi G, Pupi A, et al. Papillary carcinoma of the thyroid. A clinicopathologic study of 241 cases treated at the University of Florence, Italy. Cancer 1985;55(4): 805–28.

[31] Hay ID, McConahey WM, Goellner JR. Managing patients with papillary thyroid carcinoma: insights gained from the Mayo Clinic's experience of treating 2,512 consecutive patients during 1940 through 2000. Trans Am Clin Climatol Assoc 2002;113:241–60.

[32] DeGroot LJ, Kaplan EL, McCormick M, et al. Natural history, treatment, and course of papillary thyroid carcinoma. J Clin Endocrinol Metab 1990;71(2):414–24.

[33] Gemsenjager E, Heitz PU, Seifert B, et al. Differentiated thyroid carcinoma. Follow-up of 264 patients from one institution for up to 25 years. Swiss Med Wkly 2001;131(11–12): 157–63.

[34] McHenry CR, Rosen IB, Walfish PG. Prospective management of nodal metastases in differentiated thyroid cancer. Am J Surg 1991;162(4):353–6.

[35] Morris DM, Boyle PJ, Stidley CA, et al. Localized well-differentiated thyroid carcinoma: survival analysis of prognostic factors and (131)I therapy. Ann Surg Oncol 1998;5(4):329–37.

[36] Tseng LM, Lee CH, Wang HC, et al. The surgical treatment and prognostic factors of well-differentiated thyroid cancers in Chinese patients: a 20-year experience. Zhonghua Yi Xue Za Zhi (Taipei) 1996;58(2):121–31.

[37] Davis NL, Gordon M, Germann E, et al. Efficacy of 131I ablation following thyroidectomy in patients with invasive follicular thyroid cancer. Am J Surg 1992;163(5):472–5.

[38] Saadi H, Kleidermacher P, Esselstyn C Jr. Conservative management of patients with intrathyroidal well-differentiated follicular thyroid carcinoma. Surgery 2001;130(1):30–5.

[39] Sanders LE, Silverman M. Follicular and Hürthle cell carcinoma: predicting outcome and directing therapy. Surgery 1998;124(6):967–74.

[40] Tsang RW, Brierley JD, Simpson WJ, et al. The effects of surgery, radioiodine, and external radiation therapy on the clinical outcome of patients with differentiated thyroid carcinoma. Cancer 1998;82(2):375–88.

[41] Chow SM, Law SC, Au SK, et al. Changes in presentation, management, and outcome in 1348 patients with differentiated thyroid carcinoma: experience in a single institute in Hong Kong, 1960–2000. Clin Oncol (R Coll Radiol) 2003;15:329–36.

[42] Chow SM, Yau S, Kwan CK, et al. Local and regional control in patients with papillary thyroid carcinoma: specific indications of external radiotherapy and radioactive iodine according to T and N categories in AJCC 6th edition. Endocr Relat Cancer 2006;13:1159–72.

[43] Chow SM, Law SCK, Chan JKC, et al. Papillary microcarcinoma of the thyroid—Prognostic significance of lymph node metastasis and multifocality. Cancer 2003;98:31–40.

[44] Hay ID. Selective use of radioactive iodine in the postoperative management of patients with papillary and follicular thyroid carcinoma. J Surg Oncol 2006;94:692–700.

[45] Hackshaw A, Harmer C, Mallick U, et al. I-131 activity for remnant ablation in patients with differentiated thyroid cancer: a systematic review. J Clin Endocrinol Metab 2007;92:28–38.

[46] Pilli T, Brianzoni E, Capoccettti F, et al. A comparison of 1859 (50 mCi) and 3700 MBq (100 mCi) 131-iodine administered doses for recombinant thyrotropin-stimulated postoperative thyroid remnant ablation in differentiated thyroid cancer. J Clin Endocrinol Metab 2007; 92:3542–6.

[47] Swaka AM, Goldstein DP, Thabane L, et al. Basis for physician recommendations for adjuvant radioactive iodine in early stage thyroid carcinoma: principal findings of the CAM-ThyrCa Survey. Endocr Prac 2008;14(2):175–84.

ELSEVIER
SAUNDERS

Endocrinol Metab Clin N Am
37 (2008) 481–496

ENDOCRINOLOGY
AND METABOLISM
CLINICS
OF NORTH AMERICA

Management of Medullary Thyroid Carcinoma

Camilo Jiménez, MD[a], Mimi I-Nan Hu, MD[a],
Robert F. Gagel, MD[b],*

[a]*Department of Endocrine Neoplasia and Hormonal Disorders, The University
of Texas M. D. Anderson Cancer Center, Unit 435, 1515 Holcombe Boulevard,
Houston, TX 77030-4009, USA*
[b]*Division of Internal Medicine, Department of Endocrine Neoplasia and Hormonal Disorders,
The University of Texas M. D. Anderson Cancer Center, Unit 433, 1515 Holcombe Boulevard,
Houston, TX 77030-4009, USA*

Medullary thyroid carcinoma (MTC) is an uncommon malignant neuroendocrine tumor derived from the calcitonin-producing parafollicular cells of the thyroid gland. This tumor was first described in 1959 by Hazard and colleagues [1], who differentiated MTC from other poorly differentiated or anaplastic forms of thyroid carcinoma. Since the publication of this description almost 50 years ago, intense investigation has brought our understanding of the pathogenesis of this unusual tumor to a remarkable level. In 1961, Sipple [2] described the association between MTC and pheochromocytoma, an association that we know now as multiple endocrine neoplasia type 2 syndrome (MEN2). Then several groups of investigators demonstrated that MTC was derived from the thyroid parafollicular cells and consequently was able to produce excessive amounts of calcitonin, which would help with the biochemical diagnosis and follow-up of patients affected by this condition [3,4]. This concept was also the basis of the development of calcitonin stimulation tests using calcium or pentagastrin for early identification of individuals at risk for hereditary MTC [5,6]. In a series of studies conducted since the early 1970s, investigators have performed prophylactic thyroidectomy on a large number of people on the basis of pentagastrin-stimulated calcitonin measurements. These studies, some now having lasted for almost 40 years, have accomplished several things. First, they identified nearly all gene carriers who participated in the studies. Second, a retrospective look at these study results clearly showed a significant

---

* Corresponding author.
E-mail address: rgagel@mdanderson.org (R.F. Gagel).

0889-8529/08/$ - see front matter © 2008 Elsevier Inc. All rights reserved.
doi:10.1016/j.ecl.2008.03.001

incidence of false-positive calcitonin stimulation test results, indicating the difficulties associated with these tests in differentiating normal individuals from those with C-cell hyperplasia, the precursor lesion to hereditary MTC. Third, long-term follow-up demonstrated that most, but not all, of these individuals continue to have no evidence of metastatic MTC. Many of these affected persons are now middle aged, the point at which a previous generation began to die from MTC or pheochromocytomas, but very few deaths have been attributable to either when compared with times when the knowledge about MTC was much more limited.

A period of intense discovery came in 1993, when activating mutations of the RET proto-oncogene [7,8], a tyrosine kinase receptor [9], were found in patients with hereditary MTC. Since then, several germline RET proto-oncogene activating mutations have been found to cause almost 100% of hereditary MTCs. In addition, somatic RET proto-oncogene mutations have been found in approximately 25% of patients with sporadic MTC [10]. These findings indicate the importance of this gene in the development of both sporadic and hereditary tumors.

The recognition of RET as the major cause of MTC led to the identification of the major components of the RET receptor system, an understanding of the role of that receptor system in the normal developmental biology of the sympathetic nervous system, and the beginnings of an understanding of how mutations of RET cause transformation. These discoveries created a new paradigm for the management of genetic malignancy: identification of gene carriers and removal of the organ containing cells at risk for transformation early in life, constituting perhaps the most nearly perfect example of primary prevention of cancer in human beings to date. Another very important contribution of the understanding of the RET receptor system is the development of promising medications that may help to control and cure both hereditary and sporadic MTCs.

The RET receptor

The RET gene, which is located on chromosome 10q11.2, consists of 21 exons with 55,000 base pairs [11]. RET encodes a transmembrane receptor with a large extracellular portion containing four calcium-dependent cell-adhesion (cadherin) domains that mediate the conformational properties needed to interact with ligands and coreceptors [12]. The extracellular portion of the receptor also contains multiple glycosylation sites and a cysteine-rich region necessary for the tertiary structure of the protein and for receptor dimerization [13]. The intracellular domain of the RET receptor contains two tyrosine kinase regions that activate intracellular signal transduction pathways. RET activation requires the association of a ligand, such as glial cell line-derived neurotrophic factor (GDNF) or related molecules, including neurturin, artemin, or persephin, with a membrane surface coreceptor, glycosylphosphatidylinositol-anchored GDNF-family alpha

(GFRα). The GDNF-GFRα complex interacts with the RET receptor to permit its dimerization with another receptor. This triggers autophosphorylation of tyrosine residues on the intracellular domains of RET. The activated tyrosine residues serve as docking sites for adaptor proteins, which coordinate cellular signal transduction pathways (eg, mitogen-activated protein kinase, phosphatidylinositol 3-kinase, AKT, Jun N-terminal kinase, extracellular signal-regulated protein kinase) which are important in the regulation of cell growth, for instance [13].

The clinical syndromes

Sporadic medullary thyroid carcinoma

Sporadic MTC is the most common form of this tumor: 65% to 75% of MTCs are classified as sporadic. Sporadic MTC is most commonly not associated with germline RET proto-oncogene mutations, C-cell hyperplasia, or a family history suggestive of MTC or pheochromocytoma. Sporadic MTC arises de novo as a result of one or more somatic mutations of the RET proto-oncogene in a single parafollicular cell (monoclonal origin) or by other undefined mechanisms. Sporadic MTC is most commonly unicentric; however, multicentric disease may occur in some cases. This tumor most commonly manifests equally in women and men in the fourth decade of life. An isolated thyroid nodule is the most common manifestation. Because the parafollicular cell does not concentrate iodine, radioiodine scanning shows a "cold" thyroid nodule. The diagnosis is usually made by fine-needle aspiration biopsy. However, thyroid cytopathologic diagnosis of MTC can be challenging, and it can occasionally be incorrectly identified as a poorly differentiated carcinoma of unknown etiology, or even as a parathyroid tumor.

Metastases to local lymph nodes occur frequently: 80% of patients with a palpable MTC or a tumor bigger than 1 cm have lymph node metastases [14,15]. Furthermore, lymph node metastases are frequently inapparent to operating surgeons and may be missed by pathologists unless each node removed is carefully studied. The most common pattern of lymph node metastases is to ipsilateral nodes in areas II to VI of the neck, although metastases to the contralateral nodes may occur in up to 40% of patients with a palpable primary tumor [14,15]. Another common pattern of metastases is into mediastinal lymph nodes. Metastases to lymph nodes in the neck and mediastinum can grow, infiltrate, and compress the airway, contributing to the high rates of morbidity and mortality observed in patients with MTC. Distant metastases to the liver, skeleton, and lung parenchyma are frequently seen in patients with calcitonin values greater than 5,000 pg/mL. Hepatic and lung metastases are commonly vascular. Clinicians should be aware that even experienced radiologists will commonly report a small focus of liver metastasis as a hemangioma while reading a contrast-enhanced

CT scan. Bone metastases are most commonly lytic and can cause severe bone pain, pathologic fractures, cord compression, and, rarely, hypercalcemia.

Of patients with apparently sporadic MTCs, 6% or 7% are subsequently found to have a germline RET mutation indicative of hereditary disease [10]. Consequently, it is recommended that all patients with MTC be evaluated for RET proto-oncogene germline mutations.

Hereditary medullary thyroid carcinoma

Hereditary MTC is associated with activating germline mutations of the RET proto-oncogene. Hereditary MTC is multifocal and present in the context of simple, diffuse, and nodular C-cell hyperplasia, the precursor lesion of hereditary MTC. Hereditary MTC may manifest in various age groups, but unlike the case in sporadic MTC, the hereditary form commonly occurs in individuals younger than 20 years of age. Frequently, a positive family history suggestive of MTC or pheochromocytoma is also present. Similar to sporadic MTC, hereditary MTC can also spread to neck and mediastinal lymph nodes, liver, skeleton, and lungs, predisposing the patient to high rates of morbidity and mortality.

Hereditary MTC manifests as part of the MEN2 syndrome, which was first defined as a discrete syndrome in 1961 [2]. MEN2 is transmitted as an autosomal dominant trait. In the subsequent decades, subvariants have been defined. MEN type 2A (MEN2A) is the most common form of hereditary MTC, accounting for approximately 80% of MEN2 cases. MEN2A is characterized by bilateral, multicentric MTC in more than 90% of gene carriers, unilateral or bilateral pheochromocytomas in 50% of gene carriers, and primary hyperparathyroidism in 10% to 20% of carriers.

There are three variants of MEN2A. The first is MEN2A with Hirschsprung disease [16]. Children with this variant develop Hirschsprung disease in childhood. Kindreds with this variant are uncommon, with fewer than 25 reported, although perhaps this phenotypic expression is underreported. In the second variant, found in 20 to 30 families, MEN2A is associated with cutaneous lichen amyloidosis [17]. Patients with this variant develop a pruritic cutaneous form of amyloid located over the upper back. Most commonly, this lesion develops in the second or third decade of life, although in some reported examples, localized pruritus was an indicator of MEN2A in childhood [18]. The third variant, familial MTC (FMTC) [19], is characterized by MTC but no other manifestations of MEN2. In general, FMTC tends to be the least aggressive form of hereditary MTC.

MEN type 2B (MEN2B) is less common than MEN2A (approximately 20% of cases of MEN2), but it is the most distinctive form of this syndrome [20]. MEN2B is characterized by MTC in 100% of carriers; pheochromocytomas in 50% of carriers; mucosal ganglioneuromas localized in the distal tongue, the eyelids, and the gastrointestinal tract in more than 90% of carriers; and a marphanoid habitus in nearly all affected individuals. Early identification of MTC in MEN2B is important because metastases have been described during the first year of life.

In this order of ideas, MTC associated with MEN2B is generally the most aggressive form of MTC described in human beings. Most examples of this disease represent de novo mutations with no prior family history. Cure of MTC is difficult because the phenotype is not often recognized. Local lymph node metastases are common during the first decade of life, and distant metastases are seen with some regularity during the second decade. Death from metastatic MTC generally occurs during the third or fourth decade, though there are examples of kindreds with three or more generations of affected members still living [21,22].

Genotype-phenotype correlation in hereditary medullary thyroid carcinoma

During the 15 years since the initial discovery of RET mutations in MEN2, there has been a gradual refinement of the phenotypes associated with particular activating mutations of RET. Fig. 1 shows an overview of the current understanding of RET mutations and presents the clinical syndromes associated with different mutations of RET.

The most commonly identified mutations in hereditary MTC are localized in the extracellular cysteine-rich domain of the RET receptor. Codon 634 is mutated in 80% of all cases of MEN2, and a single cysteine-to-arginine substitution is found in more than half of kindreds with classic MEN2A. Mutation of codon 634 is also the only one associated with the cutaneous lichen amyloidosis variant of MEN2A in the few families that express this phenotype [23]. Between 10% and 15% of kindreds with MEN2A have mutations of codons 609, 611, 618, or 620; kindreds with these mutations may have either MEN2A or one of its variants (MEN2A with Hirschsprung disease or FMTC) [24]. The most common mutations associated with the MEN2B phenotype affect codons 883, 918, and 922, and account for 3% to 5% of all RET mutations [23,25–28]. These mutations are localized in the intracellular tyrosine kinase domain of the RET receptor. Mutation of codon 918 is the most common mutation associated with MEN2B [23], and mutations of codons 768 and V804M are invariably associated with FMTC [23,29]. Intracellular domain mutations that may be associated with either MEN2A or FMTC phenotypes include codons 790, 791 [30], V804L [31], and 891 [32]. The remaining mutations (codons 532, 533, 777, 912) are rare and, although they apparently exhibit a clear genotype-phenotype correlation associated with FMTC, their presence should be interpreted with caution [33–36].

Somatic RET proto-oncogene mutations in sporadic medullary thyroid carcinoma

Approximately 25% of sporadic MTCs have somatic RET proto-oncogene mutations. The most commonly identified mutation is codon met918thr [37],

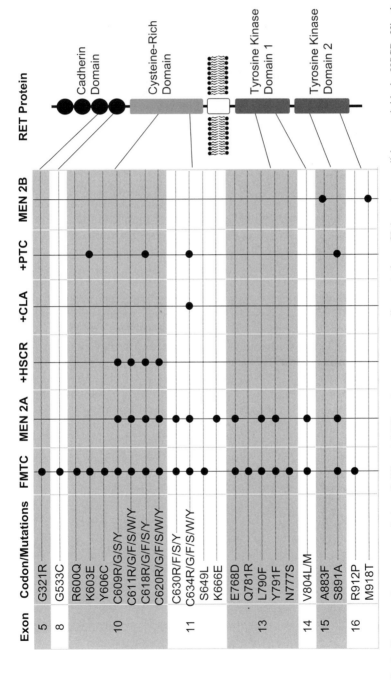

Fig. 1. Genotype-phenotype correlation of different RET proto-oncogene germline mutations. CLA, cutaneous lichen amyloidosis; HSCR, Hirschprungs disease; PTC, papillary thyroid carcinoma.

which is identical to the germline mutation that causes MEN2B. This mutation is associated with a very aggressive form of sporadic MTC. Reports from several groups have indicated that this mutation is associated with a greater extent of disease and a significant reduction in survival when compared with other mutations [38,39]. These tumors usually manifest with extensive lymph node metastasis in the neck and mediastinum and distant spread to the liver, lungs, and skeleton. The 10-year survival rate in patients with a codon 918 mutation is 50%, which is much lower than that observed in patients without this mutation (approximately 85%) [39]. Other RET codons noted to be mutated in sporadic MTC are 631, 634, 766, 768, 876, 804, 883, 884, 901, 922, and 930 [37,40–44].

It is important to recognize that somatic mutations are heterogeneous. For instance, in the context of metastatic sporadic MTC, some metastatic foci have a codon 918 mutation, whereas the primary tumor or another focus may be devoid of this mutation [45]. This finding suggests that acquisition of RET mutations is one element involved in the progression of metastatic disease.

Treatment of medullary thyroid carcinoma

Preventive surgical management of hereditary medullary thyroid carcinoma

The penetrance of hereditary MTC is almost 100%. Consequently, all individual carriers of a RET mutation should be evaluated and treated for MTC. The information collected since 1993 on RET mutations and their respective clinical expression has provided researchers studying MEN2 with enough knowledge to develop a consensus on using the genetic information to establish proper treatment to prevent morbidity and mortality associated with hereditary MTC. Some idea of the relative aggressiveness of MTC has been gained by an examination of the earliest age at which MTC has been identified with a specific mutation. Based on this information, mutations of RET have been classified as highest, high, and intermediate in risk, depending on the aggressiveness observed in the respectively associated MTCs [46].

The highest-risk mutations predispose to very aggressive MTCs, characterized by the initiation of tumor development and even metastases before the first year of life: these are the mutations of codons 883, 918, and 922 associated with the MEN2B phenotype. Consequently, carriers of these mutations are candidates for a total thyroidectomy, with central node dissection in the first month of life or as soon as the phenotype is identified. High-risk mutations predispose to aggressive MTCs that have been identified in a small but important group of children, younger than 5 years old, in whom metastases occur as early as age 6 [47]. Mutations of codons 611, 618, 620, 634, and 891 are classified as high-risk mutations. These individuals are therefore candidates for total thyroidectomy with or without central node dissection by age 5 years.

Intermediate-risk mutations are localized in codons 768, 790, 791, and 804. In certain large kindreds with these mutations, a death has never been caused by MTC; in others, metastases and death attributable to MTC have occurred infrequently [48]. If there has never been a death attributable to MTC in one of these kindreds (and the kindred is of sufficient size and the follow-up encompasses multiple generations), delaying total thyroidectomy with or without central lymph node dissection to a later age may be a reasonable course [48]. Some practitioners continue to perform pentagastrin-stimulated calcitonin measurements with removal of the thyroid gland when abnormalities in serum calcitonin appear.

Genetic information can also be used to assess risk for pheochromocytoma. Individuals with RET mutations of codons 609, 611, 618, 620, 630, 634, 790, V804L, 883, 891, 918, or 922 should be routinely screened for pheochromocytoma [49]. According to current information, it is reasonable to conclude that development of a pheochromocytoma is unlikely in kindreds with codon 768 and V804M mutations [23]. However, although pheochromocytomas have not been identified in kindreds with mutations of codons 532, 533, or 912, the experience is limited to a handful of families, and it would be prudent to consider periodic measurements of plasma metanephrines in members of these kindreds [49]. In adolescents or adults recently diagnosed with hereditary MTC associated with one of the previously mentioned pheochromocytoma-related RET proto-oncogene mutations, screening for pheochromocytoma should be performed before resection of the MTC takes place.

Hereditary or sporadic medullary thyroid carcinoma presenting as a thyroid nodule

At present, the only possible curative treatment against MTC is its complete surgical resection when the disease is confined to the neck. However, as suggested in previous sections, complete resection of MTC could be very difficult. A high percentage of MTCs manifesting as a palpable thyroid nodule may already have metastasized to ipsilateral (80%) and contralateral (40%) cervical lymph nodes [14], and frequently may present with distant metastatic disease to the liver, bones, and lung parenchyma. Consequently, for surgical purposes, patients with MTC can be classified into one of three groups. The first group is comprised of those with localized disease (no evidence of metastases to regional lymph nodes as indicated by sonography, no disease outside of the neck as indicated by CT scans of the chest and abdomen with liver protocol and bone scan, and serum calcitonin values usually less than 500 pg/mL) in which cure is possible. The second group includes those with metastatic disease limited to the neck, in which cure may be possible. The third group is comprised of those with metastatic disease outside of the neck, in which surgical cure is unlikely.

The appropriate surgical procedure for a patient with localized MTC is a total thyroidectomy with central (levels VI and VII) and bilateral lateral (levels II to V) lymph node dissections. Although surgical cure (calcitonin concentration of less than 5 pg/mL in a two-site immunoassay) in this clinical context is difficult to establish, it is believed that up to 25% of selected patients can be cured by this approach [50–53].

Patients with documented local metastatic disease should also be treated with a total thyroidectomy, with central and bilateral lateral neck lymph node dissection [54]. A question that arises in this group of patients is how thoroughly one should look for distant metastatic disease. Guidance may be provided by a combination of a serum calcitonin measurement with high-quality sonography of the neck. If the serum calcitonin concentration exceeds 500 pg/mL and there is no evidence of metastasis to the neck lymph nodes on sonography, it would be appropriate to perform chest and abdominal CT scans and bone scanning. The challenge is to differentiate between patients in whom surgical cure is possible and those with distant metastasis in whom extensive neck surgery will, in most cases, not affect long-term outcomes. In patients for whom surgical cure is not possible, the goals change. In this situation, it is appropriate to perform a total thyroidectomy with surgical resection of identifiable disease to protect the airway.

Patients with clear evidence of distant metastasis are more straightforward to identify. These patients may have substantial elevations of serum calcitonin (greater than 5,000 pg/mL), metastatic disease easily identifiable on imaging studies, and frequently diarrhea and flushing. In these patients, total thyroidectomy with removal of identifiable disease to protect the airway is indicated. When there are lymph nodes with metastasis in the upper mediastinum or perihilar area that are likely to affect the airway, consideration should be given to a mediastinal lymph node dissection [54].

It is important to understand that this is an area of flux. Recent studies (addressed later in this article) showing evidence of response to tyrosine kinase inhibitors that target RET or vascular endothelial growth factor (VEGF) receptor open a potential new treatment paradigm of long-term chronic suppressive treatment for distant metastases.

Persistent elevation of serum calcitonin and carcinoembryonic antigen after surgery

MTC produces excessive amounts of calcitonin and carcinoembryonic antigen (CEA). Consequently, measurement of these molecules may help to monitor the growth rate of MTC. Sequential measurements of calcitonin over extended periods are useful for quantification of tumor mass. Doubling times of less than 2 years are generally associated with a poor prognosis; however, there are several points to keep in mind about calcitonin measurements. First, the calcitonin concentration can be abnormally elevated in the context of pregnancy, use of oral contraceptives, goiter, and the presence of other tumors, such as breast and lung cancer. Second, calcitonin is a secretory peptide, the secretion of which is episodic and may be affected by plasma calcium concentration, exercise, or gastrin stimulation. Third, dedifferentiated MTC may lose the ability to produce calcitonin. Consequently, a decrease in plasma calcitonin in someone with advanced MTC may suggest a poor prognosis [55].

CEA is a useful tumor marker for monitoring the growth rate of MTC [56]. However, CEA is made throughout the gastrointestinal tract and liver, and its concentration may be elevated in cigarette smokers and persons with several other tumors. As such, there is a broad range of normality, making it an insensitive marker for detection of early MTC but a useful long-term indicator of disease progression when elevated.

After initial thyroidectomy and lymph node dissection, it is necessary to allow 3 to 4 months before concluding that an elevated calcitonin or CEA concentration is related to the presence of MTC and not to the postoperative inflammatory effects on calcitonin synthesis [57], or a failure of circulating CEA to clear because of its prolonged half-life [58]. Frequently, patients with MTC undergo a total thyroidectomy with limited or no lymph node dissection. In these patients, and in patients treated with total thyroidectomy and bilateral lateral neck lymph node dissection, persistent elevation of calcitonin and CEA is likely associated with residual disease in the cervical lymph nodes. Because the patient has undergone a total thyroidectomy, the decision to perform a neck lymph node dissection should be based on a realistic estimate of the probability of surgical cure. In patients with calcitonin concentrations of less than 100 pg/mL, it is unusual to find any detectable radiographic abnormalities in the neck, and long-term clinical surveillance with periodic sonography of the neck is then indicated. In patients with higher calcitonin values without radiographic evidence of macroscopic disease, close follow-up with periodic imaging (sonography of the neck, chest X-rays, CT scans of the chest and abdomen) is necessary [59]. In most circumstances, reoperating on the neck will not normalize serum calcitonin concentrations. Conversely, the risk of hypoparathyroidism is much higher than that observed if the neck dissection is performed during the initial surgical intervention [50].

Patients with calcitonin concentrations higher than 5,000 pg/mL after total thyroidectomy and lymph node dissection generally have metastatic disease outside of the neck. Neck, mediastinal, and lung parenchymal disease is almost always detected by sonography of the neck or CT scanning of the chest. Liver metastasis is usually found on high-quality CT scanning of the abdomen, and skeletal metastases are usually detected on bone scanning [59]. When the results of these radiographic studies are inconclusive, the most likely site of metastasis is the liver, where microscopic metastases are difficult to detect. Some investigators propose undertaking laparoscopic exploration of the liver to finally confirm the presence of metastases [60]. Nuclear medicine studies, such as those using octreotide or ^{131}I iobenguane (MIBG) have a very a limited value in localizing MTC, and the experience with positron-emission tomographic (PET) scanning is—at least for now—very limited [61]. Unpublished experience from recent clinical trials of tyrosine kinase inhibitors suggest PET scanning is of limited usefulness.

Radiotherapy, chemotherapy, and other treatments for bone metastases and paraneoplastic syndromes

Radiotherapy is routinely used as adjunctive, palliative treatment for extensive neck or mediastinal disease or for localized bony metastasis. Although radiotherapy seems to be effective in preventing and controlling complications associated with MTC activity in the neck and mediastinum, there is no evidence that such therapy has an effect on improving survival time [62]. Targeted radiotherapy with somatostatin analogs [63] or MIBG has a very limited value [64].

Chemotherapy based on dacarbazine has been associated with a significant reduction in tumor size in approximately 30% of patients treated with this agent in combination with others. However, a complete remission has never been observed, and it apparently has no effect on survival rates [61].

Lytic bony metastases may also be the target of parenterally administered bisphosphonates, although no study results are available to demonstrate a potential benefit of these agents against metastatic MTC bone disease. However, in the context of hypercalcemia induced by bone osteolysis, the use of bisphosphonates adequately controls this complication and improves the symptoms.

Ectopic Cushing syndrome is a rare endocrine complication of MTC associated with excessive tumor production of adrenocorticotropic hormone or its precursor peptides. When this complication is associated with a localized tumor, curative resection of the tumor will cure this paraneoplastic syndrome. In the context of ectopic Cushing syndrome secondary to a broadly metastatic disease, bilateral adrenalectomy after adequate adrenal inhibition with ketoconazol or metyrapone, followed by adrenal replacement therapy with glucocorticoids and mineralocorticoids, may be necessary.

Tyrosine kinase inhibitors

Tyrosine kinase inhibitors are small molecules that compete with the adenosine triphosphate-binding site of the catalytic domain of a tyrosine kinase. Occupation of this site inhibits autophosphorylation and activation of the tyrosine kinase, and prevents further activation of intracellular signaling pathways. A tyrosine kinase inhibitor can be specific to one or many homologous tyrosine kinases. Two promising tyrosine kinase inhibitors against MTC are ZD6474 and AMG-706. ZD6474 (Zactima; vandetanib) is a selective tyrosine kinase inhibitor of RET, VEGF receptor 2 and, to a lesser extent, of epidermal growth factor receptor. ZD6474 inhibits VEGF-mediated endothelial cell migration and proliferation. Two phase II clinical trials are evaluating the use of ZD6474 in MTC: one trial of a 100-mg daily dosage and the other of 300 mg daily. The latter, an open-label trial of ZD6474 in subjects with hereditary MTC, has provided promising initial data [65]. As of November 2005, 16 subjects had been treated orally with 300 mg of ZD6474 daily. Fifteen of the subjects could be evaluated for tumor response and for calcitonin and CEA levels. Objective partial tumor responses were seen in three subjects, stabilized disease in ten subjects (duration of 8 to more than 24 weeks), and progressive disease in two subjects. Calcitonin concentrations dropped by more than 50% for at least 4 weeks in 12 of the subjects, and a similar magnitude of decline in CEA was seen in six subjects. Side effects included diarrhea, nausea, rash, fatigue, hypertension, and asymptomatic QTc prolongation [65].

The second promising tyrosine kinase inhibitor against MTC, motesanib diphosphate (AMG-706), is a multikinase inhibitor targeting VEGF, platelet-derived growth factor, and Kit receptors, which lead to antiangiogenic and direct antitumor activity. In a phase I trial with AMG-706, one patient with MTC exhibited an objective partial response. Adverse events included diarrhea, hypertension, fatigue, dizziness, nausea, vomiting, and headache [66]. In a phase II trial with AMG 706 ($n = 83$), after a median follow-up of 32 weeks, most patients experienced some decline in tumor growth, with 80% of cases showing stable disease by RECIST (Response Evaluation Criteria in Solid Tumors) criteria [67]. Data presentation of a longer follow-up is expected in the near future [68].

RET synthesis or activation can also be targeted at various other points: biosynthesis or expression of the RET receptor, ligand binding of the GDNF ligand to the GFRα coreceptor, dimerization, recruitment of adaptor proteins, and activation of intracellular signaling pathways [13]. In the article by Sherman elsewhere in this issue, more detailed analyses and descriptions of all these therapeutic targets and other potential tyrosine kinase inhibitors against MTC are presented.

Summary

The introduction of genetic testing into the clinical management of medullary thyroid carcinoma has provided greater precision regarding diagnosis, follow-up, prognosis, and treatment against this disease. Thanks to this knowledge, new therapeutic approaches against medullary thyroid carcinoma are under development. However, more research is needed to finally identify therapies able to control and to cure this disease. This is the welcome to the future and the hope for many patients.

Acknowledgments

The authors thank Karen Phillips, ELS, for her editorial assistance, and Dr. Gilbert Cote for his academic support.

References

[1] Hazard JB, Hawk WA, Crile G Jr. Medullary (solid) carcinoma of the thyroid; a clinicopathologic entity. J Clin Endocrinol Metab 1959;19(1):152–61.

[2] Sipple J. The association of pheochromocytoma with carcinoma of the thyroid gland. Am J Med 1961;31:163–6.

[3] Melvin KE, Miller HH, Tashjian AH Jr. Early diagnosis of medullary carcinoma of the thyroid gland by means of calcitonin assay. N Engl J Med 1971;285(20):1115–20.

[4] Melvin KE, Tashjian AH Jr. The syndrome of excessive thyrocalcitonin produced by medullary carcinoma of the thyroid. Proc Natl Acad Sci USA 1968;59(4):1216–22.

[5] Graze K, Spiler IJ, Tashjian AH Jr, et al. Natural history of familial medullary thyroid carcinoma: effect of a program for early diagnosis. N Engl J Med 1978;299(18): 980–5.

[6] Gagel RF, Tashjian AH Jr, Cummings T, et al. The clinical outcome of prospective screening for multiple endocrine neoplasia type 2a. An 18-year experience. N Engl J Med 1988;318(8): 478–84.

[7] Donis-Keller H, Dou S, Chi D, et al. Mutations in the RET proto-oncogene are associated with MEN 2A and FMTC. Hum Mol Genet 1993;2(7):851–6.

[8] Mulligan LM, Kwok JB, Healey CS, et al. Germ-line mutations of the RET proto-oncogene in multiple endocrine neoplasia type 2A. Nature 1993;363(6428):458–60.

[9] Takahashi M, Ritz J, Cooper GM. Activation of a novel human transforming gene, RET, by DNA rearrangement. Cell 1985;42(2):581–8.

[10] Wohllk N, Cote GJ, Bugalho MM, et al. Relevance of RET proto-oncogene mutations in sporadic medullary thyroid carcinoma. J Clin Endocrinol Metab 1996;81(10): 3740–5.

[11] Pasini B, Hofstra RM, Yin L, et al. The physical map of the human RET proto-oncogene. Oncogene 1995;11(9):1737–43.

[12] Anders J, Kjar S, Ibanez CF. Molecular modeling of the extracellular domain of the RET receptor tyrosine kinase reveals multiple cadherin-like domains and a calcium-binding site. J Biol Chem 2001;276(38):35808–17.

[13] de Groot JW, Links TP, Plukker JT, et al. RET as a diagnostic and therapeutic target in sporadic and hereditary endocrine tumors. Endocr Rev 2006;27(5):535–60.

[14] Moley JF, DeBenedetti MK. Patterns of nodal metastases in palpable medullary thyroid carcinoma: recommendations for extent of node dissection. Ann Surg 1999;229(6):880–7 [discussion: 887–8].

[15] Moley JF, Wells SA. Compartment-mediated dissection for papillary thyroid cancer. Langenbecks Arch Surg 1999;384(1):9–15.

[16] Verdy M, Weber AM, Roy CC, et al. Hirschsprung's disease in a family with multiple endocrine neoplasia type 2. J Pediatr Gastroenterol Nutr 1982;1(4):603–7.

[17] Gagel RF, Levy ML, Donovan DT, et al. Multiple endocrine neoplasia type 2a associated with cutaneous lichen amyloidosis. Ann Intern Med 1989;111(10):802–6.

[18] Nunziata V, Giannattasio R, Di Giovanni G, et al. Hereditary localized pruritus in affected members of a kindred with multiple endocrine neoplasia type 2A (Sipple's syndrome). Clin Endocrinol (Oxf) 1989;30(1):57–63.

[19] Farndon JR, Leight GS, Dilley WG, et al. Familial medullary thyroid carcinoma without associated endocrinopathies: a distinct clinical entity. Br J Surg 1986;73(4):278–81.

[20] Williams ED, Pollock DJ. Multiple mucosal neuromata with endocrine tumours: a syndrome allied to von Recklinghausen's disease. J Pathol Bacteriol 1966;91(1):71–80.

[21] Vasen HF, van der Feltz M, Raue F, et al. The natural course of multiple endocrine neoplasia type IIb. A study of 18 cases. Arch Intern Med 1992;152(6):1250–2.

[22] Sizemore GW, Carney JA, Gharib H, et al. Multiple endocrine neoplasia type 2B: eighteen-year follow-up of a four-generation family. Henry Ford Hosp Med J 1992; 40(3–4):236–44.

[23] Eng C, Clayton D, Schuffenecker I, et al. The relationship between specific RET proto-oncogene mutations and disease phenotype in multiple endocrine neoplasia type 2. International RET mutation consortium analysis. JAMA 1996;276(19):1575–9.

[24] Angrist M, Bolk S, Thiel B, et al. Mutation analysis of the RET receptor tyrosine kinase in Hirschsprung disease. Hum Mol Genet 1995;4(5):821–30.

[25] Eng C, Smith DP, Mulligan LM, et al. Point mutation within the tyrosine kinase domain of the RET proto-oncogene in multiple endocrine neoplasia type 2B and related sporadic tumours. Hum Mol Genet 1994;3(2):237–41.

[26] Maruyama S, Iwashita T, Imai T, et al. Germ line mutations of the ret proto-oncogene in Japanese patients with multiple endocrine neoplasia type 2A and type 2B. Jpn J Cancer Res 1994;85(9):879–82.

[27] Hofstra RM, Landsvater RM, Ceccherini I, et al. A mutation in the RET proto-oncogene associated with multiple endocrine neoplasia type 2B and sporadic medullary thyroid carcinoma. Nature 1994;367(6461):375–6.

[28] Gimm O, Marsh DJ, Andrew SD, et al. Germline dinucleotide mutation in codon 883 of the RET proto-oncogene in multiple endocrine neoplasia type 2B without codon 918 mutation. J Clin Endocrinol Metab 1997;82(11):3902–4.

[29] Bolino A, Schuffenecker I, Luo Y, et al. RET mutations in exons 13 and 14 of FMTC patients. Oncogene 1995;10(12):2415–9.

[30] Berndt I, Reuter M, Saller B, et al. A new hot spot for mutations in the ret protooncogene causing familial medullary thyroid carcinoma and multiple endocrine neoplasia type 2A. J Clin Endocrinol Metab 1998;83(3):770–4.

[31] Nilsson O, Tisell LE, Jansson S, et al. Adrenal and extra-adrenal pheochromocytomas in a family with germline RET V804L mutation. JAMA 1999;281(17):1587–8.

[32] Jiménez C, Habra MA, Huang SC, et al. Pheochromocytoma and medullary thyroid carcinoma: a new genotype-phenotype correlation of the RET protooncogene 891 germline mutation. J Clin Endocrinol Metab 2004;89(8):4142–5.

[33] Jiménez C, Dang GT, Schultz PN, et al. A novel point mutation of the RET protooncogene involving the second intracellular tyrosine kinase domain in a family with medullary thyroid carcinoma. J Clin Endocrinol Metab 2004;89(7):3521–6.

[34] Pigny P, Bauters C, Wemeau JL, et al. A novel 9-base pair duplication in RET exon 8 in familial medullary thyroid carcinoma. J Clin Endocrinol Metab 1999;84(5):1700–4.

[35] Da Silva AM, Maciel RM, Da Silva MR, et al. A novel germ-line point mutation in RET exon 8 (Gly(533)Cys) in a large kindred with familial medullary thyroid carcinoma. J Clin Endocrinol Metab 2003;88(11):5438–43.

[36] D'Aloiso L, Carlomagno F, Bisceglia M, et al. Clinical case seminar: in vivo and in vitro characterization of a novel germline RET mutation associated with low-penetrant nonaggressive familial medullary thyroid carcinoma. J Clin Endocrinol Metab 2006;91(3):754–9.

[37] Uchino S, Noguchi S, Adachi M, et al. Novel point mutations and allele loss at the RET locus in sporadic medullary thyroid carcinomas. Jpn J Cancer Res 1998;89(4):411–8.

[38] Zedenius J, Larsson C, Bergholm U, et al. Mutations of codon 918 in the RET proto-oncogene correlate to poor prognosis in sporadic medullary thyroid carcinomas. J Clin Endocrinol Metab 1995;80(10):3088–90.

[39] Schilling T, Burck J, Sinn HP, et al. Prognostic value of codon 918 (ATG–>ACG) RET proto-oncogene mutations in sporadic medullary thyroid carcinoma. Int J Cancer 2001; 95(1):62–6.

[40] Scurini C, Quadro L, Fattoruso O, et al. Germline and somatic mutations of the RET proto-oncogene in apparently sporadic medullary thyroid carcinomas. Mol Cell Endocrinol 1998; 137(1):51–7.

[41] Shirahama S, Ogura K, Takami H, et al. Mutational analysis of the RET proto-oncogene in 71 Japanese patients with medullary thyroid carcinoma. J Hum Genet 1998;43(2): 101–6.

[42] Marsh DJ, Learoyd DL, Andrew SD, et al. Somatic mutations in the RET proto-oncogene in sporadic medullary thyroid carcinoma. Clin Endocrinol (Oxf) 1996;44(3):249–57.

[43] Uchino S, Noguchi S, Yamashita H, et al. Somatic mutations in RET exons 12 and 15 in sporadic medullary thyroid carcinomas: different spectrum of mutations in sporadic type from hereditary type. Jpn J Cancer Res 1999;90(11):1231–7.

[44] Jindrichova S, Kodet R, Krskova L, et al. The newly detected mutations in the RET proto-oncogene in exon 16 as a cause of sporadic medullary thyroid carcinoma. J Mol Med 2003; 81(12):819–23.

[45] Eng C, Thomas GA, Neuberg DS, et al. Mutation of the RET proto-oncogene is correlated with RET immunostaining in subpopulations of cells in sporadic medullary thyroid carcinoma. J Clin Endocrinol Metab 1998;83(12):4310–3.

[46] Brandi ML, Gagel RF, Angeli A, et al. Guidelines for diagnosis and therapy of MEN type 1 and type 2. J Clin Endocrinol Metab 2001;86(12):5658–71.

[47] Gill JR, Reyes-Mugica M, Iyengar S, et al. Early presentation of metastatic medullary carcinoma in multiple endocrine neoplasia, type IIA: implications for therapy. J Pediatr 1996;129(3):459–64.

[48] Lombardo F, Baudin E, Chiefari E, et al. Familial medullary thyroid carcinoma: clinical variability and low aggressiveness associated with RET mutation at codon 804. J Clin Endocrinol Metab 2002;87(4):1674–80.

[49] Jiménez C, Cote G, Arnold A, et al. Review: Should patients with apparently sporadic pheochromocytomas or paragangliomas be screened for hereditary syndromes? J Clin Endocrinol Metab 2006;91(8):2851–8.

[50] Fleming JB, Lee JE, Bouvet M, et al. Surgical strategy for the treatment of medullary thyroid carcinoma. Ann Surg 1999;230(5):697–707.

[51] Saad MF, Ordonez NG, Rashid RK, et al. Medullary carcinoma of the thyroid. A study of the clinical features and prognostic factors in 161 patients. Medicine (Baltimore) 1984;63(6): 319–42.

[52] Cohen MS, Moley JF. Surgical treatment of medullary thyroid carcinoma. J Intern Med 2003;253(6):616–26.

[53] Machens A, Hinze R, Thomusch O, et al. Pattern of nodal metastasis for primary and reoperative thyroid cancer. World J Surg 2002;26(1):22–8.

[54] Evans DB, Fleming JB, Lee JE, et al. The surgical treatment of medullary thyroid carcinoma. Semin Surg Oncol 1999;16(1):50–63.

[55] Mendelsohn G. Markers as prognostic indicators in medullary thyroid carcinoma. Am J Clin Pathol 1991;95(3):297–8.

[56] DeLellis RA, Rule AH, Spiler I, et al. Calcitonin and carcinoembryonic antigen as tumor markers in medullary thyroid carcinoma. Am J Clin Pathol 1978;70(4):587–94.

[57] Muller B, White JC, Nylen ES, et al. Ubiquitous expression of the calcitonin-i gene in multiple tissues in response to sepsis. J Clin Endocrinol Metab 2001;86(1):396–404.

[58] Saad MF, Fritsche HA Jr, Samaan NA. Diagnostic and prognostic values of carcinoembryonic antigen in medullary carcinoma of the thyroid. J Clin Endocrinol Metab 1984; 58(5):889–94.

[59] Sherman SI, Angelos P, Ball DW, et al. Thyroid carcinoma. J Natl Compr Canc Netw 2007; 5(6):568–621.

[60] Tung WS, Vesely TM, Moley JF. Laparoscopic detection of hepatic metastases in patients with residual or recurrent medullary thyroid cancer. Surgery 1995;118(6):1024–9 [discussion: 1029–30].

[61] Kaltsas GA, Besser GM, Grossman AB. The diagnosis and medical management of advanced neuroendocrine tumors. Endocr Rev 2004;25(3):458–511.

[62] Brierley J, Tsang R, Simpson WJ, et al. Medullary thyroid cancer: analyses of survival and prognostic factors and the role of radiation therapy in local control. Thyroid 1996;6(4): 305–10.

[63] Diez JJ, Iglesias P. Somatostatin analogs in the treatment of medullary thyroid carcinoma. J Endocrinol Invest 2002;25(9):773–8.

[64] Monsieurs M, Brans B, Bacher K, et al. Patient dosimetry for 131I-MIBG therapy for neuroendocrine tumours based on 123I-MIBG scans. Eur J Nucl Med Mol Imaging 2002; 29(12):1581–7.

[65] Wells SA Jr. A phase II trial of ZD6474 in patients with hereditary metastatic medullary thyroid cancer. ASCO Annual Meeting Proceedings 2006. J Clin Oncol 2006; 24(18S):5533.

[66] Boughton D. Safety and antitumor activity of AMG 706 in patients with thyroid cancer: A subset analysis from a phase 1 dose-finding study. ASCO Annual Meeting Proceedings Part I. 2006. J Clin Oncol 2006;24(18S):3030.

[67] Therasse P, Arbuck SG, Eisenhauer EA, et al. New guidelines to evaluate the response to treatment in solid tumors. European Organization for Research and Treatment of Cancer, National Cancer Institute of the United States, National Cancer Institute of Canada. J Natl Cancer Inst 2000;92(3):205–16.

[68] Schlumberger M, Elise R, Sherman SI, et al. Initial Results from a Phase 2 Trial of Motesanib Diphosphate (AMG 706) in Patients (pts) with Medullary Thyroid Cancer (MTC). Presented at the 89th Annual Meeting of the Endocrine Society (Endo 07). Toronto (ON), Canada, June 2–5, 2007.

ELSEVIER
SAUNDERS

Endocrinol Metab Clin N Am
37 (2008) 497–509

ENDOCRINOLOGY
AND METABOLISM
CLINICS
OF NORTH AMERICA

External Beam Radiation Therapy for Thyroid Cancer

James D. Brierley, MBBS, FRCP, FRCR, FRCP(C)*,
Richard W. Tsang, MD, FRCP(C)

*Department of Radiation Oncology, University of Toronto, Princess Margaret Hospital,
Toronto, ON M5G 2M9, Canada*

Differentiated thyroid cancer

The prognostic factors for well-differentiated thyroid cancer (WDTC) cancer are well known [1,2]. Older age, large tumor size, and extrathyroid extension are major prognostic factors for decreased survival and increased risk of local recurrence, especially the combination of increased age and extrathyroid extension (ETE). Although surgery, radioactive iodine (RAI) ablation, and thyroid-stimulating hormone (TSH) suppression are well established and very effective treatments for the majority of patients who have WDTC, there are a minority of patients (especially older patient who have ETE) who recur despite such treatment. It has been demonstrated that patients who recur locally after presenting with ETE are less likely to take up RAI and more likely to die from thyroid cancer than patients who recur with lymph node involvement [3]. It is, therefore, important to consider all available therapies in patients who have a high risk of local recurrence and, thus, a high risk of succumbing to their disease from ETE.

In the latest edition of the American Joint Committee on Cancer staging manual, the definition of T3 and T4 has changed to reflect the extent of ETE [4]. T3 represents minimal extrathyroidal extension to sternothyroid or peri-thyroid tissue or any tumor greater than 4 cm. T4a includes invasion into subcutaneous soft tissue, larynx, trachea, esophagus, and recurrent laryngeal nerve. T4b includes invasion into prevertebral fascia or mediastinal vessels or encasement of the carotid artery (Fig. 1). A review of 262 patients who had invasive papillary cancer found the site of invasion to be the muscle in 53% of cases, the laryngeal nerve in 47%, the trachea in 37%, the

---

* Corresponding author.
 E-mail address: james.brierley@rmp.uhn.on.ca (J.D. Brierley).

0889-8529/08/$ - see front matter © 2008 Elsevier Inc. All rights reserved.
doi:10.1016/j.ecl.2008.02.001

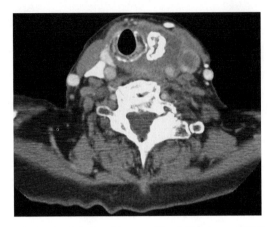

Fig. 1. CT scan (axial) showing left thyroid mass with calcification and ETE with tumor encasing the carotid artery (T4b lesion). Biopsy showed a poorly differentiated (insular) carcinoma.

esophagus in 21%, and the larynx in 12% [5]. In a retrospective review of 1067 patients who had ETE treated with surgery alone, Ito and colleagues [6] reported that "minimal" ETE (T3) did not have a deleterious effect on relapse free survival compared with no extrathyroidal extension, but "massive" ETE (T4) did have an effect on relapse free survival. These data suggest that only patients who have more extensive ETE or T4 disease are at risk, and these patients may benefit from external beam radiotherapy (XRT). Frequently, patients who have extensive extrathyroid disease that involves the tracheoesophageal groove or that is adherent to the neurovascular bundle are at high risk of having at least microscopic residual disease after resection and subsequent recurrence after RAI alone. Therefore, these patients may benefit from adjunctive postoperative XRT.

Adjuvant therapy

Adjuvant XRT has not been studied in randomized trials, and, therefore, its benefit can be determined only from retrospective reviews of patients at risk who were treated with or without XRT. In the authors' study from the Princess Margaret Hospital (Toronto, Ontario, Canada), patients who underwent XRT for microscopic residual disease had a better 10-year actuarial local control rate than those who did not (93% versus 78%, $P = .01$) [7]. A subsequent study found a higher 10-year cause-specific mortality (81% versus 65%) and local-regional relapse-free rate (86% versus 66%) among patients over 60 years of age who had ETE, but it found no gross residual disease in patients who were treated with XRT (Fig. 2) [8]. There have been a number of studies that demonstrated the benefit of XRT in high-risk patients, and these are summarized in Table 1. Because these studies are retrospective, included patients treated over a prolonged time period, and some studies might not have selected patients who were at high risk of recurrence

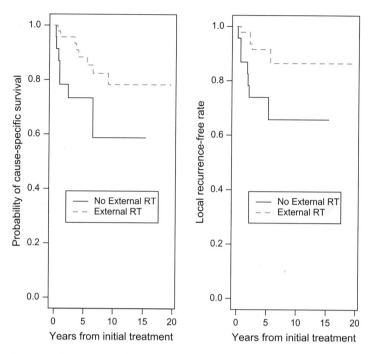

Fig. 2. Cause specific survival and local-regional relapse-free rates for patients over the age of 60 years who have completely resected differentiated thyroid cancer and evidence of ETE, with or without XRT. (*From* Brierley J, Tsang R, Panzarella T, et al. Prognostic factors and the effect of treatment with radioactive iodine and external beam radiation on patients with differentiated thyroid cancer seen at a single institution over 40 years. Clinical Endocrinology 2005;63:425; with permission.)

in the thyroid bed despite standard management (thyroidectomy, RAI, and TSH suppression), the reported results with XRT were somewhat variable. A noted exception is a study from Germany in which 137 patients over 40 years of age who had ETE were treated with total thyroidectomy and RAI [9]. Eighty-five of the 137 patients had XRT to the thyroid bed and cervical and upper mediastinal lymph nodes. The patients in the radiotherapy group had fewer local and regional recurrences ($P = .004$). More recently Chow and colleagues [10] reported their experience that XRT improved local failure free survival in patients who had pathologically confirmed positive resection margins ($P < .001$) and reduced local failures in patients who had T4 disease ($P = .002$). In 131 patients who had T4a disease, the 10-year local failure free survivals were 41% with surgery alone, 60% with surgery and XRT, 72.4% with surgery and RAI, but 88.4% with surgery, RAI, and XRT ($P = .01$). They also reported that XRT improved 10-year lymph node failure free survival in patients who had N1b disease ($P = .005$) and patients who had lymph node metastasis of a size greater than 2 cm ($P = .02$).

Table 1
Ten-year local recurrence rates after adjuvant external radiation therapy for high-risk disease

	Treatment	
Study	Surgery with RAI (%)	Surgery, RAI, and XRT (%)
Tubiana et al [15]	21	14
Simpson et al [53]	18	14
Phlips et al [54]	21	3
Farahati et al [9] (includes distant failures)	50	10
Tsang et al [7] (papillary only)	22	7
Kim et al [55] (papillary only, 5 year rates)	37.5	4.8
Keum et al [56]	89	38
Brierley et al [20] (patients over 60 who have ETE)	34.3	13.6
Chow et al [14] (papillary only with T4a)	17.6	11.6

Given the data from these studies, the authors believe XRT plays a definite role in treating some patients who have ETE, but this is probably beneficial only in patients who have extensive ETE (T4 disease) and not T3 disease. We recommend XRT in addition to total thyroidectomy, RAI, and TSH suppression in older patients (aged 50 or more) who have cT4 disease (ie, gross ETE), but the authors also consider XRT in highly selected younger patients who have T4b or extensive T4a disease and poor histologic features (insular or poor differentiation) [11]. The authors believe lymph node involvement by itself (in contrast to Chow and colleagues) is not an indication for XRT, because regional control usually is achieved with initial neck dissection in combination with postoperative RAI. However, it is of value in patients who have extracapsular extension of the lymph node and who are at high risk of recurrence [12] after previous node dissection and RAI for nodal disease. The current American Thyroid Association guidelines suggest that "XRT should be considered in patients over the age of 45 with grossly visible extrathyroid extension at the time of surgery and a high likelihood of microscopic residual disease and for patients with gross residual tumor in whom further surgery or RAI would likely be ineffective" [13].

Gross residual disease

Surgery is the mainstay of treatment for differentiated thyroid cancer. Occasionally the tumor is so locally advanced that complete resection of all gross disease is not possible. This is the case in patients who have T4b disease (tumor invading prevertebral fascia, mediastinal vessels, or an encased carotid artery). RAI is unlikely to eradicate grossly palpable disease in the thyroid bed after surgery, and, therefore, patients could benefit from planned combination RAI, assuming a total thyroidectomy was performed and was followed by XRT. In one series of 126 patients, patients who had gross residual disease and who were treated with XRT (69 patients) had significantly better local regional control than those who did not (56%

local regional control at 10 years with XRT versus 24% without; $P = .002$) [14]. Other authors have reported disease control rates of 30% to 65% [7,15–18]. Recently the authors analyzed their own patients who had post-operative gross residual disease and who were treated with radiotherapy; the 10-year cause-specific survival and local relapse free rates were 48% and 90%, respectively. Even if local control is achieved, patients who have such locally advanced disease also have a poor outcome, because they die from uncontrolled metastatic disease (J. Brierly, MBBS, unpublished data, 2007).

Medullary thyroid cancer

For patients presenting with local-regional medullary thyroid cancer (MTC), surgery is the main curative treatment modality, with removal of all known disease in the thyroid gland and regional lymph nodes. For patients who have gross residual disease after surgery, the local control rate after XRT is unsatisfactorily low (20%–25%) [19,20]. Therefore, every attempt should be made to diagnose MTC at an early stage, and surgical management should be planned to achieve complete excision of the disease. As lymph node involvement is common, meticulous neck and superior mediastinal dissections often are required. RAI has no role in the management of MTC. For patients achieving complete resection of disease, with normal or undetectable calcitonin and carcinoembryonic antigen (CEA) post-surgery, the prognosis is excellent [21]. However, a significant proportion of patients will have postoperative residual disease as evidenced by high serum calcitonin and CEA levels [22] or on imaging studies (anatomic and functional). Traditional poor prognostic factors include extrathyroidal invasion, postoperative gross residual disease [20], and high clinical stage [21,22]. Patients can be investigated further to locate regional and metastatic sites of disease by using CT scans, somatostatin, bone scans, and fluorine-18fluorodeoxyglucose–positron emission tomography (FDG-PET) [23,24]. Subclinical nodal disease in the neck and superior mediastinum is relatively common [25,26]. For disease persisting in the thyroid bed or lymph nodes despite a meticulous surgical clearance procedure (often evidenced by FDG-PET uptake and a moderate elevation of calcitonin level) and no systemic spread of disease, adjuvant XRT to the thyroid bed and regional nodal tissue may be considered. Without further treatment, approximately half of these high-risk patients will recur clinically or progress with gross disease in the neck. Radiation doses of 40–50 Gy in 20–25 fractions to the neck and upper mediastinum followed by a boost to the thyroid bed for a total of 50 Gy resulted in a locoregional control rate of 86% at 10 years [20]. If gross disease is present, a higher dose in the range of 60–66 Gy should be given for optimal control. The technique is similar to that outlined for differentiated thyroid cancer. The treatment does not impact overall survival, but locoregional control of the disease is important, because cervical relapse can have a negative impact on the patient's quality of life. Other studies have shown similar results [19,27–29]. There is no established role for adjuvant chemotherapy.

In metastatic MTC, the most frequent tumor sites are the liver, lung, and bone. The treatment is palliative, and conventional chemotherapy has a response rate of 15%–30%, including doxorubicin either as a single agent or drug combinations with cisplatin, 5-fluorouracil (5-FU) [30]. Hormonal therapy consists of somatostatin analogs (eg, octreotide) with or without interferon alpha [31]. Local radiation is indicated for symptomatic osseous metastasis, but it has a limited role for diffuse liver and bone metastasis. Typically, a dose of 20 Gy in 5 fractions or 30 Gy in 10 fractions to bone metastasis would result in pain relief. Single large lung or mediastinal metastasis causing hemoptysis or obstruction also may respond to XRT. Radioimmunotherapy approaches (eg, anti-CEA, or [111]Indium-octreotide) are under active study [32]. Some patients who have metastatic disease will have an indolent course over many years and may not require cytotoxic therapy for prolonged periods of time.

Anaplastic thyroid cancer

Patients who have anaplastic thyroid cancer (ATC) typically present with symptoms of a rapidly enlarging neck mass with extrathyroidal invasion. Metastastic disease frequently is diagnosed at presentation (30%–50%) and usually in the lung. It is important to evaluate the integrity of the upper airway and the need for tracheostomy. Complete surgical resection is rarely possible or beneficial. Patients amenable to thyroidectomy usually have predominately differentiated thyroid carcinoma and only a small focus of ATC, which is discovered at pathology evaluation [33]. Radical surgery is not warranted in patients who have extensive extrathyroidal extension of the disease [34].

The treatment for ATC is unsatisfactory, because RAI is ineffective, and XRT (given with the aim of improving local control) has toxicity and often does not even achieve this goal. The 5-year survival rate is approximately 5% with any currently available treatments [33–36]. The suboptimal result with conventional radiation therapy alone has led to the development of novel fractionation regimens and concurrent radiation-chemotherapy approaches. Hyperfractionated and accelerated radiation has been used sometimes in sequence with chemotherapy and surgical resection. A phase two study (n = 19) of hyperfractionated XRT (57.6 Gy given in 1.6 Gy fractions, twice a day, three days a week over 6 weeks) combined with weekly low-dose doxorubicin achieved a local control rate of 68% [37], but a similar approach using accelerated XRT (30–45 Gy given in 1.1 Gy fractions given four fractions a day) and low-dose doxorubicin gave a 22% local control rate [38]. Another study of hyperfractionated XRT in 17 patients (60.8 Gy in 32 fractions, given twice a day, over 20 to 24 days) documented a complete response in 3 patients (17.6%) and a partial response in 7 patients (41.2%)

[39]. Despite this response, the majority of patients developed grade 3 or 4 toxicity, and in 5 patients, death occurred before the toxicity resolved.

A Swedish group [40,41] has described a multimodality regimen that maximizes local control by combining preoperative XRT, chemotherapy, followed by surgical resection. However, despite a local control rate of 60%, only 5 of 55 patients (9%) survived for two years or longer [41], which casts doubt on the merits of such an aggressive approach in all patients who have ATC. The problem has been the rapid development of metastatic disease in the majority of patients, whether local control is achieved or not [35,37,41]. The median survival in most series is 3–6 months [35,39,41]. Unfortunately, chemotherapy for this cancer has not been greatly effective, hence innovation approaches are needed for this disease and patients should be encouraged to participate in clinical trials.

Since a radical course of XRT is associated with significant acute toxicity, often lasting 1–3 months, careful patient selection should be exercised for this treatment. For those patients who have a good performance status and no metastasis, a reasonable regimen is to use standard fractionation to total doses of 50–60 Gy or accelerated hyperfractionated XRT (without chemotherapy), 60 Gy in 40 fractions (1.5 Gy/fraction given twice a day) over 4 weeks. To minimize toxicity, regional lymph nodes may not be covered if uninvolved. Such an approach has been adopted at the Princess Margaret Hospital in Toronto. A recent review of this treatment policy showed that approximately 50% of patients were found eligible for "radical" high dose radiotherapy (n = 23), with an actuarial local progression-free rate of 94% at 6 months and 74% at two years [35]. The corresponding survival rates were 80% and 9%, respectively, with a median survival of 11 months. For others not treated radically (n = 24), palliative XRT was given for local symptom relief (eg, 20 Gy in 5 fractions) with the option of a second course 4 weeks later for responding patients. Palliative XRT resulted in a 6-month local progression-free rate of 65%, and all patients died within 9 months [35]. Similar outcomes also have been documented in British Columbia, Canada, again distinguishing the slightly better prognosis for patients treated with radical XRT, which will result in a rare long term survivor and the dismal prognosis for patients treated palliatively [36].

Palliative radiation therapy in metastatic thyroid cancer

Survival of patients who have metastatic disease is dependent on age, histology, site of involvement, tumor burden, and iodine avidity of the disease. Patients under the age of 20 have a 100% survival rate at 10 years [42], but for those who are over the age of 40 years, the rate falls to 20%. Survival is longer with diffuse lung metastasis concentrating RAI [43–45]. The mainstay of therapy for those who have differentiated thyroid cancer is RAI, but this will be effective only if a total thyroidectomy has been performed. For diffuse lung metastasis, the complete response rate to RAI is 50% and the

10-year survival is 60%, compared with bone metastasis, where the rates are 10% and 20%, respectively [44]. Occasionally, surgical resection of a solitary bone lesion may be appropriate [46,47]. Patients who present with distant metastatic disease may have prolonged survival. In one series of 111 such patients, the 10-year cause-specific survival was 31% [48], and in another series of 49 patients, the 5-year survival was 50% [45].

Many patients will benefit from XRT in addition to RAI. Lung metastasis is best treated with RAI. Occasionally dominant lesions causing hemoptysis, if reliably identified, can be radiated with good effect. Central disease in the mediastinum or lung hila causing bronchial obstruction can be relieved by XRT. More frequently, painful bone metastasis will require radiotherapy because of a lack of long-term benefits from RAI [44,46]. When palliative XRT is considered, a distinction should be made between attempts to achieve prolonged local control of the disease (ie, radical XRT given for local control in a noncurative situation or XRT given purely for the relief of symptoms). In view of indolent disease in younger patients, if the intention is local control, a higher dose of XRT is given to maximize the duration of local disease control (eg, 45–50 Gy in 1.8–2 Gy fractions). For palliation of symptoms, a variety of regimens may be suitable (eg, 20 Gy in 5 fractions, 30 Gy in 10 fractions, or 40–45 Gy in 15–20 fractions). Generally, the choice is based on the specific anatomic area, the volume of tissue being treated, and whether radiation sensitive normal organs are located adjacent to the disease. An example of radiation field arrangement and isodose distribution for the radiotherapy of bone metastasis in the sacroiliac areas is illustrated in Fig. 3. In general, XRT is given following suboptimal or incomplete symptom relief from RAI. To avoid the theoretic problem of "stunting," (ie, the XRT causing impaired uptake of RAI administered subsequently) it has been common practice to try and sequence the treatments to deliver the RAI first and the XRT afterward. However, this "stunting" effect has

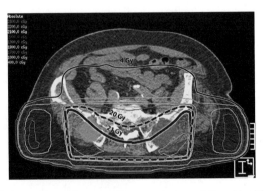

Fig. 3. Metastatic bone disease from papillary carcinoma of thyroid with two destructive lesions in the sacroiliac area and associated soft tissue mass (shaded gray), despite two doses of RAI therapy. The main symptom was pain, which improved after XRT 20 Gy (*dashed line*) and 21 Gy (*solid line*) given in 5 fractions.

not been studied adequately, and recent in vitro data reported the opposite, with increased RAI uptake following exposure to radiation in cell culture [49]. Occasionally, it is important to consider administering XRT first, (eg, in the setting of impending or actual spinal cord compression from vertebral metastasis, particularly in a situation where a patient presents with metastatic disease before thyroidectomy) to treat the primary lesion.

External beam radiation therapy

Traditionally, the thyroid bed has been a difficult area to treat with radiotherapy, because of the shape of the thyroid bed itself curving around the vertebral body, the presence of an air column (the trachea), the changes in contours of the neck, the necessity to spare normal structures, and especially the difficulty of ensuring that the dose of radiotherapy to the spinal cord is within tolerance. A variety of different techniques have been employed (none without some degree of compromise), and these techniques have become outdated with the advent of intensity modulated radiotherapy (IMRT) [50,51] and will not be discussed further [52]. IMRT involves treating a well-defined target volume with multiple radiation beams, each beam having a variable intensity, which allows for more precise delivery of the radiation to the area at risk of recurrence while allowing for more normal tissue sparing (Fig. 4). Advances in imaging with CT, MRI, and positron emission tomography scans aid the accurate definition of the target volume and normal structures to be avoided. Some investigators advocate avoiding contrast CT scan in WDTC because of concerns about subsequent RAI uptake, but the authors believe good quality imaging (including intravenous contrast CT scan) before surgery is important in patients who have clinical advanced tumors, because it will not only aid the surgeon in planning surgery, but it also will help the radiation oncologist by identifying the anatomic extent of disease, and thus help in planning any subsequent radiotherapy.

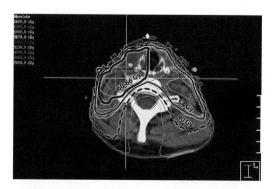

Fig. 4. Isodose distribution achieved with intensity modulated radiation therapy. Thyroid bed and cervical lymphoma nodes: 54 Gy (*solid line*), right paratracheal tissues boosted to 60–66 Gy (*thick solid line*), and spinal cord dose limited to less than 40 Gy (*dashed line*).

One of the major toxicities associated with XRT is xerostomia. Because patients are at high risk of developing this as a consequence of RAI treatment already, the additional impact of XRT can be a major concern. The risk can be reduced with IMRT designed to avoid the salivary glands as much as possible. However, since the majority of patients who may benefit from XRT do not require the whole neck to be treated, significant xerostomia can be avoided even without IMRT. For patients who have gross residual disease or are at high risk of recurrence in the thyroid bed because of ETE, XRT can be confined to the thyroid bed, jugular, and posterior cervical lymph nodes between the hyoid and sternal notch, including levels III, IV, VI, and partial level V nodal regions. This target volume is adjusted according to the clinical, surgical, and pathological findings, thus sparing the salivary glands in the majority of patients. The usual radiation dose to the thyroid bed is 50 Gy in 20 fractions or 60–66 Gy in 30–33 fractions.

The authors reserve large volume treatment (that includes the cervical and superior mediastinal lymph nodes and the thyroid bed) for WDTC that either persists after neck dissection and RAI or that has extensive nodal extracapsular extension. This large volume treatment also would apply to ATC if regional nodes were involved (in addition to the local thyroid disease) and to MTC. Usually a large volume of disease is treated with a dose of 50 Gy in 2 Gy fractions in the first phase, and in the second phase, the thyroid bed is treated with a dose of 10–16 Gy also in 2 Gy fractions. With IMRT, this can be given concurrently as a single phase treatment: 56 Gy in 33 fractions to the cervical lymph nodes, and 66 Gy in 33 fractions to the thyroid bed.

Toxicity

Well-planned XRT therapy rarely produces serious complications, and one must be aware that it does not preclude future surgical intervention, especially in the hands of experienced head and neck surgeons. Acute skin toxicity is common, and depending on the volume being treated, mucositis of the esophagus, trachea, and larynx can occur toward the end of the course of radiation, but it usually resolves shortly after completion. However, more serious late toxicity with esophageal or tracheal stenosis is extremely rare. Tsang and colleagues [7] reported no grade IV toxic effects (using the Radiation Therapy Oncology Group scale) and Farahati and colleagues [9] observed no irreversible late toxic effects in patients given high doses of XRT in addition to RAI.

Summary

Evidence demonstrates that XRT can control gross residual WDTC. Also, in selected patients who have high risk features, XRT improves local control after surgery and RAI. There is a more limited role for XRT in medullary thyroid cancer, but it remains the most effective single agent in the management of patients who have ATC. Its value in the management of symptomatic metastatic thyroid cancer should not be forgotten.

References

[1] Brierley JD, Asa SL. Thyroid cancer. In: Gospodarowicz MK, O'Sullivan B, Sobin LH, editors. Prognostic factors in cancer. Hoboken (NJ): John Wiley and Sons, Inc; 2006. p. 119–22.

[2] Baloch ZW, LiVolsi VA. Prognostic factors in well-differentiated follicular-derived carcinoma and medullary thyroid carcinoma. Thyroid 2001;11(7):637–45.

[3] Vassilopoulou-Sellin R, Schultz PN, Haynie TP. Clinical outcome of patients with papillary thyroid carcinoma who have recurrence after initial radioactive iodine therapy. Cancer 1996; 78(3):493–501.

[4] Greene FL, Page DL, Flemming ID, et al. AJCC cancer staging manual. 6th edition. New York: Springer-Verlag; 2002.

[5] McCaffrey TV, Bergstralh EJ, Hay ID. Locally invasive papillary thyroid carcinoma: 1940–1990. Head Neck 1994;16(2):165–72.

[6] Ito Y, Tomoda C, Uruno T, et al. Prognostic significance of extrathyroid extension of papillary thyroid carcinoma: massive but not minimal extension affects the relapse-free survival. World J Surg 2006;30(5):780–6.

[7] Tsang RW, Brierley JD, Simpson WJ, et al. The effects of surgery, radioiodine and external radiation therapy on the clinical outcome of patients with differentiated thyroid cancer. Cancer 1998;82:375–88.

[8] Brierley J, Tsang R, Panzarella T, et al. Prognostic factors and the effect of treatment with radioactive iodine and external beam radiation on patients with differentiated thyroid cancer seen at a single institution over 40 years. Clin Endocrinol (Oxf) 2005;63(4):418–27.

[9] Farahati J, Reiners C, Stuschke M, et al. Differentiated thyroid cancer. Impact of adjuvant external radiotherapy in patients with perithyroidal tumor infiltration (stage pT4). Cancer 1996;77(1):172–80.

[10] Chow SM, Yau S, Kwan CK, et al. Local and regional control in patients with papillary thyroid carcinoma: specific indications of external radiotherapy and radioactive iodine according to T and N categories in AJCC 6th edition. Endocr Relat Cancer 2006;13(4): 1159–72.

[11] Sanders EM Jr, LiVolsi VA, Brierley J, et al. An evidence-based review of poorly differentiated thyroid cancer. World J Surg 2007;31(5):934–45.

[12] Ito Y, Hirokawa M, Jikuzono T, et al. Extranodal tumor extension to adjacent organs predicts a worse cause-specific survival in patients with papillary thyroid carcinoma. World J Surg 2007;31(6):1196–203.

[13] Cooper DS, Doherty GM, Haugen BR, et al. Management guidelines for patients with thyroid nodules and differentiated thyroid cancer. Thyroid 2006;16(2):109–42.

[14] Chow S-M, Law SCK, Mendenhall WM, et al. Papillary thyroid carcinoma: prognostic factors and the role of radioiodine and external radiotherapy. Int J Radiat Oncol Biol Phys 2002;52(3):784–95.

[15] Tubiana M, Haddad E, Schlumberger M, et al. External radiotherapy in thyroid cancers. Cancer 1985;55(Suppl 9):2062–71.

[16] Sheline GE, Galante M, Lindsay S. Radiation therapy in the control of persistent thyroid cancer. Am J Roentgenol Radium Ther Nucl Med 1966;97(4):923–30.

[17] Garcia-Serra A, Amdur RJ, Morris CG, et al. Thyroid function should be monitored following radiotherapy to the low neck. Am J Clin Oncol 2005;28(3):255–8.

[18] O'Connell ME, A'Hern RP, Harmer CL. Results of external beam radiotherapy in differentiated thyroid carcinoma: a retrospective study from the Royal Marsden Hospital. Eur J Cancer 1994;30A(6):733–9.

[19] Fife KM, Bower M, Harmer CL. Medullary thyroid cancer: the role of radiotherapy in local control. Eur J Surg Oncol 1996;22(6):588–91.

[20] Brierley JD, Tsang RW, Gospodarowicz MK, et al. Medullary thyroid cancer—analyses of survival and prognostic factors and the role of radiation therapy in local control. Thyroid 1996;6:305–10.

[21] Modigliani E, Cohen R, Campos JM, et al. Prognostic factors for survival and for biochemical cure in medullary thyroid carcinoma: results in 899 patients. The GETC Study Group. Groupe d'etude des tumeurs a calcitonine. Clin Endocrinol (Oxf) 1998;48(3):265–73.

[22] Dottorini ME, Assi A, Sironi M, et al. Multivariate analysis of patients with medullary thyroid carcinoma. Prognostic significance and impact on treatment of clinical and pathologic variables. Cancer 1996;77(8):1556–65.

[23] Gotthardt M, Battmann A, Hoffken H, et al. 18F-FDG PET, somatostatin receptor scintigraphy, and CT in metastatic medullary thyroid carcinoma: a clinical study and an analysis of the literature. Nucl Med Commun 2004;25(5):439–43.

[24] Crippa F, Alessi A, Gerali A, et al. FDG-PET in thyroid cancer. Tumori 2003;89(5):540–3.

[25] Raue F. German medullary thyroid carcinoma/multiple endocrine neoplasia registry. German MTC/MEN Study Group. Medullary thyroid carcinoma/multiple endocrine neoplasia type 2. Langenbecks Arch Surg 1998;383(5):334–6.

[26] Samaan NA, Schultz PN, Hickey RC. Medullary thyroid carcinoma: prognosis of familial versus sporadic disease and the role of radiotherapy. J Clin Endocrinol Metab 1988;67(4):801–5.

[27] Mak A, Morrison W, Garden A, et al. The value of postoperative radiotherapy for regional medullary carcinoma of the thyroid. Int J Radiat Oncol Biol Phys 1994;30(Suppl):234.

[28] Nguyen TD, Chassard JL, Lagarde P, et al. Results of postoperative radiation therapy in medullary carcinoma of the thyroid: a retrospective study by the French Federation of Cancer Institutes–the Radiotherapy Cooperative Group. Radiother Oncol 1992;23(1):1–5.

[29] Fersht N, Vini L, A'Hern R, et al. The role of radiotherapy in the management of elevated calcitonin after surgery for medullary thyroid cancer. Thyroid 2001;11(12):1161–8.

[30] Schlumberger M, Abdelmoumene N, Delisle MJ, et al. Treatment of advanced medullary thyroid cancer with an alternating combination of 5 FU-streptozocin and 5 FU-dacarbazine. The Groupe d'Etude des Tumeurs a Calcitonine (GETC). Br J Cancer 1995;71(2):363–5.

[31] Vitale G, Tagliaferri P, Caraglia M, et al. Slow release lanreotide in combination with interferon-alpha2b in the treatment of symptomatic advanced medullary thyroid carcinoma. J Clin Endocrinol Metab 2000;85(3):983–8.

[32] Chatal JF, Campion L, Kraeber-Bodere F, et al. Survival improvement in patients with medullary thyroid carcinoma who undergo pretargeted anti-carcinoembryonic-antigen radioimmunotherapy: a collaborative study with the French Endocrine Tumor Group. J Clin Oncol 2006;24(11):1705–11.

[33] Voutilainen PE, Multanen M, Haapiainen RK, et al. Anaplastic thyroid carcinoma survival. World J Surg 1999;23(9):975–8 [discussion: 978–79].

[34] Passler C, Scheuba C, Prager G, et al. Anaplastic (undifferentiated) thyroid carcinoma (ATC). A retrospective analysis. Langenbecks Arch Surg 1999;384(3):284–93.

[35] Wang Y, Tsang R, Asa S, et al. Clinical outcome of anaplastic thyroid carcinoma treated with radiotherapy of once- and twice-daily fractionation regimens. Cancer 2006;107(8):1786–92.

[36] Goutsouliak V, Hay JH. Anaplastic thyroid cancer in British Columbia 1985–1999: a population-based study. Clin Oncol (R Coll Radiol) 2005;17(2):75–8.

[37] Kim JH, Leeper RD. Treatment of locally advanced thyroid carcinoma with combination doxorubicin and radiation therapy. Cancer 1987;60(10):2372–5.

[38] Wong CS, Van Dyk J, Simpson WJ. Myelopathy following hyperfractionated accelerated radiotherapy for anaplastic thyroid carcinoma. Radiother Oncol 1991;20:3–9.

[39] Mitchell G, Huddart R, Harmer C. Phase II evaluation of high dose accelerated radiotherapy for anaplastic thyroid carcinoma. Radiother Oncol 1999;50(1):33–8.

[40] Nilsson O, Lindeberg J, Zedenius J, et al. Anaplastic giant cell carcinoma of the thyroid gland: treatment and survival over a 25-year period. World J Surg 1998;22(7):725–30.

[41] Tennvall J, Lundell G, Wahlberg P, et al. Anaplastic thyroid carcinoma: three protocols combining doxorubicin, hyperfractionated radiotherapy and surgery. Br J Cancer 2002; 86(12):1848–53.

[42] La Quaglia MP, Black T, Holcomb GW III, et al. Differentiated thyroid cancer: clinical characteristics, treatment, and outcome in patients under 21 years of age who present with distant metastases. A report from the Surgical Discipline Committee of the Children's Cancer Group. J Pediatr Surg 2000;35(6):955–9 [discussion: 960].

[43] Vassilopoulou-Sellin R, Goepfert H, Raney B, et al. Differentiated thyroid cancer in children and adolescents: clinical outcome and mortality after long-term follow-up. Head Neck 1998; 20(6):549–55.

[44] Schlumberger M, Challeton C, De Vathaire F, et al. Radioactive iodine treatment and external radiotherapy for lung and bone metastases from thyroid carcinoma. J Nucl Med 1996;37(4):598–605.

[45] Sampson E, Brierley JD, Le LW, et al. Clinical management and outcome of papillary and follicular (differentiated) thyroid cancer presenting with distant metastasis at diagnosis. Cancer 2007;110(7):1451–6.

[46] Proye CA, Dromer DH, Carnaille BM, et al. Is it still worthwhile to treat bone metastases from differentiated thyroid carcinoma with radioactive iodine? World J Surg 1992;16(4): 640–5 [discussion: 645–46].

[47] Zettinig G, Fueger BJ, Passler C, et al. Long-term follow-up of patients with bone metastases from differentiated thyroid carcinoma—surgery or conventional therapy? Clin Endocrinol (Oxf) 2002;56(3):377–82.

[48] Haq M, Harmer C. Differentiated thyroid carcinoma with distant metastases at presentation: prognostic factors and outcome. Clin Endocrinol (Oxf) 2005;63(1):87–93.

[49] Meller B, Deisting W, Wenzel BE, et al. Increased radioiodine uptake of thyroid cell cultures after external irradiation. Strahlenther Onkol 2006;182(1):30–6.

[50] Nutting CM, Convery DJ, Cosgrove VP, et al. Improvements in target coverage and reduced spinal cord irradiation using intensity-modulated radiotherapy (IMRT) in patients with carcinoma of the thyroid gland. Radiother Oncol 2001;60(2):173–80.

[51] Rosenbluth BD, Serrano V, Happersett L, et al. Intensity-modulated radiation therapy for the treatment of nonanaplastic thyroid cancer. Int J Radiat Oncol Biol Phys 2005;63(5): 1419–26.

[52] Wilson PC, Millar BM, Brierley JD. The management of advanced thyroid cancer. Clin Oncol (R Coll Radiol) 2004;16(8):561–8.

[53] Simpson WJ, Panzarella T, Carruthers JS, et al. Papillary and thyroid cancer: impact of treatment in 1578 patients. Int J Radiat Oncol Biol Phys 1998;14:1063–75.

[54] Phlips P, Hanzen C, Andry G, et al. Postoperative irradiation for thyroid cancer. Eur J Surg Oncol 1993;19:399–404.

[55] Kim TH, Yang DS, Jung KY, et al. Value of external irradiation for locally advanced papillary thyroid cancer. In J Radiat Oncol Biol Phys 2003;55:1006–12.

[56] Keum KC, Suh YG, Koom WS, et al. The role of postoperative external-beam radiotherapy in the management of patients with papillary thyroid cancer invading the trachea. Int J Radiat Oncol Biol Phys 2006;65:474–80.

ELSEVIER
SAUNDERS

Endocrinol Metab Clin N Am
37 (2008) 511–524

ENDOCRINOLOGY
AND METABOLISM
CLINICS
OF NORTH AMERICA

Early Clinical Studies of Novel Therapies for Thyroid Cancers

Steven I. Sherman, MD

*Department of Endocrine Neoplasia and Hormonal Disorders, Division of Internal Medicine,
The University of Texas M. D. Anderson Cancer Center, 1515 Holcombe Boulevard, Unit 435,
Houston, TX 77030, USA*

Historically, systemic therapies for advanced, metastatic thyroid carcinomas have been poorly effective, with response rates typically 25% or less [1]. Despite (or perhaps because of) such poor outcomes with chemotherapy, results from few prospective clinical trials of new drugs or combinations of drugs for thyroid carcinomas were published during the latter half of the twentieth century [2]. Thus, patients with metastatic disease unresponsive to or unsuitable for surgery, radioiodine (for tumors derived from differentiated carcinomas), and external beam radiotherapy, have generally been treated with cytotoxic chemotherapy only when they became symptomatic or rapidly progressive, using a wide variety of single- and combination-agent regimens. Doxorubicin was frequently administered, largely based upon a small uncontrolled study that reported a surprisingly high rate of short lived responses [3]. The addition of platinum-based drugs to doxorubicin was studied in two cooperative group trials in the early 1980s, with quite contrasting results; in a randomized comparative trial, 5 of 43 subjects treated with combination doxorubicin and cisplatinum experienced durable complete responses, whereas in a single arm study, subjects treated with the combination demonstrated few, transient partial responses [4,5].

Plaguing these and similar trials was the practice of lumping patients with all histologies of thyroid carcinoma (differentiated, medullary, and anaplastic) in treatment cohorts as if these were identical diseases. Taxanes were introduced to the thyroid carcinoma armamentarium, with reports suggesting clinical responses first in medullary and subsequently anaplastic carcinomas [6,7], and use spread into the treatment of advanced differentiated carcinoma as well [8]. Although use data are lacking, these three types

E-mail address: sisherma@mdanderson.org

of drugs—doxorubicin, platinum-derivatives, and taxanes—are probably the most commonly employed cytotoxic agents against thyroid carcinomas.

During the past 10 to 15 years, several opportunities have arisen that have led to a relative plethora of clinical trials testing novel therapies for advanced thyroid carcinomas. Of prime importance has been the discovery of key etiologic, oncogenic mutations in papillary and medullary carcinomas (see article by Castellone and Santoro in this issue). Somatic mutations in the signaling kinases BRAF and RAS, and the unique RET/PTC rearrangements seen in papillary carcinomas, lead to constitutive activation of upstream signaling via the mitogen-activated protein kinase pathway. Evidence from transgenic animal models, as well as analysis of papillary microcarcinomas and radiation-induced chromosomal changes, all support the contention that most papillary carcinomas arise as a result of a single activating mutation in one of these three genes [9]. For medullary carcinomas, almost all familial forms of the disease arise because of an inheritable germline-activating mutation in RET, and identical somatic mutations occurring in C cells can cause sporadic medullary carcinomas as well. Consistent with the "oncogene addiction" hypothesis, in vitro evidence suggests that inhibition or loss of these etiologic-activating mutations leads to either tumor stabilization or regression. Therefore, interest arose in the therapeutic potential of inhibitors of these key etiologic mutant kinases.

A second development was the recognition of the importance of physiologic processes that facilitate tumor growth, processes that either reflect normal (such as hypoxia-inducible angiogenesis) or frankly abnormal (such as epigenetic modifications of chromosomal DNA and histones) adaptations. Angiogenesis plays a critical role in tumor cell growth and metastasis, and neovascularization is essential to get nutrients and oxygen, remove waste products, and establish distant metastasis [10]. Several proangiogenic factors have been identified, including basic fibroblast growth factor, platelet-derived growth factor (PDGF), and vascular endothelial growth factor (VEGF). VEGF-A belongs to the VEGF-PDGF supergene family, along with five other members, including VEGF-B, -C, -D, -E, and placental growth factor. VEGF-A angiogenic activities are mediated through binding to two receptor tyrosine kinases, VEGFR-1 (Flt-1) and VEGFR-2 (Flk-1/KDR). VEGFR-3 is also a member of the same family as VEGFR-1 and -2; however, it preferentially binds VEGF-C and VEGF-D, and is associated with lymphangiogenesis [11]. In thyroid carcinoma, the intensity of VEGF-A expression in papillary thyroid carcinoma (PTC) correlates with a higher risk of metastasis and recurrence, as well as a shorter disease-free survival period [12,13].

Thirdly, there has been recognition by key sources of investigational drugs and research funding (ie, the United States National Cancer Institute and multinational pharmaceutical companies) that effective treatment for advanced thyroid cancers remains an unmet need. The routes leading to drugs being tested for thyroid cancer in clinical trials have been varied, ranging from logical extension of in vitro studies that identify a rationale for a particular drug's use, to empiric observations in phase I trials that certain therapies yielded clinical benefit in participating patients with thyroid cancers. Once clinical trials became available, awareness among patients grew rapidly, fueled by access to Internet-based clinical trial databases as well as by well-organized patient support networks and associations.

As a result of this confluence of increasing knowledge of the biologic basis for thyroid cancer development and progression, identification of therapeutic agents that could target these biologic abnormalities, and enthusiasm for research by both funding agencies as well as patients, multiple clinical trials have been initiated and successfully completed during the past several years. Consensus guidelines from professional organizations for the treatment of thyroid carcinoma emerged that explicitly recommend referral of patients with advanced disease for participation in such studies [14,15]. The remainder of this article focuses on findings from key studies that reflect this new paradigm for treatment.

Kinase inhibitors

Small molecule inhibitors capable of targeting signaling kinases have been of keen interest for thyroid carcinomas, given the oncogenic roles of mutations in BRAF, RET, and RAS, and the contributory roles of various growth factor receptors, such as VEGFR [9,16,17]. These drugs are generally partially selective, capable of inhibiting multiple kinases, and often affecting multiple signaling pathways (Table 1). Oral administration typically produces nanomolar drug concentrations, with common side effects including hypertension, diarrhea, skin lesions, and fatigue. As of the date of this article, the results of most of the phase II trials that have focused on the efficacy of these drugs in thyroid carcinomas have not been published, except in abstract form arising from presentations at scientific meetings.

Motesanib diphosphate

Motesanib diphosphate (AMG 706; Amgen Inc.) is an oral, small molecule tyrosine kinase inhibitor targeting the VEGF receptors 1, 2, and 3; PDGF receptor, and KIT [18]. Using both in vitro and cell-based assays, nanomolar concentrations of motesanib diphosphate effectively inhibited autophosphorylation of wild type RET, as well as the C634W mutant associated with familial medullary carcinoma; growth of xenografts of TT cells bearing the C634W RET mutation was inhibited by dosages of 75 mg/kg twice daily [19]. In a phase 1 study, motesanib diphosphate, up to 125 mg once daily, demonstrated antitumor activity in patients with advanced solid malignancies, including five patients with differentiated thyroid carcinoma (DTC) and one with medullary thyroid carcinoma (MTC); three thyroid patients experienced greater than 30% reductions in tumor diameters,

Table 1
Kinase inhibitors recently in clinical trials for advanced or metastatic thyroid carcinomas

Drug category/ drug	VEGFR1 IC50 (nM)	VEGFR2 IC50 (nM)	VEGFR3 IC50 (nM)	RET IC50 (nM)	RET/PTC3 IC50 (nM)	BRAF IC50 (nM)	PDGFRβ IC50 (nM)	Other IC50 (nM)	Refs
Axitinib	1.2	0.25	0.29	—	—	—	2.5	C-KIT 1.7	[42]
Gefitinib	—	—	—	—	—	—	—	EGFR 33	[51]
Imatinib	—	>10,000	—	3,700	—	—	100	BCR-ABL 25 C-KIT 150	[47]
Motesanib diphosphate	2	3	6	59	—	—	84	C-KIT 8	[18]
Sorafenib	—	90	20	47	50	22	57	C-KIT 68	[32]
Sunitinib	2	9	17	41	224	—	2	—	[71,72]
Vandetanib	1600	40	110	130	100	—	—	EGFR 500	[25,26]
XL184	—	0.035	—	4	—	—	234	C-MET 1.8	[55]

qualifying as partial responders [20]. The most common toxicities included fatigue, nausea, diarrhea, and hypertension, all typical of this class of drugs.

On the basis of these findings, a multicenter, open-label phase II trial was initiated in July 2005, testing the efficacy of motesanib diphosphate therapy in separate cohorts of subjects with progressive DTC [21] and subjects with progressive or symptomatic MTC [22]. The starting oral dosage for all patients was 125 mg daily. Enrolled in fewer than 8 months, 93 DTC subjects initiated therapy, of whom one-third were still on the drug after 48 weeks. Partial response was confirmed in 14% of the DTC subjects, and another 35% of these previously progressive disease subjects maintained stable disease for at least 24 weeks. The median progression-free survival was 40 weeks. Among the 91 subjects with progressive or symptomatic MTC who initiated therapy, only 2% had confirmed partial response, but another 47% experienced stable disease for at least 24 weeks. Unexpectedly, the maximum and trough plasma concentrations of the drug in MTC subjects were lower than reported with other solid tumor subjects, including DTC, and these differing pharmacokinetics may have contributed to the lower response rate. In both cohorts, the drug was well tolerated, with similar side effects to what was reported in the phase I trial. An unanticipated side effect of motesanib diphosphate therapy was an average 30% increase in the doses of levothyroxine that were were required to maintain either thyroid stimulating hormone suppression or euthyroidism, respectively, in the DTC and MTC cohorts, and 60% to 70% of the subjects experienced peak thyroid stimulating hormone concentrations out of the therapeutic ranges [23].

Vandetanib

Vandetanib (ZD 6474; AstraZeneca) is an oral, small molecule tyrosine kinase inhibitor that targets VEGF receptors 2 and 3, RET, and at higher concentrations, the EGF receptor [24,25]. One of the first small molecule inhibitors to be studied in thyroid cancer cell lines, vandetanib was shown to inhibit effectively RET/PTC3 mutations found in some PTC and M918T RET mutations occurring in MEN2B-associated and some sporadic MTC [26]. Growth of cell lines containing RET/PTC1 or RET/PTC3 was inhibited. However, the drug was not able to block RET when a hydrophobic amino acid substitution occurs at V804, as in some inherited forms of MTC [27]. In a phase I trial in 77 subjects with various solid tumors other than thyroid carcinoma, dosages up to 300 mg daily were tolerated, with the most common dose-limiting side effects of diarrhea, hypertension, and skin rash [28].

On the basis of the preclinical demonstration that vandetanib inhibited most RET point mutations, a multicenter, open-label phase II trial was initiated to study the efficacy of the drug in patients with metastatic familial forms of MTC [29]. Thirty subjects were enrolled, starting therapy with vandetanib, 300 mg daily. Confirmed partial response was reported in

17% of these subjects, and stable disease lasting at least 24 weeks was seen in another 33%. Calcitonin levels dropped by more than 50% in almost two-thirds of the subjects, but recent findings suggest that blocking RET may lead to a direct inhibition of calcitonin gene expression, independent of tumor volume changes [30]. In this trial, the most common side effects included rash, diarrhea, fatigue, and nausea, whereas the most severe toxicities included asymptomatic QT interval prolongation, rash, and diarrhea.

Currently ongoing studies with vandetanib include: (1) a two-site, open-label phase II trial in patients under the age of 18 with familial MTC (open for recruitment); (2) a European multicenter, open-label phase II trial in patients with metastatic papillary or follicular carcinoma (open for recruitment); (3) a multicenter, randomized, double-blind phase II trial comparing vandetanib with placebo in patients with metastatic MTC, either sporadic or inherited (fully recruited); and (4) a multicenter, open-label phase II trial of low dose (100 mg) vandetanib in patients with hereditary MTC (not open for recruitment) [31].

Sorafenib

Sorafenib (BAY 43-9006; Bayer Pharmaceuticals Corporation) is an oral, small molecule tyrosine kinase inhibitor targeting VEGF receptors 2 and 3, RET (including most mutant forms that have been examined), and the serine kinase B-RAF, along with c-KIT, PDGFR, and Flt-3 [32]. In preclinical studies, sorafenib prevented the growth of the TPC1 and TT cell lines, which contain the oncogenic RET/PTC1 and C634W RET mutations, respectively, at concentrations as low as 100 nM [33]. In four phase I trials of varying doses and administration schedules of sorafenib in 173 subjects with solid tumors, the optimal therapeutic dosage was found to be 400 mg twice daily [34]. The most common or significant toxicities included hand-foot syndrome, rash, fatigue, diarrhea, and hypertension.

Although no thyroid cancer patients were reported in these phase I trials, tumor shrinkage was reported in one thyroid cancer patient included in a large randomized discontinuation phase II trial for advanced solid tumors [35]. Subsequently, two phase II trials were performed specifically in subjects with metastatic PTC. Sponsored by the National Cancer Institute, an open-label phase II trial was performed at Ohio State University and recruited 58 subjects in a 10-month period [36]. Of 36 evaluable subjects, confirmed partial response was seen in 8%, and minor response (defined as 23%–29% reduction in tumor diameters) was described in another 19%. More encouraging were the results of a smaller open-label phase II study performed at University of Pennsylvania, in which partial responses were reported in 5 of 15 subjects [37]. Tumor specimens obtained while on sorafenib therapy were available from two subjects, demonstrating decreased levels of pERK (which transduces signals from both VEGFR2 and B-RAF), pAKT (which transduces signals from VEGFR2), and Ki-67 labeling index (which indicates reduced tumor proliferation), despite the absence of B-RAF mutations. Why such seemingly dissimilar results were seen in these two studies remains unclear.

The anti-RET activity of sorafenib makes MTC a potential therapeutic target for this drug as well [17]. In a small pilot study recently reported, five subjects with metastatic MTC were treated with sorafenib, and responses were described in two (including one complete response) after 6 months of treatment [38]. A larger, open-label phase II study has been initiated in patients with metastatic MTC, and recruitment is still ongoing [31]. With a partial response seen in an MTC patient, a phase I study of the combination of sorafenib and the farnesyltransferase inhibitor tipifarnib is actively recruiting thyroid cancer patients as well [39]. Preclinical data also suggest that sorafenib might be active against anaplastic thyroid carcinoma, and a phase II study is also ongoing for this aggressive subtype [31,40].

Sorafenib was approved by the US Food and Drug Administration as treatment for advanced renal cell carcinoma and unresectable hepatocellular carcinoma. Although not specifically approved for thyroid carcinomas, sorafenib is being used in selected patients with progressive metastatic papillary thyroid carcinoma for whom clinical trials are not appropriate. As with any new medication, further experience with the drug is leading to identification of less common but significant toxicities, which for sorafenib include keratoacanthomas and other malignant cutaneous squamous cell lesions [41]. Thus, only physicians familiar with management of adverse events of such therapies should consider their use in thyroid cancer patients.

Axitinib

Axitinib (AG-013736; Pfizer) is an oral, small molecule tyrosine kinase inhibitor that effectively blocks all of the VEGF receptors at subnanomolar concentrations, along with PDGFR and c-KIT, but notably not RET [42]. In a phase I study of 36 subjects with advanced solid malignancies, one of five thyroid cancer subjects experienced tumor shrinkage that did not qualify as a partial response [43]. A multicenter, open-label phase II study was initiated to determine the efficacy of axitinib in advanced or metastatic thyroid carcinoma, starting at a dosages of 5 mg twice daily [44]. Of the 60 subjects who started therapy, 48% had PTC, 25% had follicular thyroid carcinoma (FTC) (including Hürthle cell variants), and 20% had MTC. Partial response was reported in 22%, including subjects in all three histologic subgroups. Overall, the median progression-free survival was 18 months. Common adverse events included fatigue, stomatitis, proteinuria, diarrhea, hypertension, and nausea.

Based on these data, a pivotal multicenter, open-label phase II study has been initiated to determine the efficacy of axitinib in patients with metastatic DTC refractory to doxorubicin, or for whom doxorubicin therapy is contraindicated [31].

Imatinib

Imatinib (STI571; Novartis) is an oral, small molecule tyrosine kinase inhibitor of BCR-ABL and c-KIT that inhibits RET autophosphorylation and RET-mediated cell growth [45–47]. Two small open-label phase II studies have been completed that examined a total of 24 subjects with metastatic MTC treated with imatinib, starting at 600 mg daily [48,49]. No objective tumor responses were reported, and a minority of subjects achieved stable disease as their best tumor response. Toxicities included diarrhea, laryngeal edema, rash, and nausea; increased thyroid hormone dose requirements were reported in 9 of 15 subjects in the larger trial [49]. No objective responses were seen in a phase I study of imatinib combined with dacarbazine and capecitabine that included seven subjects with MTC [50].

Gefitinib

Gefitinib (ZD1839; AstraZeneca) is an oral, small molecule inhibitor of the EGF receptor (EGFR) that was initially introduced for therapy of nonsmall cell lung carcinoma [51]. Subsequent studies have demonstrated that the drug is only effective in the presence of a mutant EGFR and has no clinical activity in the presence of the wild type receptor [52]. Because many papillary and anaplastic thyroid carcinomas display activated EGFR signaling, and inhibitors have had demonstrated efficacy in preclinical models, an open-label phase II study was initiated, examining the effectiveness of gefitinib in a mixed cohort of thyroid cancer patients [53]. The starting daily dosage was 250 mg. Of 27 enrolled subjects, 41% had PTC, 22% FTC, 19% had anaplastic carcinoma, and 15% had MTC. There were no complete or partial responses in the 25 evaluable subjects, although eight had tumor reduction that did not qualify as partial response. One subject with anaplastic carcinoma had stable disease beyond 12 months of therapy, similar to that reported in a phase I trial of gefitinib and docetaxel [54]. Overall, median progression-free survival was just under 4 months, and under 3 months in the MTC cohort. Whether erlotinib, an EGFR inhibitor more efficacious in the treatment of nonsmall cell lung carcinoma, would be more effective than gefitinib for thyroid cancer remains to be examined.

XL184

XL184 (Exelixis) is an oral, small molecule inhibitor of VEGF receptors 1 and 2, C-MET, RET, C-KIT, FLT3, and Tie-2 [55]. The inhibitory activity against C-MET, the cognate receptor for the hepatocyte growth factor, may provide additional synergistic benefit in thyroid carcinomas, given the enhanced expression of the receptor and frequent mutations seen in both PTC and MTC [56–58]. An ongoing phase I dose-escalation study has examined the safety and pharmacokinetics of XL184 in patients with metastatic solid malignancies. Preliminary results were reported at a recent conference, summarizing the experience of the first 44 subjects enrolled [59]. Whereas the maximum tolerated dose had not yet been identified, three MTC subjects had achieved partial responses, and two were stable after 9 and 13 months of therapy, respectively; two other MTC subjects had not been treated long enough to undergo response evaluation. Because of these early responses, the phase I study has been amended to permit cohort expansion of at least 20 MTC subjects to be enrolled once the maximum tolerated dose is identified, in anticipation of an eventual phase II or phase III trial [31].

Antivascular agents

Beyond direct inhibitors of angiogenic kinases such as VEGFR, other drugs are capable of either inhibiting angiogenesis or disrupting existing tumor vasculature. Two of these agents, thalidomide and combretastatin A4 phosphate, have been of particular interest following reported responses in individual patients with anaplastic thyroid carcinoma.

Thalidomide was found to be an angiogenesis inhibitor decades after it achieved notoriety as a teratogenic cause of neonatal dysmelia [60]. However, the exact mechanism by which thalidomide exerts its antiangiogenic effects remains unknown. In the article that described the efficacy of paclitaxel for treatment of anaplastic thyroid carcinoma, one patient who had progressed on the taxane was subsequently stabilized for at least 6 months while taking thalidomide [7]. Building upon this experience, an open label, phase II trial was initiated to examine the efficacy of thalidomide in patients with progressive, metastatic thyroid carcinoma of varying histologies [61]. Starting at 200 mg daily, the dose of drug was progressively increased as tolerated, with a median maximum daily dosage of about 600 mg. Of 28 evaluable subjects, 18% achieved a partial response and 32% had stable disease as their best response. Histology-specific partial response rates were not reported, but partial response or durable stable disease was seen in three PTC subjects, two FTC subjects, three Hürthle cell cancer subjects, and one MTC subject, along with four subjects with either tall cell or insular variants. Toxicities were dose limiting in the majority of subjects, and the most common adverse events included somnolence, peripheral neuropathy, constipation, dizziness, and infection. Given the suggested efficacy but high rate of adverse events with thalidomide, a subsequent phase II study has been initiated using the presumably less-toxic lenalidomide [31].

Combretastatin A4 phosphate is a tubulin inhibitor whose dephosphorylated metabolite selectively inhibits proliferating endothelial cells in tumors [62]. Of four phase I studies that were performed, one patient with anaplastic thyroid carcinoma was reported to have a complete response of more than four years duration. Interim results of an open-label phase II trial of combretastatin A4 phosphate were recently presented, describing 21 subjects with metastatic anaplastic carcinoma treated with 45 mg/m^2 intravenously on days 1, 8, and 15 of every 28 day cycle [63]. Median survival was 4.4 months, and the 12-week progression free survival was 29%, results probably comparable with those reported in the paclitaxel trial [7]. A randomized phase III trial is now underway, comparing the survival of subjects treated with combretastatin A4 phosphate in addition to paclitaxel and carboplatin with that of subjects treated with paclitaxel and carboplatin alone [31].

Intranuclear targeting

Gene expression abnormalities are common contributors to the progression of thyroid malignancies, and therefore therapies have been developed attempting to target such alterations. The possible role of retinoid receptors to regulate iodine uptake by thyroid follicular cells was suggested by data from in vitro studies that incubation of thyroid cancer cells that do not concentrate iodine with 13 cis-retinoic acid could partially restore radioiodine uptake [64]. Subsequent clinical trials yielded conflicting results, however [65]. Recently, a synthetic agonist of the retinoid X receptor, bexarotene, was tested in a phase II trial in patients with radioiodine-unresponsive metastatic disease [66]. After 6 weeks of therapy with bexarotene, 300 mg daily, radioiodine uptake was partially restored in 8 of 11 subjects, but a clinical response with measurable tumor reduction was lacking. A similar rationale was the basis of studies of the histone deacetylase inhibitor depsipeptide [67]. In a phase II trial in subjects with radioiodine-unresponsive metastatic DTC, one of 14 subjects exhibited dramatic restoration of uptake, permitting therapeutic radioiodine administration. Significant cardiac toxicities were seen, however, including sudden death in one subject. The orally available histone deacetylase inhibitor SAHA was studied in 16 subjects; no objective responses were reported, and most subjects discontinued therapy because of adverse events [68]. In a phase I trial, combining valproic acid, a histone deacetylase inhibitor, with 5-azacytidine, a DNA methylation inhibitor, the therapy was well tolerated; two subjects with metastatic PTC demonstrated prolonged stable disease, but radioiodine uptake was not assessed [69]. Finally, the peroxisome proliferator-activated receptor gamma agonist rosiglitazone was evaluated for the potential of restoring radioiodine uptake in 10 patients with unresponsive metastases [70]. In four patients, radioiodine uptake was visualized following 8 weeks of therapy with oral dosages up to 8 mg daily, but clinical response was limited.

Overall, these various studies of therapies targeting nuclear mechanisms of gene regulation indicate that reversal of epigenetic or nuclear receptor abnormalities can potentially re-establish the cellular capacity to take up radioiodine, but the actual clinical significance of such an effect appears limited.

Summary

Compared with the dismal historical track record, the recent proliferation of clinical trials for thyroid cancer has been remarkable. Clearly, targeting angiogenesis (and specifically VEGF receptors) has produced the most impressive clinical responses to date in both DTC and MTC. Although most small molecule VEGF receptor antagonists also inhibit RET, the efficacy of axitinib to induce objective responses in the absence of any anti-RET activity suggests that RET may not be as important a target for therapy as VEGFR. Nonetheless, the low rate of partial response, and the absence of complete responses in all of the various trials of monotherapy, identify the need to develop either more effect single agents or to identify rational combinations of therapeutic targets that have synergistic effectiveness without enhanced cross-toxicities.

References

[1] Haugen BR. Management of the patient with progressive radioiodine non-responsive disease. Semin Surg Oncol 1999;16:34–41.

[2] Sherman SI. Clinical trials for thyroid carcinoma: past, present, and future. In: Mazzaferri EL, Harmer C, Mallick UK, et al, editors. Practical management of thyroid cancer: a multidisciplinary approach. London: Springer-Verlag; 2006. p. 429–34.

[3] Gottlieb JA, Hill CS Jr. Chemotherapy of thyroid cancer with adriamycin: experience with 30 patients. N Engl J Med 1974;290(4):193–7.

[4] Shimaoka K, Schoenfeld DA, DeWys WD, et al. A randomized trial of doxorubicin versus doxorubicin plus cisplatin in patients with advanced thyroid carcinoma. Cancer 1985;56(9): 2155–60.

[5] Williams SD, Birch R, Einhorn LH. Phase II evaluation of doxorubicin plus cisplatin in advanced thyroid cancer: a Southeastern Cancer Study Group Trial. Cancer Treat Rep 1986;70(3):405–7.

[6] Stein R, Juweid M, Zhang CH, et al. Assessment of combined radioimmunotherapy and chemotherapy for treatment of medullary thyroid cancer. Clin Cancer Res 1999;5(10 Suppl):3199s–206s.

[7] Ain KB, Egorin MJ, DeSimone PA. Treatment of anaplastic thyroid carcinoma with paclitaxel: phase 2 trial using ninety-six-hour infusion. Thyroid 2000;10(7):587–94.

[8] Sherman SI, Lopez-Penabad L, Garden A, et al. Preliminary report on the use of paclitaxel as a sensitizer to the effects of external beam radiotherapy (EBRT) for control of locoregional disease in thyroid carcinoma. Presented at 84th Annual Meeting of The Endocrine Society. San Francisco, June 2002.

[9] Fagin JA. How thyroid tumors start and why it matters: kinase mutants as targets for solid cancer pharmacotherapy. J Endocrinol 2004;183(2):249–56.

[10] Carmeliet P. Mechanisms of angiogenesis and arteriogenesis. Nat Med 2000;6:389–95.

[11] Ferrara N, Kerbel RS. Angiogenesis as a therapeutic target. Nature 2005;438:967–74.

[12] Klein M, Vignaud JM, Hennequin V, et al. Increased expression of the vascular endothelial growth factor is a pejorative prognosis marker in papillary thyroid carcinoma. J Clin Endocrinol Metab 2001;86(2):656–8.

[13] Lennard CM, Patel A, Wilson J, et al. Intensity of vascular endothelial growth factor expression is associated with increased risk of recurrence and decreased disease-free survival in papillary thyroid cancer. Surgery 2001;129:552–8.

[14] Cooper DS, Doherty GM, Haugen BR, et al. Management guidelines for patients with thyroid nodules and differentiated thyroid cancer. Thyroid 2006;16(2):109–42.

[15] Sherman SI, Angelos P, Ball DW, et al. Thyroid carcinoma. J Natl Compr Canc Netw 2007; 5(6):568–621.

[16] Laird AD, Cherrington JM. Small molecule tyrosine kinase inhibitors: clinical development of anticancer agents. Expert Opin Investig Drugs 2003;12(1):51–64.

[17] Ball DW. Medullary thyroid cancer: therapeutic targets and molecular markers. Curr Opin Oncol 2007;19(1):18–23.

[18] Polverino A, Coxon A, Starnes C, et al. AMG 706, an oral, multikinase inhibitor that selectively targets vascular endothelial growth factor, platelet-derived growth factor, and kit receptors, potently inhibits angiogenesis and induces regression in tumor xenografts. Cancer Res 2006;66(17):8715–21.

[19] Coxon A, Bready J, Fiorino M, et al. Anti-tumor activity of AMG 706, an oral multi-kinase inhibitor, in human medullary thyroid carcinoma xenografts. Thyroid 2006;16(9):920.

[20] Rosen LS, Kurzrock R, Mulay M, et al. Safety, pharmacokinetics, and efficacy of AMG 706, an oral multikinase inhibitor, in patients with advanced solid tumors. J Clin Oncol 2007; 25(17):2369–76.

[21] Sherman SI, Schlumberger MJ, Droz J, et al. Initial results from a phase II trial of motesanib diphosphate (AMG 706) in patients with differentiated thyroid cancer (DTC). J Clin Oncol 2007;25(18 Suppl):6017.

[22] Schlumberger MJ, Elisei R, Sherman SI, et al. Phase 2 trial of motesanib diphosphate (AMG 706) in patients with medullary thyroid cancer (MTC). Presented at 89th Annual Meeting of the Endocrine Society. Toronto (ON), June 2007.

[23] Sherman SI, Schlumberger MJ, Elisei R, et al. Exacerbation of postsurgical hypothyroidism during treatment of thyroid carcinoma with motesanib diphosphate (AMG 706). Presented at 89th Annual Meeting of the Endocrine Society. Toronto (ON), June 2007.

[24] Herbst RS, Heymach JV, O'Reilly MS, et al. Vandetanib (ZD6474): an orally available receptor tyrosine kinase inhibitor that selectively targets pathways critical for tumor growth and angiogenesis. Expert Opin Investig Drugs 2007;16(2):239–49.

[25] Wedge SR, Ogilvie DJ, Dukes M, et al. ZD6474 inhibits vascular endothelial growth factor signaling, angiogenesis, and tumor growth following oral administration. Cancer Res 2002; 62(16):4645–55.

[26] Carlomagno F, Vitagliano D, Guida T, et al. ZD6474, an orally available inhibitor of KDR tyrosine kinase activity, efficiently blocks oncogenic RET kinases. Cancer Res 2002;62:7284–90.

[27] Carlomagno F, Guida T, Anaganti S, et al. Disease associated mutations at valine 804 in the RET receptor tyrosine kinase confer resistance to selective kinase inhibitors. Oncogene 2004; 23(36):6056–63.

[28] Holden SN, Eckhardt SG, Basser R, et al. Clinical evaluation of ZD6474, an orally active inhibitor of VEGF and EGF receptor signaling, in patients with solid, malignant tumors. Ann Oncol 2005;16(8):1391–7.

[29] Wells SA Jr, Gosnell JE, Gagel RF, et al. Vandetanib in metastatic hereditary medullary thyroid cancer: follow-up results of an open-label phase II trial. J Clin Oncol 2007; 25(18 suppl):6018.

[30] Akeno-Stuart N, Croyle M, Knauf JA, et al. The RET kinase inhibitor NVP-AST487 blocks growth and calcitonin gene expression through distinct mechanisms in medullary thyroid cancer cells. Cancer Res 2007;67(14):6956–64.

[31] ClinicalTrials.gov. National Institutes of Health. Available at: www.clinicaltrials.gov/ct2/home. Accessed January 11, 2008.

[32] Wilhelm SM, Carter C, Tang L, et al. BAY 43-9006 exhibits broad spectrum oral antitumor activity and targets the RAF/MEK/ERK pathway and receptor tyrosine kinases involved in tumor progression and angiogenesis. Cancer Res 2004;64(19):7099–109.

[33] Carlomagno F, Anaganti S, Guida T, et al. BAY 43-9006 inhibition of oncogenic RET mutants. J Natl Cancer Inst 2006;98(5):326–34.

[34] Strumberg D, Clark JW, Awada A, et al. Safety, pharmacokinetics, and preliminary antitumor activity of sorafenib: a review of four phase I trials in patients with advanced refractory solid tumors. Oncologist 2007;12(4):426–37.

[35] Ratain MJ, Eisen T, Stadler WM, et al. Phase II placebo-controlled randomized discontinuation trial of sorafenib in patients with metastatic renal cell carcinoma. J Clin Oncol 2006; 24(16):2505–12.

[36] Kloos R, Ringel M, Knopp M, et al. Significant clinical and biologic activity of RAF/VEGF-R kinase inhibitor BAY 43-9006 in patients with metastatic papillary thyroid carcinoma (PTC): updated results of a phase II study. J Clin Oncol 2006;24(18 Suppl):5534.

[37] Gupta V, Puttaswamy K, Lassoued W, et al. Sorafenib targets BRAF and VEGFR in metastatic thyroid carcinoma. J Clin Oncol 2007;25(18 Suppl):6019.

[38] Kober F, Hermann M, Handler A, et al. Effect of sorafenib in symptomatic metastatic medullary thyroid cancer. J Clin Oncol 2007;25(18 Suppl):14065.

[39] Hong DS, Camacho L, Ng C, et al. Phase I study of tipifarnib and sorafenib in patients with biopsiable advanced cancers (NCI protocol 7156 supported by NCI grant UO1 CA062461). J Clin Oncol 2007;25(18 Suppl):3549.

[40] Kim S, Yazici YD, Calzada G, et al. Sorafenib inhibits the angiogenesis and growth of orthotopic anaplastic thyroid carcinoma xenografts in nude mice. Mol Cancer Ther 2007; 6(6):1785–92.

[41] Kong HH, Cowen EW, Azad NS, et al. Keratoacanthomas associated with sorafenib therapy. J Am Acad Dermatol 2007;56(1):171–2.

[42] Inai T, Mancuso M, Hashizume H, et al. Inhibition of vascular endothelial growth factor (VEGF) signaling in cancer causes loss of endothelial fenestrations, regression of tumor vessels, and appearance of basement membrane ghosts. Am J Pathol 2004;165(1): 35–52.

[43] Rugo HS, Herbst RS, Liu G, et al. Phase I trial of the oral antiangiogenesis agent AG-013736 in patients with advanced solid tumors: pharmacokinetic and clinical results. J Clin Oncol 2005;23(24):5474–83.

[44] Cohen EE, Vokes EE, Rosen LS, et al. A phase II study of axitinib (AG-013736 [AG]) in patients (pts) with advanced thyroid cancers. J Clin Oncol 2007;25(18 Suppl): 6008.

[45] de Groot JW, Plaza Menacho I, Schepers H, et al. Cellular effects of imatinib on medullary thyroid cancer cells harboring multiple endocrine neoplasia Type 2A and 2B associated RET mutations. Surgery 2006;139(6):806–14.

[46] Skinner MA, Safford SD, Freemerman AJ. RET tyrosine kinase and medullary thyroid cells are unaffected by clinical doses of STI571. Anticancer Res 2003;23(5A):3601–6.

[47] Buchdunger E, O'Reilley T, Wood J. Pharmacology of imatinib (STI571). Eur J Cancer 2002;38(Suppl 5):S28–36.

[48] Frank-Raue K, Fabel M, Delorme S, et al. Efficacy of imatinib mesylate in advanced medullary thyroid carcinoma. Eur J Endocrinol 2007;157(2):215–20.

[49] de Groot JW, Zonnenberg BA, Quarles van Ufford-Mannesse P, et al. A phase-II trial of imatinib therapy for metastatic medullary thyroid carcinoma. J Clin Endocrinol Metab 2007;92(9):3466–9.

[50] Hoff PM, Hoff AO, Phan AT, et al. Phase I/II trial of capecitabine (C), dacarbazine (D) and imatinib (I) (CDI) for patients (pts) metastatic medullary thyroid carcinomas (MTC). J Clin Oncol 2006;24(18 Suppl):13048.

[51] Wakeling AE, Guy SP, Woodburn JR, et al. ZD1839 (Iressa): an orally active inhibitor of epidermal growth factor signaling with potential for cancer therapy. Cancer Res 2002;62: 5749–54.

[52] Lynch TJ, Bell DW, Sordella R, et al. Activating mutations in the epidermal growth factor receptor underlying responsiveness of non-small-cell lung cancer to gefitinib. N Engl J Med 2004;350(21):2129–39.

[53] Pennell NA, Daniels GH, Haddad RI, et al. A phase II study of gefitinib in patients with advanced thyroid cancer. Thyroid 2008;18(3):317–23.

[54] Fury MG, Solit DB, Su YB, et al. A phase I trial of intermittent high-dose gefitinib and fixed-dose docetaxel in patients with advanced solid tumors. Cancer Chemother Pharmacol 2007; 59(4):467–75.

[55] Cui JJ. Inhibitors targeting hepatocyte growth factor receptor and their potential therapeutic applications. Expert Opin Ther Pat 2007;17(9):1035–45.

[56] Mineo R, Costantino A, Frasca F, et al. Activation of the hepatocyte growth factor (HGF)-Met system in papillary thyroid cancer: biological effects of HGF in thyroid cancer cells depend on Met expression levels. Endocrinology 2004;145(9):4355–65.

[57] Wasenius VM, Hemmer S, Karjalainen-Lindsberg ML, et al. MET receptor tyrosine kinase sequence alterations in differentiated thyroid carcinoma. Am J Surg Pathol 2005;29(4):544–9.

[58] Papotti M, Olivero M, Volante M, et al. Expression of hepatocyte growth factor (HGF) and its receptor (MET) in medullary carcinoma of the thyroid. Endocr Pathol 2000;11(1):19–30.

[59] Salgia R, Hong D, Sherman S, et al. A phase I dose-escalation study of the safety and pharmacokinetics of XL184, a VEGFR and MET kinase inhibitor administered orally to patients with advanced malignancies. In: 19th AACR-NCI-EORTC International Conference on Molecular Targets and Cancer Therapeutics. San Francisco (CA), October 22–26, 2007.

[60] D'Amato RJ, Loughnan MS, Flynn E, et al. Thalidomide is an inhibitor of angiogenesis. Proc Natl Acad Sci U S A 1994;91(9):4082–5.

[61] Ain KB, Lee C, Williams KD. Phase II trial of thalidomide for therapy of radioiodine-unresponsive and rapidly progressive thyroid carcinomas. Thyroid 2007;17(7):663–70.

[62] Cooney MM, Ortiz J, Bukowski RM, et al. Novel vascular targeting/disrupting agents: combretastatin A4 phosphate and related compounds. Curr Oncol Rep 2005;7(2):90–5.

[63] Cooney MM, Savvides P, Agarwala S, et al. Phase II study of combretastatin A4 phosphate (CA4P) in patients with advanced anaplastic thyroid carcinoma (ATC). J Clin Oncol 2006; 24(18 suppl):5580.

[64] Van Herle AJ, Agatep ML, Padua DN, et al. Effects of 13 cis-retinoic acid on growth and differentiation of human follicular carcinoma cells (UCLA R0 82 W-1) in vitro. J Clin Endocrinol Metab 1990;71(3):755–63.

[65] Gruning T, Tiepolt C, Zophel K, et al. Retinoic acid for redifferentiation of thyroid cancer—does it hold its promise? Eur J Endocrinol 2003;148(4):395–402.

[66] Liu YY, Stokkel MP, Pereira AM, et al. Bexarotene increases uptake of radioiodide in metastases of differentiated thyroid carcinoma. Eur J Endocrinol 2006;154(4):525–31.

[67] Su YB, Tuttle RM, Fury M, et al. A phase II study of single agent depsipeptide (DEP) in patients (pts) with radioactive iodine (RAI)-refractory, metastatic, thyroid carcinoma: preliminary toxicity and efficacy experience. J Clin Oncol 2006;24(18 Suppl):5554.

[68] Ringel MD, Kloos RT, Arbogast D, et al. Phase II study of oral histone deacetylase inhibitor SAHA in patients with metastatic thyroid cancer. Thyroid 2006;14(9):928–9.

[69] Soriano AO, Braiteh F, Garcia-Manero G, et al. Combination of 5-azacytidine (5-AZA) and valproic acid (VPA) in advanced solid cancers: a phase I study. J Clin Oncol 2007; 25(18 Suppl):3547.

[70] Kebebew E, Peng M, Reiff E, et al. A phase II trial of rosiglitazone in patients with thyroglobulin-positive and radioiodine-negative differentiated thyroid cancer. Surgery 2006;140(6):960–6 [discussion: 966–7].

[71] Kim DW, Jo YS, Jung HS, et al. An orally administered multitarget tyrosine kinase inhibitor, SU11248, is a novel potent inhibitor of thyroid oncogenic RET/papillary thyroid cancer kinases. J Clin Endocrinol Metab 2006;91(10):4070–6.

[72] Sun L, Liang C, Shirazian S, et al. Discovery of 5-[5-fluoro-2-oxo-1,2- dihydroindol-(3Z)-ylidenemethyl]-2,4- dimethyl-1H-pyrrole-3-carboxylic acid (2-diethylaminoethyl)amide, a novel tyrosine kinase inhibitor targeting vascular endothelial and platelet-derived growth factor receptor tyrosine kinase. J Med Chem 2003;46(7):1116–9.

ELSEVIER
SAUNDERS

Endocrinol Metab Clin N Am
37 (2008) 525–538

ENDOCRINOLOGY
AND METABOLISM
CLINICS
OF NORTH AMERICA

Anaplastic Thyroid Cancer

Ryan L. Neff, MD[a], William B. Farrar, MD[a],
Richard T. Kloos, MD[b,c],*

Kenneth D. Burman, MD, Guest Editor[d]

[a]Department of Surgery, Division of Surgical Oncology, The Ohio State University,
The Arthur G. James Cancer Hospital and Richard J. Solove Research Institute, N 924 Doan
Hall, 410 West 10th Avenue, Columbus, OH 43210-1228, USA
[b]Departments of Internal Medicine and Radiology, Divisions of Endocrinology, Metabolism,
and Diabetes, and Nuclear Medicine, The Ohio State University, The Arthur G. James Cancer
Hospital and Richard J. Solove Research Institute, A458 Starling Loving Hall,
320 W. 10th Avenue, Columbus, OH 43210-1228, USA
[c]The Ohio State University Comprehensive Cancer Center, Columbus, Ohio, USA
[d]Endocrine Section, Washington Hospital Center, 110 Irving Street, NW, Room 2A-72,
Washington, DC 20010-2975, USA

Anaplastic thyroid cancer (ATC) is an uncommon, usually lethal malignancy of older adults with no effective systemic therapy. The mean survival time is frequently less than 6 months from diagnosis (Fig. 1) [1], an outcome that may not be significantly altered by our largely ineffective treatment. While the diagnosis and treatment of ATC should be considered a medical urgency, end-of-life planning to optimize the patient's quality of remaining life must also be given a high priority. A few fortunate patients with completely resectable disease demonstrate long-term survival.

Epidemiology and tumor characteristics

Wordwide experience

The annual incidence of ATC is about one to two cases per million, with the overall incidence being higher in areas of endemic goiter [2]. From a sample of 53,856 thyroid carcinomas registered in the United States between 1985 and 1995 in the National Cancer database, 80% were papillary

---

* Corresponding author. The Ohio State University, 446 McCampbell Hall, 1581 Dodd
Drive, Columbus, OH 43210-1296.
E-mail address: richard.kloos@osumc.edu (R.T. Kloos).

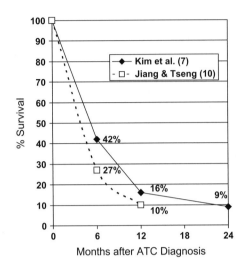

Fig. 1. Percentage of patients surviving over time after ATC diagnosis.

(PTC), 11% follicular (FTC), 3% Hürthle cell, 3% medullary (MTC), and 2% were undifferentiated or anaplastic [3]. Similar rates and incidence of ATC were reported in Japan and Norway [4,5]. However, with the rising detection of previous subclinical small PTCs increasing the incidence of differentiated thyroid carcinomas (DTC), the percentage of ATC cases is expected to decrease [6]. Furthermore, the incidence of ATC has been declining worldwide [1], possibly related to reclassification of small cell ATC as lymphoma or undifferentiated MTC, the removal of insular carcinoma as an ATC variant, the decreased incidence of FTC from dietary iodine supplementation, and the overall earlier diagnosis and treatment of DTC at a lower stage of disease, which may eliminate the opportunity for it to undergo dedifferentiation.

Although children with ATC have been reported [7,8], the disease typically presents in the seventh decade of life [1,7,9–13], with more than 90% of patients older than 50 years (Fig. 2) [14]. The female to male ratio is often between 1.5–2 to 1 [1,7,10–13]. The mean tumor size is usually 6 cm to 9 cm [1,7,11,12], and confined to the thyroid in only 0% to 9% of cases [7,12,13,15]. Lymph node metastases or extrathyroidal extension in the absence of distant metastases are present in 53% to 64% of cases [7,12,15], and distant metastases are present in a quarter to two-thirds of patients [11,15]. About a quarter of patients subsequently develop distant metastases during their course [1]. The most common sites of distant metastases in descending order are the lungs (approximately 80%), then bone, skin, and brain (each about 5%–15%) [16]. Less common metastatic sites include the heart and abdomen [2,7,8,12,13].

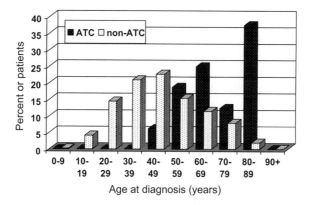

Fig. 2. Age distribution of the last 1,184 consecutive thyroid cancer cases, including 16 ATC and 1,168 non-ATC cases. (*Adapted from* Kloos RT. Anaplastic thyroid carcinoma. In: Hay I, Turner H, Wass J, editors. Clinical endocrine oncology. 2nd edition. Oxford (UK): Blackwell Publishing; 2008; with permission.)

The Ohio State University and Arthur G. James Cancer Hospital experience

ATC has represented 1.4% of the last 1,184 patients who underwent all or part of their first course of treatment at the authors' medical center (R.T. Kloos, MD, unpublished data, 2006). Women outnumbered men 3 to 1 and 70 years was the mean age at diagnosis. For non-ATC cases, women outnumbered men 2.6 to 1 and 45 years was the mean age at diagnosis (see Fig. 2). Indeed, none of the ATC cases at the Arthur G. James Cancer Hospital were less than 45 years old and only 25% were less than 60 years old, compared with 52% and 79%, respectively, for the non-ATC cases. One quarter of the ATC cases were less than 7 cm, compared with 82% for the non-ATC cases, and 44% of the ATC cases presented with distant metastases, compared with only 5% for the non-ATC cases.

Etiology

While it is possible that ATC may arise de novo (but not proven), it is generally accepted that ATC can develop from pre-existing DTC (PTC or FTC). Indeed, in a study of patients who died from thyroid cancer, 99 had ATC at the time of death while only two-thirds had this diagnosis at their initial thyroid cancer presentation [17]. About one-quarter to one-half of patients with ATC have a previous or concurrent DTC history [1,11–13,17,18]. Unique molecular signature events support the notion that ATC may derive from PTC or FTC. For example, PTC initiating BRAF mutations are present in approximately 44% of PTC and are absent in FTC, MTC, and benign neoplasms, while they are present in 24% of ATC [19].

Presentation

ATC almost always presents as a rapidly growing fixed and hard neck mass, often with metastatic local lymph nodes appreciable on examination, and vocal cord paralysis [8,12]. Symptoms may reflect rapid growth of the tumor with local invasion or compression. Tenvall and colleagues [15] reported that the median duration of symptoms before diagnosis was 1.5 months (range, 0–8 months). The most frequent presenting signs and symptoms included hoarseness (77%), dysphagia (56%), vocal cord paralysis (49%), neck pain (29%), weight loss (24%), dyspnea (19%), and stridor (11%) [2]. Local tissue necrosis resulting from these quickly growing neoplasms occasionally causes thyrotoxicosis [20]. About one-quarter of cases present as the sudden enlargement of a pre-existing thyroid mass or goiter over the previous few weeks or months [11,12,15]. In a series of 84 consecutive ATC patients, Giuffrida and Gharib [2] reported that a single nodule was present in 58%, multiple nodules in 36%, bilateral involvement in 24%, and a hard and fixed lesion was present in 75%.

Cause of death

From a series of patients who presented with ATC and died of their disease, a single specific cause of death could not be identified in 40% because either serious conditions developed simultaneously in multiple organs, or general weakness progressed gradually without specific verified organ failure (cachexia) [17]. In those with a specific cause of death, 35% died from replacement of lung tissue by extensive pulmonary metastases (while 86% had or developed pulmonary metastases), airway obstruction in 16%, tumor related hemorrhage in 14%, cardiac failure in 11%, 5% from tumor related pneumonia or disseminated intravascular coagulation from necrotic tumor infection, and 3% from circulatory failure because of vena cava stenosis, cardiac metastases, treatment-related neutropenic sepsis, renal failure, or humoral hypercalcemia of malignancy [17]. The tumor sites mainly responsible for death included concomitant local and distant metastases in 40%, local disease in 34%, distant metastases in 24%, and treatment in 2%.

Diagnosis and histology

ATC histologic patterns include giant cell, spindle cell, and squamoid cell [2]. These subtypes frequently coexist and are not predictive of patient outcome. Areas of necrosis and hemorrhage are common, and mitotic activity is high. Two uncommon variants of ATC include the paucicellular variant, which may be confused with Riedel's struma, and a carcinosarcoma variant that includes large regions of osteosarcomatous differentiation [8].

Fine needle aspiration can diagnose ATC by the demonstration of spindled or giant cells, bizarre neoplastic cells that may be multinucleated, or atypical cells with high mitotic activity. However, histologic confirmation is recommended if the diagnosis is not absolutely certain to exclude tumors with better prognoses or that require different therapy, including poorly differentiated thyroid cancer, MTC, primary thyroid lymphoma, poorly differentiated metastasis to the thyroid, primary squamous cell carcinoma, and angiomatoid thyroid neoplasms [8]. Tennvall and colleagues [15] reported that 4% of patients referred for ATC based on fine needle aspiration cytology were found to have discrepant histologic findings at surgery (although they argue that surgical biopsy unnecessarily delays initiation of neoadjuvant chemoradiation therapy).

Dedifferentiation, a hallmark of ATC, is manifested by a loss of specific thyroid cell characteristics and functions, including expressions of thyroglobulin, thyroid peroxidase, thyroid stimulating hormone (TSH) receptor, and the Na/I symporter expression. Consequently, thyroglobulin cannot be used as a tumor marker for diagnosis or monitoring. Cytokeratin (keratin) may be the most useful epithelial immunohistochemical marker, and is present in 40% to 100% of tumors [2,21]. Other markers suggesting the epithelial origin of the tumor may be epithelial membrane antigen and carcinoembryonic antigen [2]. Other immunohistochemical markers that may be helpful include vimentin, alpha-1-chymotrypsin, and desmin. The spindle cell variant may be differentiated from sarcoma with immunostaining to anticytokeratin antibodies [1]. Lymphomas do not have the marked cellular pleomorphism that is typical of ATC, and MTC may be recognized by immunohistochemical staining for neuron-specific enolase, chromogranin, and calcitonin [9].

Staging and prognostic features

All ATCs are classified as T4 and Stage IV tumors by the American Joint Committee on Cancer Cancer Staging Manual, 6th edition, because of their aggressive behavior. T4a tumors are intrathyroidal surgically resectable, while T4b tumors are extrathyroidal- surgically unresectable. Stage IV is subdivided as Stage IVA, which is T4a, any N, M0; Stage IVB, which is T4b, any N, M0; and Stage IVC, which is any T, any N, M1.

Kim and colleagues [7] reported that the median survival time was 5.1 months in a series of 121 ATC subjects. The overall cause-specific survival was 42%, 16%, and 9% at 6, 12, and 24 months, respectively (see Fig. 1). Age less than 60 years, tumor size less than 7 cm, and lesser extent of disease were independent predictors of lower cause-specific mortality on multivariate analysis. Others have also reported that smaller tumor size (less than 5 cm–6 cm) is prognostically important [22–26]. Hundahl and colleagues [3] reported that the survival rates among 893 undifferentiated or anaplastic carcinomas were 23%, 18%, 15%, and 14% at 1, 2, 3, and 5 years, respectively. Among those who survived greater than or equal to 5 years, age less than 45 years and small tumor sizes (and possibly the absence of extrathyroidal extension) were more common. For example, the 5-year survival rate for those aged less than 45 years was 55%, while the 5-year survival rate was 13% for all age groups above age 45. Pierie and colleagues [23] reported that age less than or equal to 70 years was an independent predictor of survival. Venkatesh and colleagues [18] also reported that younger patients survived longer than older patients, and noted that patients who presented with only local disease had a median survival of 8 months, compared with just over 3 months when distant metastases were present. In contrast, however, Haigh and colleagues [11] found that neither age nor tumor size were associated with survival. Rather, potentially curative surgery was their only variable associated with prolonged survival after multivariate analysis.

Jiang and Tseng [10] described a series of 45 ATC patients from Taiwan whose overall survival was 27% and 10% at 6 and 12 months, respectively (see Fig. 1). Significantly shorter survival was seen in patients with leukocytosis, hypoalbuminemia, or hypothyroxinemia.

Treatment

Therapy options include surgery, external beam radiation therapy (EBRT), tracheostomy, chemotherapy, and investigational clinical trials. The value of these treatment options, and the order and combination in which they are used, must be carefully evaluated for their ability to promote quality of life, prolong survival, and to reduce tumor-specific mortality. Unfortunately, the data are not convincing that any treatment strategy reduces tumor-specific mortality beyond the rare patient cured by surgical resection. Furthermore, it is not clear that survival is prolonged by therapy other than palliative treatments, such as those that prevent strangulation. It is impossible to accurately discern the benefits of the many uncontrolled treatment trials because of the potential confounding influences of age, gender [1,26], tumor size, extent of local invasion and resectability, influence of surgical resection, and the overall extent of disease.

Surgery

Surgical treatment of local disease offers the best opportunity for prolonged survival if the tumor is intrathyroidal. When the tumor is extrathyroidal, the surgical approach to ATC is controversial, as some have found that neither the extent of the operation nor the completeness of the tumor resection affect survival [13]. The aggressive nature of this disease results in a high rate of local recurrence, despite morbid surgical resections [11,12], and distortion of the normal anatomy can even prohibit the safe placement of a tracheostomy. Still, complete surgical resection is recommended whenever possible if excessive morbidity can be avoided [1,27]. Lateral neck dissections should be performed only in the setting of complete macroscopic resection. Resections of the larynx, pharynx, and esophagus are generally discouraged [1,18,28].

Multimodal or combination therapy

Local tumor surgical debulking, combined with EBRT and chemother-apy as neoadjuvant (before surgery) or adjuvant (after surgery) therapy, may prevent death from local airway obstruction and at best may slightly prolong survival [1,2,13,29]. Tracheostomy should be performed in patients with impending airway obstruction when death is not imminent from other sites of disease, and who are not candidates for local resection or chemora-diation [1,17]. Prophylactic tracheostomy in the absence of impending risk to the airway is discouraged [8].

Schlumberger and colleagues [30] investigated two protocols in 20 ATC subjects using different chemotherapy regimens combined with EBRT, with or without surgery. Treatment toxicity was high and was a limiting fac-tor. The investigators concluded that gross tumor resection should be per-formed whenever possible, and that combined treatment may prevent death from suffocation because of local tumor growth. The investigators also concluded that this treatment was effective in terms of survival. Yet there was no control group on which to base these conclusions, and the im-pact of the treatment beyond surgery may be questioned based on historical controls. Of the seven subjects in the series with neck disease remaining after surgery, four experienced a best response in the neck of a complete remis-sion, while three had a partial remission. Of the eight subjects who did not undergo surgery, one experienced a best response of complete remission in the neck that lasted 8 months, four had a partial remission, and three demonstrated tumor progression. Unfortunately, survival exceeding 20 months was seen in only three of the original 20 subjects (15%). Two of these three subjects to survive more than 20 months were among four sub-jects with no evidence of disease after surgery. These four subjects had a mean duration of response of 20 months (range 2–40 months), which may be no different than expected without additional treatment in patients without demonstrable residual disease postoperatively [3,7,12]. The third subject to survive more than 20 months was one of four subjects with resid-ual disease confined to the neck after surgery. These 4 subjects had an un-usually low mean age of 38 years (range 27–42 years) and their mean survival of 10 months (range 4–22 months) may be no different than ex-pected without additional treatment in young patients [3,7,12]. The nine subjects in this series that had distant metastases at the time of treatment all experienced tumor progression during therapy that resulted in death.

Of additional disappointment is that therapy has not been shown to in-dependently improve overall cause-specific mortality in multivariate analysis that include patient, tumor, and treatment variables [7,13]. For example, Kim and colleagues [7] found that only patient and tumor factors predicted lower cause-specific mortality. In subjects with unresectable disease who were considered candidates only for supportive care, palliative EBRT, or palliative chemotherapy, the 12-month survival was 3% with a median survival of 2.9 months. As all 11 of their subjects who survived longer than 24 months received bilateral surgery with curative intent, they performed a subanalysis of their 71 subjects who received this same treatment. The 12-month survival rate in this group of subjects was 64%, with a median survival of 12.3 months. On multivariate analysis, age less than 60 years, female gender, tumor less than 7 cm, and intrathyroidal disease were identified as independent predictors of lower cause-specific mortality, while treatment variables including EBRT and chemotherapy were not. Similarly, others have been unable to clearly demonstrate a benefit of therapy including hyperfractionated EBRT and chemo-radiosensitization [2,8]. Some have reported improved survival with higher doses of radiotherapy [23,31,32], while others have demonstrated no survival advantage despite an 80% tumor response rate [33]. Aggressive hyperfractionated EBRT protocols that have reported complete or partial local tumor responses have also been associated with high rates of treatment toxicity [34,35].

In a series of 47 ATC subjects, Chang and colleagues [12] reported that in their subjects with unresectable disease, the median survival was 2 to 3 months, regardless of additional therapies. Those subjects that underwent complete tumor resection combined with chemoradiotherapy had a median survival of 6 months, a difference in survival that was not statistically significant. Thus, regardless of treatment provided, most subjects demonstrated rapid disease progression and distant metastases, with a mean survival of 4.3 months (range, 1–21 months), and no significant difference in survival time was observed between the various types of treatment. Neither neoadjuvant nor adjuvant chemotherapy demonstrated an increase in survival. These disappointing results of local and systemic treatment to diminish mortality are consistent with the report of Kitamura and colleagues [17], who reported that distant metastases were not initially present in 71% of their 62 patients initially diagnosed with ATC who eventually died of their disease.

Unlike Chang and colleagues [12], others have suggested that neoadjuvant chemo-radiotherapy may be superior to adjuvant therapy [1,16]. Perhaps the most compelling data for neoadjuvant multimodal therapy come from Tenvall and colleagues [15], who studied 55 subjects treated with hyperfractionated (twice daily, 5 days per week) radiotherapy, doxorubicin, and whenever possible, surgery. Subjects were not randomized, but rather the three protocols were comprised of subjects treated at different time periods who received daily radiotherapy doses of 1 Gy in protocol A, 1.3 Gy in protocol B, and 1.6 Gy in protocol C. Twenty milligrams of doxorubicin was administered intravenously weekly, starting before radiotherapy. Protocols A and B received 30 Gy before surgery and 16 Gy after surgery. Protocol C received the entire 46 Gy before surgery. There was no evidence of local recurrence in 31% of protocol A, 65% of protocol B, and 77% of protocol C. In those that underwent surgery, there was no evidence of local recurrence in 56% of protocol A, 79% of protocol B, and 100% of protocol C. While these results are encouraging in regards to local disease control with protocol C, the overall survival data were sobering in that the median survival was 3.5, 4.5, and 2 months for protocols A, B, and C, respectively. Patients surviving more than 2 years were 13% of protocol A, 12% of protocol B, and 5% of protocol C.

Haigh and colleagues [11] reported a series of 24 ATC subjects with a median survival of 43 months for the 8 patients that underwent potentially curative surgery, with no residual or minimal residual disease, compared with 3 months survival in the 18 subjects who underwent palliative surgery ($P = .001$). There was no difference in survival between those treated with only chemotherapy and EBRT without surgery (survival 3.3 months), and those that underwent palliative surgery defined as neck surgery in which macroscopic extrathyroidal disease or persistent distant disease remained postoperatively. These findings raise questions about the benefits of surgery for a patient whose airway is not an immediate risk, yet who is not a candidate for a potentially curable procedure.

Ain and colleagues [36] evaluated the activity of paclitaxel against ATC. Eleven of 19 patients demonstrated a partial response (nine), complete response (one), or disease stabilization (one) that lasted at least 2 weeks. Responders tended to be younger and female. Disappointingly, the median survival of all 19 evaluable patients was 25 weeks from diagnosis, and 24 weeks from initiation of paclitaxel. Potentially encouraging, however, was that the 10 patients with a partial or complete response to paclitaxel had a median survival of 32 weeks from starting treatment, compared with 10 weeks for the others, although this difference was not a statistically significant ($P = .40$).

Investigational therapies

Gefitinib is the first selective inhibitor of epidermal growth factor receptor's tyrosine kinase domain. A phase I study investigating if gefitinib could sensitize various tumors to subsequent treatment with docetaxel reported a partial response in one patient with ATC [37].

Dowlati and colleagues [38] performed a phase I study of the anti-angiogenic prodrug combretastatin A-4 phosphate in patients with various advanced cancers, including three with ATC. One patient with ATC that extended into the mediastinum and had palpable nodal involvement experienced a complete response after eight cycles of therapy and underwent an exploratory neck dissection where no tumor was found. An additional two cycles of treatment were given and he was alive 30 months after treatment. In the treatment cohort, tumor pain occurring shortly after dosing was a unique side effect of the drug, and dynamic contrast-enhanced MRI demonstrated a significant decline in gradient peak tumor blood flow consistent with vascular activity.

A preliminary report of an international multicenter two-stage, phase II trial of irofulven and capecitabine to evaluate the objective response rate of

patients with advanced thyroid cancer included four metastatic ATC subjects. Subjects received irofulven intravenously on days 1 and 15 and capecitabine orally on days 1 to 15 every 28 days. No subject with ATC
demonstrated a response [39]. Similarly, disease stabilization was not demonstrated in subjects with metastatic ATC in a phase II trial of the oral
multi-kinase inhibitor Sorafenib [40].

Radioactive iodine and thyroid stimulating hormone suppression therapy

Radioactive iodine may be considered in patients whose thyroid cancer
contains only a minor component of intrathyroidal ATC that was completely resected, although there are no data to demonstrate a benefit. However, ATC does not accumulate I-131 secondary to the loss of effective
iodine uptake, and therefore is refractory to this therapy. Patients with concomitant DTC typically do not have a better prognosis, as they unfortunately succumb to the anaplastic component of their disease [8,11].
Various strategies to "redifferentiate" ATC, including restoration I-131 uptake, have been investigated, but no method has achieved clinical utility.

TSH suppression therapy is an important part of treating metastatic
DTC [41]. Conversely, functional TSH receptors are ordinarily absent in
ATC and no role for TSH suppressive therapy has been identified.

Authors' recommendations

Fig. 3A and B suggest a diagnostic and treatment algorithm that is consistent with the guidelines of the National Comprehensive Cancer Network
[42]. CT imaging with contrast of the head, neck, chest, abdomen, and pelvis
is suggested to rapidly determine the extent of the tumor, local invasion, and
distant metastases. Data regarding the utility of fluorodeoxyglucose (FDG)-
positron emission tomography (PET) are limited [43], but the increased expression of the FDG transporter GLUT1 by ATC [44] may predict a greater
sensitivity of FDG-PET whole-body assessment for ATC, as compared with
DTC.

Patients with disease confined to the thyroid should undergo urgent complete tumor resection, generally via near-total or total thyroidectomy. The
airway must be kept in mind throughout the course of the patient's illness,
and those with impending obstruction without imminent death from other
sites of disease require an urgent procedure to secure the airway, such as a tracheostomy. Other than for these two situations, currently available treatment
options are largely futile, and therefore end-of-life issues and patient comfort
must be addressed and a treatment course of standard therapy, comfort care,
or clinical trials must be selected by a fully informed patient and supportive
clinical team. Given the poor impact of all available therapies, it is difficult to
be dogmatic regarding the necessity of any treatment modality. Clinical trials
should be given the highest priority at all decision points.

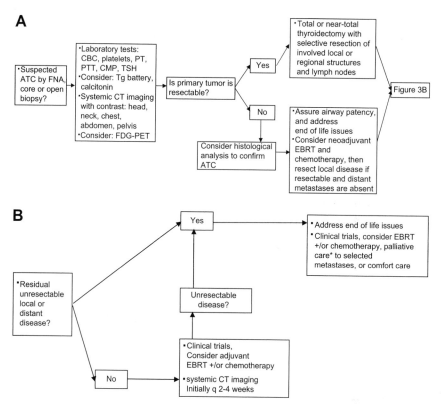

Fig. 3. Diagnostic and treatment algorithm consistent with the guidelines of the National Comprehensive Cancer Network. (*A*) CBC, complete blood count; CMP, comprehensive metabolic profile; PT, prothrombin time; PTT, partial thromboplastin time; Tg battery, thyroglobulin and antithyroglobulin antibody. (*B*) (*asterisk*) May include external beam radiation therapy, surgery, tracheostomy, tracheal stent, radiofrequency ablation, photodynamic therapy, laser thermal ablation, gamma knife, tumor embolization. (*Adapted from* Kloos RT. Anaplastic thyroid carcinoma. In: Hay I, Turner H, Wass J, editors. Clinical endocrine oncology. 2nd edition. Oxford (UK): Blackwell Publishing; 2008; with permission.)

Locally resectable disease

In the absence of an available clinical trial, patients with local disease that is potentially completely resectable should undergo surgery. If the local tumor is confined to the thyroid and completely resected with no evidence of distant metastases, then additional treatment with EBRT or chemotherapy (as outlined below) is not mandatory, as these patients may be cured, but treatment may be considered (although it may be futile). If the local tumor demonstrated local lymph node metastases or extrathyroidal extension, yet is completely resected with no evidence of distant metastases, then additional chemoradiation is often considered. Historically, the vast majority of these patients will still have persistent disease, as witnessed by eventual local or distant recurrent disease and death. If local tumor remains after surgery, then it should be resected, or multimodal therapy with chemoradiation may be elected, as discussed below. Operated patients with distant metastases are candidates for additional multimodal therapy, although those with limited residual local disease may not benefit from radiotherapy and may be spared the morbidity of this treatment, given their limited survival. Treatment with paclitaxel alone may be offered to these patients [36].

Locally unresectable disease

If after initial staging it is likely that the local disease cannot be completely resected, then neoadjuvant radiotherapy and chemotherapy may be instituted. The hyperfractionated radiotherapy protocol C of Tennvall and colleagues [15] may be combined with doxorubicin, as in their study, or a regimen of paclitaxel, as outlined by Ain and colleagues [36], may be chosen given its potential greater efficacy. This is especially pertinent if distant metastases are present (with or without doxorubicin). If after receiving the target dose of radiotherapy the patient has no distant metastases and the local disease is likely resectable, then curative surgery should be attempted if excessive morbidity can be avoided. However, if distant metastases are present after receiving radiotherapy, then it is likely that local surgery can be avoided and the airway observed, as death is likely to result shortly from distant metastases.

Summary

ATC is a rare and lethal tumor that has nearly always spread systemically by the time of diagnosis or shortly thereafter. Rare, fortunate individuals are diagnosed and treated when the tumor is small and intrathyroidal, and are cured by surgical resection. Once the tumor is extrathyroidal the disease is typically lethal and radical surgery is discouraged. End-of-life issues should be addressed promptly in all patients and optimal emotional support provided. Currently available treatments, beyond initial curative surgery, may provide limited palliation and possibly prolong patient survival to a minimal degree. Enrollment in clinical trials is highly encouraged because of the lack of effective treatments. However, all therapies (conventional and experimental) require commitments of the patient's limited remaining time and are associated with potential side effects that may impair their quality of life. Furthermore, it is likely that the patient's functional level and ability to enjoy their remaining time will only deteriorate with time. Thus, decisions to enter into an active treatment phase, or to elect comfort care only, should be made in partnership with a fully informed patient.

References

[1] Are C, Shaha AR. Anaplastic thyroid carcinoma: biology, pathogenesis, prognostic factors, and treatment approaches. Ann Surg Oncol 2006;13(4):453–64.

[2] Giuffrida D, Gharib H. Anaplastic thyroid carcinoma: current diagnosis and treatment. Ann Oncol 2000;11(9):1083–9.

[3] Hundahl SA, Fleming ID, Fremgen AM, et al. A National Cancer Data Base report on 53,856 cases of thyroid carcinoma treated in the US, 1985–1995. Cancer 1998;83: 2638–48.

[4] Akslen LA, Haldorsen T, Thoresen SO, et al. Incidence of thyroid cancer in Norway 1970–1985. Population review on time trend, sex, age, histological type and tumour stage in 2625 cases. APMIS 1990;98:549–58.

[5] Ezaki H, Ebihara S, Fujimoto Y, et al. Analysis of thyroid carcinoma based on material registered in Japan during 1977–1986 with special reference to predominance of papillary type. Cancer 1992;70(4):808–14.

[6] Davies L, Welch HG. Increasing incidence of thyroid cancer in the United States, 1973–2002. JAMA 2006;295(18):2164–7.

[7] Kim TY, Kim KW, Jung TS, et al. Prognostic factors for Korean patients with anaplastic thyroid carcinoma. Head Neck 2007;29(8):765–72.

[8] Ain KB. Anaplastic thyroid carcinoma: a therapeutic challenge. Semin Surg Oncol 1999; 16(1):64–9.

[9] Wiseman SM, Masoudi H, Niblock P, et al. Anaplastic thyroid carcinoma: expression profile of targets for therapy offers new insights for disease treatment. Ann Surg Oncol 2007;14(2): 719–29.

[10] Jiang JY, Tseng FY. Prognostic factors of anaplastic thyroid carcinoma. J Endocrinol Invest 2006;29(1):11–7.

[11] Haigh PI, Ituarte PH, Wu HS, et al. Completely resected anaplastic thyroid carcinoma combined with adjuvant chemotherapy and irradiation is associated with prolonged survival. Cancer 2001;91(12):2335–42.

[12] Chang HS, Nam KH, Chung WY, et al. Anaplastic thyroid carcinoma: a therapeutic dilemma. Yonsei Med J 2005;46(6):759–64.

[13] McIver B, Hay ID, Giuffrida DF, et al. Anaplastic thyroid carcinoma: A 50-year experience at a single institution. Surgery 2001;130(6):1028–34.

[14] Hadar T, Mor C, Shvero J, et al. Anaplastic carcinoma of the thyroid. Eur J Surg Oncol 1993; 19(6):511–6.

[15] Tennvall J, Lundell G, Wahlberg P, et al. Anaplastic thyroid carcinoma: three protocols combining doxorubicin, hyperfractionated radiotherapy and surgery. Br J Cancer 2002; 86(12):1848–53.

[16] O'Neill JP, O'Neill B, Condron C, et al. Anaplastic (undifferentiated) thyroid cancer: improved insight and therapeutic strategy into a highly aggressive disease. J Laryngol Otol 2005;119(8):585–91.

[17] Kitamura Y, Shimizu K, Nagahama M, et al. Immediate causes of death in thyroid carcinoma: clinicopathological analysis of 161 fatal cases. J Clin Endocrinol Metab 1999;84: 4043–9.

[18] Venkatesh YS, Ordonez NG, Schultz PN, et al. Anaplastic carcinoma of the thyroid. A clinicopathologic study of 121 cases. Cancer 1990;66:321–30.

[19] Xing M. BRAF mutation in thyroid cancer. Endocr Relat Cancer 2005;12(2):245–62.

[20] Kumar V, Blanchon B, Gu X, et al. Anaplastic thyroid cancer and hyperthyroidism. Endocr Pathol 2005;16(3):245–50.

[21] Ordonez NG, el Naggar AK, Hickey RC, et al. Anaplastic thyroid carcinoma. Immunocytochemical study of 32 cases. Am J Clin Pathol 1991;96(1):15–24.

[22] Sugitani I, Kasai N, Fujimoto Y, et al. Prognostic factors and therapeutic strategy for anaplastic carcinoma of the thyroid. World J Surg 2001;25(5):617–22.

[23] Pierie JP, Muzikansky A, Gaz RD, et al. The effect of surgery and radiotherapy on outcome of anaplastic thyroid carcinoma. Ann Surg Oncol 2002;9(1):57–64.

[24] Lo CY, Lam KY, Wan KY. Anaplastic carcinoma of the thyroid. Am J Surg 1999;177: 337–9.

[25] Nel CJ, van Heerden JA, Goellner JR, et al. Anaplastic carcinoma of the thyroid: a clinico-pathologic study of 82 cases. Mayo Clin Proc 1985;60:51–8.

[26] Tan RK, Finley RK III, Driscoll D, et al. Anaplastic carcinoma of the thyroid: a 24-year experience. Head Neck 1995;17(1):41–7.

[27] Green LD, Mack L, Pasieka JL. Anaplastic thyroid cancer and primary thyroid lymphoma: a review of these rare thyroid malignancies. J Surg Oncol 2006;94(8):725–36.

[28] Haigh PI. Anaplastic thyroid carcinoma. Curr Treat Options Oncol 2000;1(4):353–7.

[29] Heron DE, Karimpour S, Grigsby PW. Anaplastic thyroid carcinoma: comparison of conventional radiotherapy and hyperfractionation chemoradiotherapy in two groups. Am J Clin Oncol 2002;25(5):442–6.

[30] Schlumberger M, Parmentier C, Delisle MJ, et al. Combination therapy for anaplastic giant cell thyroid carcinoma. Cancer 1991;67:564–6.

[31] Wang Y, Tsang R, Asa S, et al. Clinical outcome of anaplastic thyroid carcinoma treated with radiotherapy of once- and twice-daily fractionation regimens. Cancer 2006;107(8): 1786–92.

[32] Levendag PC, De Porre PM, Van Putten WL. Anaplastic carcinoma of the thyroid gland treated by radiation therapy. Int J Radiat Oncol Biol Phys 1993;26:125–8.

[33] Shimaoka K, Schoenfeld DA, DeWys WD, et al. A randomized trial of doxorubicin versus doxorubicin plus cisplatin in patients with advanced thyroid carcinoma. Cancer 1985;56: 2155–60.

[34] Mitchell G, Huddart R, Harmer C. Phase II evaluation of high dose accelerated radiotherapy for anaplastic thyroid carcinoma. Radiother Oncol 1999;50:33–8.

[35] Wong CS, Van Dyk J, Simpson WJ. Myelopathy following hyperfractionated accelerated radiotherapy for anaplastic thyroid carcinoma. Radiother Oncol 1991;20(1):3–9.

[36] Ain KB, Egorin MJ, DeSimone PA. Treatment of anaplastic thyroid carcinoma with paclitaxel: phase 2 trial using ninety-six-hour infusion. Collaborative Anaplastic Thyroid Cancer Health Intervention Trials (CATCHIT) Group. Thyroid 2000;10(7):587–94.

[37] Fury MG, Solit DB, Su YB, et al. A phase I trial of intermittent high-dose gefitinib and fixed-dose docetaxel in patients with advanced solid tumors. Cancer Chemother Pharmacol 2007; 59(4):467–75.

[38] Dowlati A, Robertson K, Cooney M, et al. A phase I pharmacokinetic and translational study of the novel vascular targeting agent combretastatin a-4 phosphate on a single-dose intravenous schedule in patients with advanced cancer. Cancer Res 2002;62(12):3408–16.

[39] Droz J, Baudin E, Medvedev V, et al. Activity of irofulven (IROF) combined with capecitabine (CAPE) in patients (pts) with advanced thyroid carcinoma: Phase II international multicenter study (preliminary results). J Clin Oncol 2006;24:15511 [Meeting Abstracts].

[40] Kloos R, Ringel M, Knopp M, et al. Preliminary Results of Phase II Study of RAF/VEGF-R Kinase Inhibitor, BAY 43–9006 (Sorafenib), in Metastatic Thyroid Carcinoma. Thyroid 2005;15(S1):S-22.

[41] Cooper DS, Doherty GM, Haugen BR, et al. Management guidelines for patients with thyroid nodules and differentiated thyroid cancer. Thyroid 2006;16(2):109–41.

[42] National Comprehensive Cancer Network. Practice Guidelines in Oncology- v.1.2006. Available at: http://www.nccn.org/. Accessed May 23, 2006.

[43] Khan N, Oriuchi N, Higuchi T, et al. Review of fluorine-18-2-fluoro-2-deoxy-D-glucose positron emission tomography (FDG-PET) in the follow-up of medullary and anaplastic thyroid carcinomas. Cancer Control 2005;12(4):254–60.

[44] Kim YW, Do IG, Park YK. Expression of the GLUT1 glucose transporter, p63 and p53 in thyroid carcinomas. Pathol Res Pract 2006;202(11):759–65.

ELSEVIER
SAUNDERS

Endocrinol Metab Clin N Am
37 (2008) 539–557

ENDOCRINOLOGY
AND METABOLISM
CLINICS
OF NORTH AMERICA

Index

Note: Page numbers of article titles are in **boldface** type.

A

Adjuvant therapy, for anaplastic thyroid
cancer, 531–533
locally unresectable disease, 536
for differentiated thyroid cancer,
external beam radiation as,
498–500

Age, thyroid cancer and, as prognostic
factor, 497, 503
anaplastic, 525, 530
distributions of, 527

Age at diagnosis, in thyroid cancer death
risk, 420–422
in thyroid cancer recurrence risk, 420,
423–424

AKT activity/pathway, in thyroid
neoplasia, 375–377
intragenic gene mutations of,
350–351
novel therapies targeting, 516
PI3K pathway and, 381–383
RET point mutations and, 366

AMG-706, for thyroid cancer, early clinical
studies of, 513–515
medullary, 491–492

Anaplastic thyroid carcinoma (ATC),
525–538
death causes with, 528, 531
diagnosis of, 528–529
algorithm for, 534–535
epidemiology of, 525–527
Arthur G. James Cancer
Hospital, 526
Ohio State University, 526
worldwide, 525–526
epigenetic regulation of, 394–395
etiology of, 527
histology of, 528–529
paucicellular variant of, 302–303, 528
PI3K pathway and, 380–381
presentations of, 528
prognostic factors of, 529–530
staging of, 529–530
summary overview of, 525, 536

survival with, median time, 529
percentages over time, 525–526
rates, 529–530
therapy impact on, 531–533
TP53 gene mutations in, 346–348
treatment of, 530–536
adjuvant therapy for, 531–533
locally unresectable disease,
536
authors' recommendations for,
534–535
chemotherapy for, 445, 531–533
combination therapies for,
531–533
external beam radiation therapy
for, 445, 502–503, 531–533
investigational therapies for,
533–534
multimodal therapy for, 531–533
options for, 530
radioactive iodine for, 534
surgical approaches to, 445,
502–503, 530
thyroid stimulating hormone
suppression therapy for, 534

Aneuploidy, in thyroid cancer, 338–339

Angiogenesis, thyroid cancer and, 382
epigenetic regulation of,
394–395
novel therapies targeting, 512,
533–534

Anti-angiogenic therapies, for thyroid
cancer, anaplastic, 533–534
early clinical studies on, 512,
519–520

Antivascular agents, for thyroid cancer,
512, 519–520

Array comparative genomic hybridization
(aCGH), 319

Arthur G. James Cancer Hospital,
anaplastic thyroid cancer and, 526

Avascular plane, between thyroid and
cricothyroid muscle, 446–447

doi:10.1016/S0889-8529(08)00023-6